Nutrition in Clinical Nursing

Nutrition in Clinical Nursing

Idamarie Laquatra, Ph.D., R.D.
Nutritionist
Heinz USA
Pittsburgh, Pennsylvania

Mary Jo Gerlach, R.N., M.S.N.Ed.
Assistant Professor
Medical College of Georgia School of Nursing
Athens, Georgia

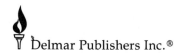
Delmar Publishers Inc.®

Cover illustration by Catherine Minnery

Delmar Staff

Executive Editor: Leslie Boyer
Editing Manager: Barbara A. Christie
Design Coordinator: Susan Mathews
Production Coordinator: Sandra Woods

For information, address Delmar Publishers Inc.
2 Computer Drive West, Box 15-015
Albany, New York 12212

Printed in the United States of America
Published simultaneously in Canada
by Nelson Canada,
a division of The Thomson Corporation

Library of Congress Cataloging in Publication Data

Laquatra, Idamarie.
    Nutrition in clinical nursing / Idamarie Laquatra, Mary Jo Gerlach.
      p. cm.
    ISBN 0-8273-3075-8 (pbk.). —ISBN 0-8273-3076-6 (instructor's guide)
    1. Diet in disease. 2. Nutrition. 3. Nursing. I. Gerlach, Mary Jo. II. Title.
    [DNLM: 1. Nutrition—nurses' instructions. QU 145 L317n]
RM217.L38 1990
615.8'54—dc20
DNLM/DLC   89-23601
for Library of Congress   10 9 8 7 6 5 4 3 2   CIP

CONTENTS

Tables vii

Preface ix

Acknowledgments ix

Part One   *Introductory Concepts in Nutrition and Metabolic Patterns* 1

Chapter 1   The Nutrition-Health Relationship 3

Chapter 2   An Overview of Nutrition Principles 27

Chapter 3   Nutrition for Pregnancy, Fetal Development, and Lactation 55

Chapter 4   Nutrition During Infancy, Childhood, and Adolescence 75

Chapter 5   Nutrition for the Adult 101

Part Two   *Clinical Aspects of Nutrition* 119

Chapter 6   Nutrition and the Patient under Physiological Stress 121

Chapter 7   Nutrition and the Patient with Gastrointestinal Disorders 141

Chapter 8   Nutrition and the Patient with Renal Disease 187

Chapter 9   Nutrition and the Patient with Cardiovascular Disease 217

Chapter 10   Nutrition and the Patient with Blood Disorders 250

Chapter 11   Nutrition and the Patient with Respiratory Disorders 266

Chapter 12   Nutrition and the Patient with Cancer 279

Chapter 13   Nutrition and the Patient with Diabetes Mellitus 297

Chapter 14   Nutrition and the Patient with Selected Metabolic
              Disorders 320

Chapter 15   Nutrition and the Patient with Eating Disorders 346

Chapter 16   Nutrition and the Patient with an Alteration in the
              Immune Response 372

Chapter 17   Selected Nursing-Care Plans 385

              Appendices 403

              Index 415

TABLES

1-1	The Basic Food Groups and Examples of Foods They Contain ...	4
1-2	Dietary Recommendations from the Surgeon General	8
1-3	Dietary Recommendations of the Committee on Diet and Health, National Academy of Sciences	9
1-4	Strengths and Weaknesses of Protein Sources	12
1-5	Food-Borne Illnesses	16
2-1	Major Food Sources of Vitamin A	34
2-2	Dietary Sources of Vitamin C	36
2-3	Dietary Sources of Folate	37
2-4	Dietary Sources of Vitamin B_{12}	38
2-5	Trace Elements	45
2-6	Stages of Iron-Deficiency Anemia	47
3-1	Recommended Dietary Allowances for Women (Revised 1989)	57
3-2	Weight Gain during Pregnancy	59
3-3	Daily Intake Food Guide	60
3-4	Caffeine Content of Common Items	62
3-5	Food Guide for the Pregnant Adolescent	66
4-1	Energy and Macronutrients in Breast Milk during the First Month of Lactation	77
4-2	Nutrient Content of Mature Human Milk, Infant Formula, and Cow's Milk	79
4-3	Sources of Macronutrients in Commercial Infant Formulas	81
4-4	Guidelines for Dietary Intake for the Preschool Years (Age 1–5 Years)	89
4-5	Characteristics of Food Commonly Accepted by Preschoolers ...	90
4-6	Food Substitutions	91
4-7	Daily Food Guide for Adolescents	92
4-8	School Lunch Patterns for Various Age/Grade Groups	93
5-1	Biological Changes with Age	105
5-2	Drug-Nutrient Interactions	110
6-1	Classification of Catabolism	122
6-2	Stages of Response Following Trauma	123
6-3	Baseline Fluid Requirements in Temperate Climate	130
6-4	Supplements Used for Patients under Metabolic Stress	137

7-1   Examples of Foods Included on Full-Liquid and Soft Diets 143
7-2   Classification of Plant Fiber 147
7-3   Sources of Fiber 147
7-4   Potential Problem Foods for the Person with an Ileostomy 160
7-5   Dietary Guidelines for Selected Liver Diseases 173

8-1   Foods High in Calcium, Oxalates, and Purines 195
8-2   Summary of Dietary Recommendations in Chronic Renal
          Failure 205
8-3   Protein Intakes at Various Levels of Renal Function 206
8-4   Protein Values of Food Groups 206

9-1   Lipoprotein Classes 220
9-2   The Hyperlipoproteinemias 222
9-3   Total Cholesterol and LDL Guidelines for Adults Aged 21
          and Older 223
9-4   Dietary Modifications for Hyperlipoproteinemia 224
9-5   Food Sources of Fats, Cholesterol, and Complex
          Carbohydrates 225
9-6   Classification of Blood Pressure 230
9-7   Kilocalories and Alcohol Content of Beverages 232
9-8   Potassium in Foods 233
9-9   Natural Sodium in Foods 235
9-10   Sodium in Foods 237

10-1   Types and Causes of Anemia 251

12-1   Indications for Use and Possible Complications of
          Enteral Feedings 287
12-2   Factors for Reduced Cancer Risk 291

13-1   Blood Glucose Values in the Normal and Diabetic State 303
13-2   Insulin Formulations 305
13-3   Dietary Recommendations for Individuals with Diabetes 307
13-4   Guidelines for Carbohydrate Supplementation During Exercise .. 309

15-1   Kilocalories in Macronutrients 347
15-2   Caloric Cost of Physical Activity 348
15-3   Height and Weight Tables for Adults (1959) 351
15-4   Height and Weight Tables for Adults (1983) 352
15-5   Current Treatments for Obesity 355

16-1   Clinical Manifestations That may Be Associated with
          Food Allergy 375

PREFACE

This text is designed to provide nursing students with an understanding of nutrition from two perspectives. First, we present current nutrition principles and theories that may help to promote and maintain optimal health throughout the life cycle. Second, we address nutritional alterations that may be required for persons who have health disorders in both the hospital and community settings.

We have provided a physiological/pathophysiological framework, because we believe it creates the rationale for nutrition management. Understanding the rationale then facilitates the development of nursing interventions that may be useful in developing a care plan. Because good nutritional status requires an interdisciplinary team effort, the nurse frequently plays a pivotal role in identifying nutritional needs of patients and coordinating the activities of the various members in order to implement a care plan.

Special features that make this text beneficial include **Nursing Diagnoses** pertaining to nutritional aspects of wellness and illness; **Nursing Interventions** for dietary management throughout the life span and for nutrition disorders; **Topics of Interest** that highlight a particular facet of nutrition pertinent to the chapter; **Spotlight on Learning,** a case-study approach that allows the student to apply the nutrition principles described in the chapter; **Activities** to reinforce learning; and **Review Questions** to enable students to test their knowledge.

An **Instructor's Guide** has been developed to accompany the text. It contains answers to the **Review Questions** and **Resources,** a listing of materials available at the local, state and national level, which may be used as adjuncts for teaching. **Transparency Masters** and a **Test Bank** are also included.

ACKNOWLEDGMENTS

A special thanks is extended to our husbands and families for their patience, understanding, and contributions during each phase in the development of the final text. It was with their support that we were able to meet our deadlines. We would like to acknowledge contributions provided by Joanne Malenock, Ph.D., R.D., Dee Adinaro, M.S.N., R.N., Pamela Chally, M.N., R.N., Martha Bramlett, M.S.N., R.N., Dereen Nolan, R.N., and Sandra Hopper, M.Ed., R.N. The assistance of Lenette O. Burrell, Ed.D., R.N., and Sarah H. Gueldner, D.S.N., R.N., was invaluable.

PART
ONE

INTRODUCTORY CONCEPTS IN NUTRITION AND METABOLIC PATTERNS

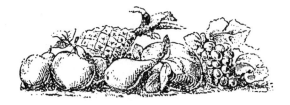

CHAPTER
1

THE NUTRITION-HEALTH RELATIONSHIP

Objectives

After studying this chapter, you will be able to

- discuss the evolution of the relationship between nutrition and health in the United States.
- identify factors that can influence dietary intake.
- describe the complications that result from hospital malnutrition.
- explain measures that can be taken to prevent hospital malnutrition.
- list methods for avoiding food-borne illness.
- discuss the nursing process as it relates to optimal nutrition and nutritional alterations.
- describe the unique role of the nurse in relation to other members of the health-care team as it pertains to the nutritional aspects of patient care.

Overview

Perceptions about the relationship between nutrition and health in the United States have changed over the years. The general public has become more educated about food choices and the effect that various foods have on the promotion of good health. Today, we have more information available than ever before, and major efforts are underway to translate complex nutritional principles into practical dietary recommendations. How did we get where we are, and what influences our decisions to follow the recommendations?

THE EVOLUTION OF THE ROLE OF NUTRITION IN HEALTH MAINTENANCE

In the late 1930s, when facing the prospect of World War II, the United States was startled to discover the high number of young service recruits who were rejected for reasons attributed to suboptimal nutrition (1). Therefore, the first Food and Nutrition Board of the National Research Council met in 1940 to establish dietary standards that were to be used as a guide for advising on nutritional problems in connection with the national defense (2). Three years later, in 1943, the first edition of the *Recommended Dietary Allowances* (RDA) was published. The publication represented the first formal effort in the United States to establish nutrient standards. Because the science of nutrition was still in its infancy, the scientists involved in the first edition fully recognized the limits of the available knowledge and expected revisions to the recommendations to be made on a regular basis. The latest edition of the RDA, 1989, is listed in Appendices A, B, and C.

As illustrated in the appendices, the RDA is a listing by age group of the quantities of nutrients that are believed to be adequate to meet the known nutritional needs of practically all healthy persons in the United States. Thus, the RDA exceed the requirements of many individuals. They are used for planning adequate diets for groups, interpreting food consumption data, and establishing standards for government intervention programs, such as the School Lunch Program. The levels of nutrients recommended take into consideration nutrient loss during preparation and storage, the range of population requirements, the stability of the nutrient, the body's capacity for storage, the availability of the nutrients in the American diet, and the hazards from excessive consumption of the particular nutrient. While the RDA are valuable for assessing the intake of population groups, the value of the recommendations is somewhat limited when evaluating the diet of individuals. In addition, the recommendations do not take into account the therapeutic needs of individuals suffering from burns, metabolic disorders, and chronic diseases. These disorders require special dietary management, which is described in detail in later chapters.

Translating the recommendations for various nutrients into a practical guide was the work of the United States Department of Agriculture (USDA). The USDA's basic food groups (Table 1-1) have

Table 1-1. THE BASIC FOOD GROUPS AND EXAMPLES OF FOODS THEY CONTAIN

BREADS, CEREALS, AND OTHER GRAIN PRODUCTS					
Whole-Grain			*Enriched*		
Brown rice	Oatmeal	Whole-wheat bread and rolls	Bagels	Farina	Muffins
Buckwheat groats	Popcorn		Biscuits	French bread	Noodles
	Pumpernickel bread	Whole-wheat crackers	Corn bread	Grits	Pancakes
Bulgur			Corn muffins	Hamburger rolls	Pasta
Corn tortillas	Ready-to-eat cereals	Whole-wheat pasta	Cornmeal		Ready-to-eat cereals
Graham crackers	Rye crackers		Crackers	Hot dog buns	
		Whole-wheat cereals	English muffins	Italian bread	Rice
Granola				Macaroni	White bread and rolls

Continued

Table 1-1. THE BASIC FOOD GROUPS AND EXAMPLES OF FOODS THEY CONTAIN
(continued)

FRUITS					
Citrus, Melons, Berries			*Other Fruits*		
Blueberries	Honeydew	Raspberries	Apple	Grapes	Pineapple
Cantaloupe	melon	Strawberries	Apricot	Guava	Plantain
Citrus juices	Kiwifruit	Tangerine	Banana	Mango	Plum
Cranberries	Lemon	Watermelon	Cherries	Nectarine	Pomegranate
Grapefruit	Orange		Dates	Papaya	Prune
			Figs	Peach	Raisins
			Fruit juices	Pear	

VEGETABLES					
Dark-Green			*Deep-Yellow*	*Starchy*	
Beet greens	Dandelion	Romaine	Carrots	Breadfruit	Lima beans
Broccoli	greens	lettuce	Pumpkin	Corn	Potatoes
Chard	Endive	Spinach	Sweet potatoes	Green peas	Rutabaga
Chicory	Escarole	Turnip greens	Winter squash	Hominy	Taro
Collard greens	Kale	Watercress			
	Mustard greens				

Dry Beans and Peas (Legumes)		*Other Vegetables*			
Black beans	Lima beans	Artichokes	Cabbage	Green beans	Radishes
Black-eyed peas	(mature)	Asparagus	Cauliflower	Green peppers	Summer squash
Chickpeas	Mung beans	Bean and	Celery	Lettuce	Tomatoes
(garbanzos)	Navy beans	alfalfa	Chinese	Mushrooms	Turnips
Kidney beans	Pinto beans	sprouts	cabbage	Okra	Vegetable juices
Lentils	Split peas	Beets	Cucumbers	Onions (mature	Zucchini
		Brussels	Eggplant	and green)	
		sprouts			

MEAT, POULTRY, FISH, AND ALTERNATES					
Meat, Poultry, and Fish				*Alternates*	
Beef	Ham	Pork	Veal	Eggs	Nuts and seeds
Chicken	Lamb	Shellfish	Luncheon	Dry beans and	Peanut butter
Fish	Organ meats	Turkey	meats,	peas	Tofu
			sausage	(legumes)	

Continued

Table 1-1. THE BASIC FOOD GROUPS AND EXAMPLES OF FOODS THEY CONTAIN
(continued)

MILK, CHEESE, AND YOGURT				
Lowfat Milk Products		*Other Milk Products with More Fat or Sugar*		
Buttermilk Lowfat milk (1%, 2%)	Lowfat plain yogurt Skim milk	American cheese Cheddar cheese	Chocolate milk Flavored yogurt	Fruit yogurt Process cheeses	Swiss cheese Whole milk

FATS, SWEETS, AND ALCOHOLIC BEVERAGES				
Fats		*Sweets*		*Alcohol*
Bacon, salt pork Butter Cream (dairy, nondairy) Cream cheese Lard Margarine	Mayonnaise Mayonnaise- type salad dressing Salad dressing Shortening Sour cream Vegetable oil	Candy Corn syrup Fruit drinks, ades Gelatin desserts Honey Frosting	Jam Jelly Maple syrup Marmalade Molasses	Popsicles and ices Sherbets Soft drinks and colas Sugar (white and brown)	Beer Liquor Wine

Source: U.S. Department of Agriculture and U.S. Department of Health and Human Services, "Nutrition and Your Health: Dietary Guidelines for Americans." *Home and Garden Bulletin No. 232-1* (Washington, D.C.: USDA and DHHS, 1986), 7.

come an easy tool for quickly assessing an individual's overall intake. It should be noted that the tool's lack of precision makes it useful as a screening method, but not for assessing nutrient inadequacy. Servings from the various food groups differ, depending on age, and more specific information is given in later chapters.

During the late 1960s and early 1970s, the conscience of the United States was again jarred. This time, the primary focus turned to diseases associated with not getting enough food to eat. "Hunger in America," a television documentary that graphically illustrated pockets of severe poverty and malnutrition in the United States, shook the nation. The government responded with the introduction of numerous assistance programs designed to improve the health and nutrition of individuals in low income brackets.

In the latter part of the 1970s, the emphasis again shifted. Attention was diverted from the diseases of undernutrition to the diseases of overnutrition: cardiovascular disease, cancer, and diabetes, since these were and continue to be the major causes of death in the United States. In 1977, the Senate Select Committee on Nutrition and Human Needs, chaired by Senator George McGovern, issued *Dietary Goals for the United States*. The goals promoted the maintenance of appropriate body weight and specified recommendations for decreasing fat, saturated fat, cholesterol, sugar, and salt in the diet, and increasing complex carbohydrate consumption (3). The goals were highly controversial, with some scientific groups applauding their appearance and other groups totally rejecting them. The momentum for taking control of our health was growing, and an increasing number of scientists and health organizations began to communicate to Americans the types of dietary changes that would maintain health. In 1980, the United States Departments of Agriculture and Health and Human Services issued its first set of dietary guidelines for Americans. The guidelines were revised in 1985:

1. Eat a variety of foods.
2. Maintain desirable weight.
3. Avoid too much fat, saturated fat, and cholesterol.
4. Eat foods with adequate starch and fiber.
5. Avoid too much sugar.
6. Avoid too much sodium.
7. If you drink alcoholic beverages, do so in moderation.

In addition to the general guidance on diet and health, various organizations were recommending dietary alterations to prevent specific chronic diseases. For example, the National Academy of Sciences published *Diet, Nutrition and Cancer* in 1982 (4). The document reviewed the relationship between dietary components and the incidence of certain types of cancer. The American Cancer Society incorporated the findings of the Academy in publications for the general public for reducing cancer risk. In addition, the American Heart Association was becoming more vocal in the specific dietary guidance it recommended for reducing the risk of cardiovascular disease (5), and the National Institutes of Health issued specific recommendations for the prevention of osteoporosis (6).

The media played a major role in disseminating the information on the relationship between diet and health. Newspaper articles, popular magazine features, and newscasts bombarded the public with sometimes conflicting messages. Americans were becoming confused on how to apply the recommendations. Should the public follow one set of rules to avoid osteoporosis and another to avoid heart disease, and still others to avoid cancer? Two major documents that were recently released have clarified the situation. In July 1988, the *Surgeon General's Report on Nutrition and Health* was issued (7). The focus of the report was the relationship of diet to the occurrence of the leading causes of death in the United States. The significance of the report is that it provided overwhelming support of the dietary guidelines; established the reduction of total fat as the primary priority for dietary change; and distinguished recommendations for the general public from those to specific population groups (8). Table 1-2 is a list of the Surgeon General's recommendations.

The second major document, *Diet and Health: Implications for Reducing Chronic Disease Risk,* was issued in 1989 by the Committee on Diet and Health, Food and Nutrition Board, Commission on Life Sciences, National Research Council (9). The Committee's charge was to review evidence concerning all major chronic health conditions influenced by diet. It was then to draw conclusions about the effects of nutrients, foods, and dietary patterns on health, propose dietary recommendations that had a potential for decreasing risk, and estimate the public health impact of the recommendations. To their credit, the Committee took into account the competing risks for different diseases as well as nutrient interactions. (See Table 1-3).

FACTORS INFLUENCING DIETARY INTAKE

The pronouncements of government organizations and health agencies can increase awareness of the general public with regard to eating patterns most conducive to good health, but changes in dietary habits require more than just the dissemination of information. Dietary habits are influenced by psychosocial, economic, religious, and cultural factors. Attempts to influence dietary change in both well and ill individuals must take these factors into consideration. Sensitivity to the specific needs of individuals will help to promote adherence to preventive and therapeutic nutritional recommendations.

Psychosocial Factors

It is well known that individuals eat food for reasons other than satisfying hunger. Many holidays feature a special meal, when members of the entire family join together to celebrate. Eating lunch or dinner with someone may be a sign of

Table 1-2. DIETARY RECOMMENDATIONS FROM THE SURGEON GENERAL

Issues for Most People

- *Fats and cholesterol.* Reduce consumption of fat (especially saturated fat) and cholesterol. Choose foods relatively low in these substances, such as vegetables, fruits, whole-grain foods, fish, poultry, lean meats, and low-fat dairy products. Use food preparation methods that add little or no fat.

- *Energy and weight control.* Achieve and maintain a desirable body weight. To do so, choose a dietary pattern in which energy (caloric) intake is consistent with energy expenditure. To reduce energy intake, limit consumption of foods relatively high in calories, fats, and sugars, and minimize alcohol consumption. Increase energy expenditure through regular and sustained physical activity.

- *Complex carbohydrates and fiber.* Increase consumption of whole-grain foods and cereal products, vegetables (including dried beans and peas), and fruits.

- *Sodium.* Reduce intake of sodium by choosing foods relatively low in sodium and limiting the amount of salt added in food preparation and at the table.

- *Alcohol.* To reduce the risk for chronic disease, take alcohol only in moderation (no more than two drinks a day), if at all. Avoid drinking any alcohol before or while driving, operating machinery, taking medications, or engaging in any other activity requiring judgment. Avoid drinking alcohol while pregnant.

Other Issues for Some People

- *Fluoride.* Community water systems should contain fluoride at optimal levels for prevention of tooth decay. If such water is not available, use other appropriate sources of fluoride.

- *Sugars.* Those who are particularly vulnerable to dental caries (cavities), especially children, should limit their consumption and frequency of use of foods high in sugars.

- *Calcium.* Adolescent girls and adult women should increase consumption of foods high in calcium, including low-fat dairy products.

- *Iron.* Children, adolescents, and women of childbearing age should be sure to consume foods that are good sources of iron, such as lean meats, fish, certain beans, and iron-enriched cereals and whole-grain products. This issue is of special concern for low-income families.

Source: U.S. Department of Health and Human Services, *The Surgeon General's Report on Nutrition and Health: Summary and Recommendations.* DHHS (PHS) Publication No. 88-50211, 1988.

friendship or an occasion to settle a business deal. Food also plays a central role in most social events.

Specific foods seem to have special meanings in our society: Cake and ice cream mean celebration, chicken soup is a remedy for illness, and sweets are often used as rewards. Some individuals find that eating food is comforting, particularly when they are under stress or angry or sad.

Economic Factors

Although income affects dietary patterns, it does not necessarily have a substantial impact on nutrient intakes in the United States (10). The Nationwide Food Consumption Survey, Continuing Survey of Food Intakes by Individuals (CSFII), indicated that women in low-income brackets had lower mean intakes of milk and milk products,

Table 1-3. DIETARY RECOMMENDATIONS OF THE COMMITTEE ON DIET AND HEALTH, NATIONAL ACADEMY OF SCIENCES

- Reduce total fat intake to 30% or less of calories. Reduce saturated fatty acid intake to less than 10% of calories and the intake of cholesterol to less than 300 mg daily. The intake of fat and cholesterol can be reduced by substituting fish, poultry without skin, lean meats, and low-fat or nonfat dairy products for fatty meats and whole-milk dairy products; by choosing more vegetables, fruits, cereals, and legumes; and by limiting oils, fats, egg yolks, and fried and other fatty foods.

- Every day, eat five or more servings of a combination of vegetables and fruits, especially green and yellow vegetables and citrus fruits. Also, increase intake of starches and other complex carbohydrates by eating six or more daily servings of a combination of breads, cereals, and legumes. (Note: An average serving is equal to a half cup for most fresh or cooked vegetables, fruits, dry or cooked cereals and legumes, one medium piece of fresh fruit, one slice of bread, or one roll or muffin.)

- Maintain protein intake at moderate levels

- Balance food intake and physical activity to maintain appropriate weight.

- The committee does not recommend alcohol consumption. For those who drink alcoholic beverages, the committee recommends limiting consumption to the equivalent of less than two ounces of pure alcohol in a single day. This is the equivalent of two cans of beer, two small glasses of wine, or two average cocktails. Pregnant women should avoid alcoholic beverages.

- Limit total daily intake of salt (sodium chloride) to six grams or less. Limit the use of salt in cooking and avoid adding it to food at the table. Salty, highly processed salty, salt-preserved, and salt-pickled foods should be consumed sparingly.

- Maintain adequate calcium intake.

- Avoid taking dietary supplements in excess of the RDA in any one day.

- Maintain an optimal intake of fluoride, particularly during the years of primary and secondary tooth formation and growth.

Source: *Diet and Health: Implications for Reducing Chronic Disease Risk,* © 1989, by the National Academy of Sciences, Washington, D.C.

vegetables, and fruits than women in the highest income bracket (11, 12). Despite the differences in food intake, intakes of nutrients below the RDA were the same across income levels. Similar findings were observed in men (13). Only in instances of severe poverty are substandard diets found in the United States (10).

Income does appear to be related to obesity, however. In the United States, the prevalence of overweight among adult women below the poverty line is greater than for women above the poverty line. In contrast to women, American men are more likely to be overweight if their incomes are above the poverty line (14). The differences may be attributed to food intake as well as exercise patterns.

The influx of women into the labor force has caused major changes in food intake and preparation. A premium has been placed on time and convenience. Today, less time is spent preparing meals, with more meals eaten out or more carry-out food brought into the home. In addition, the traditional three meals per day is fading in favor of "grazing," that is, eating many small meals and snacks throughout the day (15). Family members, other than the mother, are beginning to take a larger share of the responsibility for food purchases and preparation, and this trend shows no signs of diminishing (16).

Religious Factors

Many religions have specific dietary laws that the observant are expected to follow. Although a discussion of all religious observances is beyond the scope of this text, a sampling of some of the dietary laws illustrates the sensitivity needed when prescribing certain nutrition interventions for various diseases.

Roman Catholic. Dietary rules in the Roman Catholic Church have changed considerably over the years. Most prominent are the changes in the restrictions regarding meat eating and fasting. Today, observant Catholics are asked to refrain from eating meat on Fridays during the Lenten season. Fish or dairy products may be substituted for meat and provide adequate protein to cover needs. Fasting is practiced on Ash Wednesday and Good Friday during the Lenten season.

Jewish. Many individuals of the Jewish faith follow kosher dietary laws. According to the kosher dietary laws, there are three classes of foods: meat, dairy, and pareve (17). There must be a total segregation of meat and dairy foods during preparation (including utensils used) and at meals; the spacing between a meat and milk meal is between three to six hours. Pareve foods (breads made without dairy products, fruits, and vegetables without animal-based coatings) are considered neutral and may be eaten with either meat or dairy foods. Pork and shellfish are forbidden, and only animals that have undergone a kosher slaughter are permitted. A kosher slaughter involves the use of a very sharp knife with a quick single cut by hand of the carotid arteries, jugular veins, and windpipe by a trained religious slaughterer (17). After kosher slaughter, all meat and poultry must be soaked in cold water for one-half hour, salted with coarse salt for one hour, and rinsed before cooking. Kosher fish must have fins and scales that can be removed without tearing the skin.

Religious holidays have special requirements. For example, Passover in March or April has extensive dietary observances for its duration of eight days. Observant Jews must avoid any leavened grains and related products in commemoration of the hasty departure of the Jews from Egypt. European Jews do not eat legumes, corn, rice, mustard, or products containing these during this time (17).

Many food processors manufacture kosher products. The symbol on the food package that indicates that the product is kosher is K or Ⓤ. The symbol K indicates that the product was prepared according to requirements and under supervision of the Organized Kashrut Laboratories. The symbol Ⓤ represents preparation under supervision of the Union of Orthodox Jewish Congregations.

It should be noted that not all Jews who keep kosher do things according to one unitary Jewish custom. A continuum exists, and the level of observance is dependent on the community in which the person lives, custom, and personal preference (18).

Moslem. Moslems, followers of the Islam religion, represent another large group of individuals in the United States with specific dietary requirements. The dietary laws must be observed at all times, including while the individual is in the hospital, during pregnancy, and when traveling. As in the Jewish religion, certain foods are prohibited. For Moslems, the forbidden foods are alcohol, pork, meat from wild animals with fangs, birds with claws, animals without ears (frogs), or poison-makers (19). All meat must be slaughtered according to strict slaughtering laws. Milk is permitted at all times, as are meats, fish, fruits, vegetables, breads, and cereals. Special foods that are believed to have health benefits or religious significance include figs, olives, dates, honey, milk, and buttermilk. All food is to be eaten in moderation, according to the belief that the stomach has three compartments: one for solid food, one for liquid food, and one for air.

Fasting in the Moslem religion begins at age 10–14 years. Ramadan, the ninth month of the Moslem linear year, is a 30-day period of daylight fasting. Two meals are permitted: one is eaten before sunrise, and one is eaten at sunset. Medications should not be taken during the fasting period, and an IV is considered to break the fast if it contains glucose (19).

Seventh-Day Adventist. Seventh-Day Adventists are lacto-ovo-vegetarians. There are three groups of vegetarians: vegans, lacto-vegetarians, and lacto-ovo-vegetarians. Vegans abstain from all animal products: meat, fish, fowl, dairy products, and eggs. Lacto-vegetarians are similar to vegans except that they include milk products in the diet. In addition to milk, lacto-ovo-vegetarians include eggs.

Not all vegetarians are Seventh-Day Adventists. Individuals follow vegetarian diets for a number of reasons: health, economic, and philosophical, as well as religious reasons. Vegetarian diets are considered to be healthful and nutritionally adequate when properly planned. In fact, because most vegetarian diets in the United States are high in fiber and low in total fat, saturated fat, and cholesterol, they are associated with decreased risk of the chronic diseases of obesity, coronary artery disease, hypertension, diabetes, and colon cancer (20).

Some care needs to be directed toward intake of specific nutrients when following a vegetarian diet. Because vegans eat no animal products, they are at risk for inadequate intake of vitamin B_{12}, since this vitamin is found naturally in animal sources. Adequate intake can be ensured through the use of a supplement, fortified soy milk, and fortified breakfast cereals. Some foods, such as tempeh (fermented soybeans), were originally thought to contain substantial amounts of the vitamin; however, it has been discovered in recent years that the analytical technique for examining the presence of vitamin B_{12} does not determine the presence of the active form only, but also the inactive forms (21). The Food and Drug Administration was petitioned to change the official testing method for vitamin B_{12} so that labels for foods and supplements will be more accurate and include values for the active form only (21).

Vitamin D can also be a critical nutrient for the vegan, since food sources of the vitamin are limited to animal products. Adequate sunshine or a supplement of vitamin D is necessary. The ultraviolet rays from the sun transform a precursor of vitamin D in the skin to the active form. More information on vitamins is given in Chapter 2.

Protein needs of vegetarians have received much attention, and better understanding of protein metabolism has made dietary recommendations much more practical. The basic building blocks of protein are amino acids. The adult human body has the ability to synthesize all but eight amino acids, which must be supplied through the diet. These eight amino acids are commonly known as the essential amino acids and include tryptophan, leucine, isoleucine, lysine, valine, threonine, methionine, and phenylalanine. In addition to requiring the eight amino acids, children require histidine. All of the essential amino acids are required simultaneously in varying amounts for protein synthesis to occur. Animals products, including eggs and dairy foods such as milk and cheese, are good sources of all of the essential amino acids. Plant sources, such as grains, legumes, seeds, and nuts, contain adequate amounts of some essential amino acids and not enough of others. It is therefore recommended that vegetarians, especially those who abstain from all animal products, eat mixtures of protein from grains, vegetables, legumes, seeds, and nuts over the course of the day to complement the amino acid profiles of the foods. It is no longer considered necessary to complement the amino acid profiles in each meal or to precisely plan protein intake (20). (See Table 1-4 for sources of protein with their strengths and weaknesses.)

Culture

The United States used to be called a "melting pot." Immigrants from various cultures blended to become "American." Today, a more accurate description is a "mosaic," in which each culture retains its basic elements while still contributing to the overall profile of the United States. The recent waves of immigration have increased the numbers of Hispanics and Asians in the United States, each

Table 1-4. STRENGTHS AND WEAKNESSES OF PROTEIN SOURCES

CATEGORY	WEAKNESSES	STRENGTHS
Plant Sources		
Legumes	tryptophan methionine	lysine isoleucine
Grains	lysine isoleucine	tryptophan methionine
Seeds/nuts	lysine isoleucine	tryptophan methionine
Other vegetables	isoleucine methionine	tryptophan lysine
Animal Sources		
Meat, fish, poultry	none	contains adequate amounts of all eight essential amino acids
Eggs	none	contains adequate amounts of all eight essential amino acids
Milk	none	contains adequate amounts of all eight essential amino acids

Reprinted by permission of Francis Moore Lappé and her agents, Raines & Raines, 71 Park Avenue, NY, NY 10016. © 1971, 1975, 1982, by Francis Moore Lappé.

with their specific food patterns. The four major ethnic groups in the United States are black American, Hispanic, Asian, and native American (22).

The Black American Culture. Currently, 12.5% of America's population is black, and it is expected that the black population will grow 50% by the year 2000 (23). Just over half of black Americans live in the South, and many living elsewhere have southern origins. The diets of black Americans are similar to southern whites of the same socioeconomic level. Preferences in cooking include frying and barbecuing meats and the use of hot sauce and black pepper. Specific food preferences include hot breads, ham hocks, hominy grits, and black-eyed peas (22).

Nutritionally, the diet is high in protein (from meat intake) and rich in vitamin A due to the high intake of dark leafy green vegetables. On the negative side, the diet can be high in fat, due to reliance on frying, high in sodium, from the use of salt and cured meats, and low in calcium, due to a low intake of dairy foods (22). Additionally, because many of the vegetables are overcooked, water soluble vitamin loss can be substantial.

The Hispanic Culture. There are three major subgroups of Hispanics in the United States: Puerto Rican, Cuban, and Mexican (24). The Puerto Rican subgroup is concentrated in the Northeast, the Cubans in the Southeast, particularly Florida, and the Mexican subgroup is concentrated in the Southwest. Regardless of socioeconomic status, rice, dried peas, beans, root vegetables, dried codfish, sugar, lard, and coffee with milk are usually found in the Puerto Rican household (24). Cubans rely on foods similar to Puerto Ricans; however, they prefer black versus red beans. In Mexican cuisine, beans are used in numerous ways, and corn and maize play a prominent role in the making of tortillas and their endless variations: tacos, enchiladas, and tostadas. Rice is often coated with oil, fried with spices, and flavored with bits of meat or fish. Fruits and vegetables are plentiful at meals

(25). The Hispanic diet can be high in saturated fat due to the heavy reliance on lard for cooking.

The Asian Culture. More than 340,000 Southeast Asians (Vietnamese, Laotians, Cambodians) have immigrated to the United States since 1971, with the main population centers located in California, Texas, Illinois, and Pennsylvania (26). Traditional cuisine includes rice, fresh fruits, fish, shellfish, chicken, duck, pork, and beef. In addition, fresh, uncooked vegetables and salads are an integral part of Southeast Asian meals (27). Dishes are well seasoned with fresh herbs, particularly lemon grass, spices, and condiments. Milk intake is quite low in the adult diet, with its use usually limited to sweetened condensed milk in coffee. Food preparation techniques include simmering, stir-frying, and cooking over charcoal (26).

Since their arrival in the United States, Southeast Asians have made substitutions for traditional foods, depending on cost and availability. For example, more beef and lamb are eaten, since these items are cheaper in the United States than in Southeast Asia, and fish, shellfish, and duck are eaten less frequently. Intake of eggs, sweet snacks, sodas, butter, and margarine has also increased.

The Southeast Asian diet is rich in potassium due to the high fruit and vegetable intake. The diet is also relatively low in fat. Problem nutrients include sodium, which can be high depending on the intake of pickled vegetables and salted fish products. Calcium intake is usually quite limited, due to the low intake of milk. Because of this, secondary sources of calcium, such as the deep-green leafy vegetables low in oxalic acid and soybean curd, become more important; however, it is unlikely that the RDA for calcium will be met on the Southeast Asian diet.

The Chinese approach to cooking has been described as "famine cooking," due to the often harsh economic conditions in China (28). No part of the animal or plant is wasted, and the method of cooking, stir-frying, is a consequence of the shortage of fuel. Food cut into small pieces cooked quickly over high heat uses less energy than large pieces that are broiled or roasted. Pork is the most popular meat because pigs do not require fodder, which is expensive. Pigs can also be raised on very small land areas. The Chinese diet is characterized by small quantities of meat with large servings of rice and vegetables. Fruit is often served as dessert. Milk, dairy products, bread, butter, and margarine are not part of the daily diet. Although the elderly Chinese continue to follow their customs, the second and third generations are adopting western eating habits and customs.

The Native American Culture. American Indians account for less than 1% of the population in the United States (22). Common foods in the native American diet include mutton, game, fish, tortilla, fruits, roots, wild greens, and corn. In addition, convenience foods such as soda, salty snacks, and processed meats are consumed. The diet can be high in saturated fat, sodium, and sugar. Calcium content of the diet is usually low due to infrequent intake of dairy products (22).

Cultural Awareness in Nursing. Knowing some of the customs and traditional foods of various cultures can be critical to the nurse working in public-health settings. Adequate nutrition, especially for older immigrants in a community setting, may depend on the availability of traditional foods. Some government assistance programs have been successful in altering their menu selections to include foods from different cultures, and more supermarkets are carrying a wider variety of fruits, vegetables, and spices common to other cultures.

The realm of therapeutic nutrition must also accommodate the influence of culture. The effect of diabetes, renal disease, or cardiovascular disease on dietary intake may require major changes in traditional food-preparation techniques or food intake. Knowing and communicating the aspects of the diet that do not need to be changed can be a very positive approach. Once individuals know which traditional foods or cooking procedures can be retained, they are often more receptive to changes that must be made.

THE ROLE OF NUTRITION IN ILLNESS

Awareness of factors that influence dietary intake is especially crucial in the hospital setting, since food consumption is often affected by therapeutic procedures, diagnostic tests, and the disease process itself. Lack of attention to the nutritional well-being of patients results in preventable cases of malnutrition. It has been estimated that over 30% of patients in U.S. hospitals are malnourished, causing 50,000 preventable deaths each year and affecting approximately one-half million recoveries (29). These figures are actually an improvement over the situation in the 1970s, when hospital malnutrition was first discovered (30). Today, while there is greater recognition of the problem, it is evident that there is room for improvement. What causes malnutrition, what problems result when patients are malnourished, and what precautions can be taken to avoid the problem?

Patient Malnutrition

Malnutrition can be caused by lack of sufficient food over a period of time or lack of intake of specific nutrients (31). Patients can be admitted to the hospital in a malnourished state or become malnourished in the hospital. Malnutrition is usually manifested as serious underweight, vitamin depletion, loss of lean body mass, a decline in serum proteins (serum albumin <3.5 g/dl), and depressed immune responses (32). Illness increases the risk for malnutrition to occur because it can cause anorexia, increase nutritional needs, or result in diminished ability to ingest, digest, absorb, or metabolize nutrients. For example, individuals who have cancer have problems finding foods that taste good and do not cause nausea. Fever and infection cause energy losses in the form of heat; digestive diseases can result in energy, nitrogen, vitamin, and mineral losses in the stool; and vomiting can cause losses of potassium, sodium, and fluid, resulting in electrolyte imbalances and dehydration (33). Stroke victims often cannot take foods orally as a result of muscle paralysis, and surgical patients may not be able to ingest nutrient-dense foods for a number of days following the surgical procedure. Specialized feedings are available that provide adequate nutrition to patients who have problems that interfere with intake; however, the need for intervention must be

recognized early to avoid the consequences of malnutrition.

Malnourished patients have an increased incidence of sepsis, experience more delays in wound healing, absorb nutrients less efficiently, and have higher mortality rates than those who are not malnourished (34). Compounding the problem are the shortened hospital stays resulting from implementation of the diagnosis related groups (DRGs). Malnutrition follows the patient home, where inadequate supervision can cause the patient's condition to further deteriorate.

Nutrition support teams, which include surgeons, medical doctors, nurses, dietitians, pharmacists, and health educators, are being created to monitor the nutritional status of patients to prevent malnutrition from occurring. The teams are currently in 30% of U.S. hospitals, and the numbers are growing (31). Ideally, all hospitalized patients should undergo a basic screening process to quickly identify those who are malnourished or who are at increased risk for developing malnutrition.

When patients are admitted to a hospital, height and weight should be recorded, available laboratory test results should be reviewed, recent weight changes should be noted, and a dietary history should be taken (35). A physical exam can detect specific changes in various body systems (see Figure 1-1). Weights should be recorded on a regular basis, so that changes can be immediately noted.

The nursing staff is particularly important for identifying patients who are at special risk for developing malnutrition due to surgical procedures, physical factors such as shortness of breath, stomatitis, diarrhea, nausea and vomiting, and emotional factors such as confusion, fear, and anxiety. They can refer patients to clinical dietitians and also help to maintain regular height and weight records.

FOOD SAFETY

Not only can hospitalized individuals be at risk for developing malnutrition, but they can also be exposed to food-borne disease if special care is not given to food preparation and distribution. The Centers for Disease Control report that 6.5 million

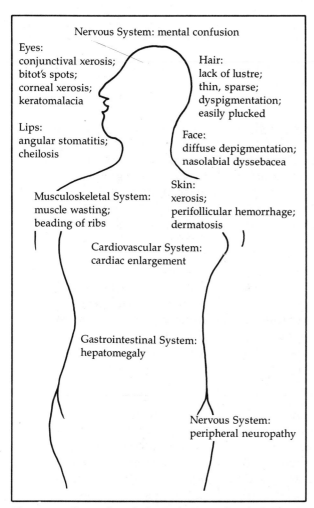

Nervous System: mental confusion

Eyes:
conjunctival xerosis;
bitot's spots;
corneal xerosis;
keratomalacia

Hair:
lack of lustre;
thin, sparse;
dyspigmentation;
easily plucked

Lips:
angular stomatitis;
cheilosis

Face:
diffuse depigmentation;
nasolabial dyssebacea

Musculoskeletal System:
muscle wasting;
beading of ribs

Skin:
xerosis;
perifollicular hemorrhage;
dermatosis

Cardiovascular System:
cardiac enlargement

Gastrointestinal System:
hepatomegaly

Nervous System:
peripheral neuropathy

Figure 1-1. Examples of physical signs of malnutrition.

cases of acute episodes of food-borne disease with 9100 fatalities occur annually in the United States (36). Of these cases, 77% are related to food-service establishments (such as restaurants and food services provided by hospitals and nursing homes), 20% can be traced to problems with food handling in the home, and 3% are a result of problems in food-processing plants. It is believed that food-borne illness is vastly underreported because the symptoms sometimes are mild, temporary, and mistaken for viral infections.

Food-borne illness can be very serious, because the organisms may affect organ systems beyond the gastrointestinal tract, including the nervous, circulatory, and skeletal systems. Diseases such as hemolytic-uremic syndrome, reactive arthritis, pericarditis and myocarditis, and Guillain-Barre syndrome may result from infection with food-borne agents (36).

In general, bacteria need food, moisture, warmth, and time to cause food-borne illness. Most bacteria experience rapid growth at a temperature range 40°F–140°F. Control measures include adequate heat treatment or cooking; avoidance of cross-contamination of cooked or ready-to-eat foods by utensils, equipment, or surfaces not cleaned and disinfected after contact with raw foods; avoidance of undercooked or contaminated raw foods; avoidance of contaminating raw foods by infected handlers; and immediate refrigeration or freezing to avoid multiplication of bacteria (37). Interestingly, the Centers for Disease Control estimate that approximately 20% of cases of food-borne illness could be reduced if hands were washed prior to food handling (38). Proper hand washing requires the use of soap and warm water and at least 20 seconds of working the soap into the hands, including the fingernail area and between the fingers (39). Jewelry should be removed before handling food, since items such as rings provide good places for bacteria to accumulate.

Most food-borne illness in North America is caused by 10 pathogenic bacteria: Salmonella, Shigella, Campylobacter jejuni, Listeria monocytogenes, Vibrio, enteropathogenic Escherichia coli, Clostridium perfringens, Clostridium botulinum, Staphylococcus aureus, and Bacillus cereus (37). (See Table 1-5, pages 16–19).

Certain populations are more vulnerable to some bacteria. For example, pregnant women (due to their high levels of immunosuppressive hormones during pregnancy), fetuses, newborns, and adults with compromised immune systems (cancer patients, patients on corticosteroids, individuals on hemodialysis, and AIDS patients) seem to be more susceptible to infection by Listeria, which has a 70% fatality rate if untreated or treated too late (36, 40). The 1% mortality rate caused by salmonella infection is confined to children younger

Table 1-5. FOOD-BORNE ILLNESSES

ILLNESS AND ORGANISM THAT CAUSES IT	SOURCES OF ILLNESS AND CONTROL METHODS	SYMPTOMS
Salmonellosis Salmonella bacteria	Improper cooling, inadequate cooking, or ingestion of contaminated or cross-contaminated raw products, particularly meats, poultry, milk and other dairy products, shrimp, and frog legs. Heat kills the salmonella bacteria.	Generally, 6–48 hours after eating, onset of nausea, vomiting, abdominal cramps, diarrhea, fever, and headache. Symptoms last 1–7 days. All age groups are susceptible, but symptoms are most severe for the elderly, infants, and the infirm.
Shigellosis Shigella bacteria	Primary route of infection: fecal-oral route. Associated with seafood and salads contaminated by infected workers coupled with improper refrigeration. The bacteria are killed by most heat treatments.	Generally, 7–36 hours after eating, onset of diarrhea, abdominal pain, fever, vomiting. Symptoms last 3–14 days.
Campylobacterosis Campylobacter jejuni	Bacteria found in the gastrointestinal tract; therefore associated with foods of animal origin, primarily raw poultry and meat and unpasteurized milk. Methods of control include proper cooking and avoidance of cross-contamination of foods, utensils, and surfaces.	Generally 2–5 days after eating, onset of diarrhea, abominal cramping, fever and sometimes bloody stools. Symptoms last 7–10 days.
Listeriosis Listeria monocytogenes	Ubiquitous in nature. Found in soil, vegetation, water. Raw or inadequately heated foods (milk, red meats, poultry, seafood, vegetables, and some fresh fruits) are major sources. To reduce risk of infection, susceptible	Pregnant women, fetuses, very young children, and immunocompromised persons are susceptible. First stage symptoms: malaise, diarrhea, mild fever, later symptoms: septicemia, abortion, stillbirth, fever,

Continued

Table 1-5. FOOD-BORNE ILLNESSES (continued)

ILLNESS AND ORGANISM THAT CAUSES IT	SOURCES OF ILLNESS AND CONTROL METHODS	SYMPTOMS
	persons should avoid contact with animals that might be affected, avoid foods that are raw or inadequately heated, and avoid foods that support Listeria during processing and storage (Camembert cheese).	possible death. Onset of symptoms may occur four days to three weeks after consuming contaminated food.
Cholera, gastroenteritis, septicemia Vibrio cholerae, Vibrio parahaemolyticus, Vibrio vulnificus	Raw seafood is the source. The bacteria are killed by heating.	Symptoms of V. cholerae: cholera epidemics, massive diarrhea with large volumes of "rice-water" stools; V. parahaemolyticus: acute gastroenteritis; V. vulnificus: serious wound infections and septicemia.
Diarrhea Enteropathogenic Escherichia coli	Major source of contamination: feces of infected humans and animals.	Significant cause of diarrhea in locales with poor sanitation.
Perfringens food poisoning Clostridium perfringens	In most instances, the actual cause of poisoning by Clostridium perfringens is improper temperature in prepared foods. Small numbers of the organisms are often present after cooking and multiply to food poisoning levels during improper cool down and storage of prepared foods. Meat and meat products are the foods most frequently implicated. These organisms grow better than other bacteria between 120°F–130°F; for this reason, food	Generally 8–24 hours (usually 12) after eating, onset of abdominal pain and diarrhea. Sometimes nausea and vomiting. Symptoms last a day or less and are usually mild. Can be more serious in older or debilitated individuals.

Continued

Table 1-5. FOOD-BORNE ILLNESSES (continued)

ILLNESS AND ORGANISM THAT CAUSES IT	SOURCES OF ILLNESS AND CONTROL METHODS	SYMPTOMS
	should be kept at temperatures above 140°. Also need to reheat cooked chilled foods to a minimum internal temperature of 167°.	
Botulism Clostridium botulinum (toxin)	Spores of these bacteria are widespread. Bacteria produce toxin only in an anaerobic environment of little acidity. Botulinum toxin has been found in a considerable variety of canned foods (primarily improperly processed home-canned foods): corn, peppers, green beans, soups, beets, asparagus, mushrooms, ripe olives, spinach, tuna fish, chicken, chicken liver, and liver pate. It has also been found in luncheon meats, ham, sausage, stuffed eggplant, lobster, and smoked and salted fish.	Generally 4–36 hours after eating, onset of neurotoxic symptoms, including double vision, inability to swallow, speech difficulty, and progressive paralysis of the respiratory system. Medical help should be sought immediately because botulism can be fatal.
Staphylococcal food poisoning Staphylococcus aureus (enterotoxin)	The toxin is produced when food contaminated with the bacteria is left too long at room temperature and when foods are inadequately cooled. Meats, poultry, egg products, tuna, potato and macaroni salads, and cream-filled pastries are good environments for these bacteria to produce toxin. Raw foods are never the source of infection. Staphylococcus aureus bacteria are commonly found	Generally ½–8 hours after eating, onset of diarrhea, vomiting, nausea, abdominal cramps, and prostration. Mimics flu. Lasts 24–48 hours. Rarely fatal.

Continued

Table 1-5. FOOD-BORNE ILLNESSES (*continued*)

ILLNESS AND ORGANISM THAT CAUSES IT	SOURCES OF ILLNESS AND CONTROL METHODS	SYMPTOMS
	in the nose, throat, hair, and skin of more than 50% of healthy individuals.	
Diarrheal and emetic illnesses Bacillus cereus (toxin)	Common in soil and on vegetation. Causes no problems at low levels; however, when cooked foods are held at 50°F–131°F for long periods, the organism grows to large numbers and releases a toxin. Cooked foods should be held at temperatures higher than 140° and cooled rapidly to temperatures below 50°. Cereal dishes, meat products, fried and boiled rice dishes have been implicated.	Onset of diarrheal illness 8–20 hours after ingestion. Onset of emetic illness 1–5 hours after ingestion. Symptoms last 24 hours.

Sources: *FDA Consumer* (June 1987), 18; *Food Technology* 42 (1988):182–99.

than four years old, the elderly, and those suffering from diseases that weaken resistance (41, 42). It is therefore apparent that precautions need to be taken to avoid infection in hospitals and nursing homes, which more than likely house the most vulnerable populations.

THE CRITICAL ROLE OF THE NURSE AS PART OF THE HEALTH-CARE TEAM

Throughout this chapter, references have been made to the importance of the interaction between the nurse and dietitian to guarantee the best possible nutritional care of the patient. As the health professional who has the most contact with the hospitalized patient, the nurse also has the responsibility for coordination of all of the patient's therapies, which extend well beyond nutrition. The nurse must interact closely with other members of the health-care team to ensure that patient needs

are met. A short description of the duties of the other members of the health-care team as they relate to nutritional needs or alterations illustrates how the nurse can best perform his or her role as an integral part of the team. (See Figure 1-2).

Physician

The overall responsibility for patient care is in the hands of the physician. The physician frequently consults with members of other disciplines when outlining a plan for care. He or she is responsible for writing orders for drug and diet therapies and diagnostic tests. The physician relies on the nurse to observe patients closely, maintain records on the patient's reactions to treatment, and report changes in the patient's condition.

Registered Dietitian

The registered dietitian performs the nutritional assessment of the patient. Based on data obtained

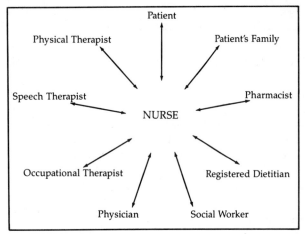

Figure 1-2. The nurse must interact with other members of the health-care team.

from the assessment, the dietitian can calculate the nutrient needs and address any special needs dictated by the patient's disease. It is the dietitian's responsibility to monitor the nutrition progress of the patient and instruct the patient and family on dietary modifications when required.

The nurse collaborates with the dietitian in implementing the plan and can help reinforce dietary teaching. In addition, the nurse is responsible for modifying care relating to nutritional needs. For example, the nurse can optimize the patient's dietary intake by providing a rest period prior to meals if the patient tires easily, ensuring that snacks and other nourishments are provided, and feeding patients who are unable to feed themselves. As stated earlier, the nurse can identify those patients who are nutritionally at risk and refer them to the dietitian. Careful documentation of height and weight, as well as nutritional intake and output in specific disease states, aid in the monitoring of nutritional progress.

Pharmacist

The pharmacist is trained to prepare and dispense drugs, monitor the drug therapy of patients, and identify drug-drug or drug-nutrient interactions. Special feedings such as enteral or parenteral solutions are available through the pharmacist at most hospitals.

Social Worker

The social worker provides assistance in the support of patients and families who have social, financial, or emotional problems that may interfere with recovery. The social worker facilitates problem solving, provides financial counseling, and arranges for referrals to other community service agencies that will be of help to the patient once he or she is discharged from the hospital. For example, the social worker may initiate contacts for services, such as Meals on Wheels, Congregate Meals, Food Stamps, and the Special Supplemental Food Program for Women, Infants and Children (WIC), that may be needed to supplement nutritional intake.

Physical, Occupational, and Speech Therapists

The physical therapist is trained to evaluate the patient's need for therapeutic exercise and assist in improving the patient's strength and coordination following, for example, strokes, amputations, burns, spinal-cord injuries, or fractures. Physical therapists also instruct patients in the use of ambulation aids and artificial limbs and institute measures to alleviate pain through application of heat, cold, light, water, electricity, sound waves, or massage (43).

Occupational therapists focus on retraining patients for activities of daily living. They are familiar with special aids that make the process of eating or dressing easier for individuals who, for example, have suffered a stroke or who have undergone an amputation.

Speech therapists retrain individuals who have lost the facility for forming or recognizing words. They also provide training to patients who have impaired swallowing as a result of neurological or physical impairments such as stroke or partial glossectomy. Successful therapy often means the difference between the patient's self-reliance and dependence on caregivers or tube feedings.

THE NURSING PROCESS

To provide the best possible nursing care for patients, and to function as a member of the health-care team, the nurse uses an approach to care called the nursing process. The nursing process is a systematic method of assessment, diagnosis, planning, implementation, and evaluation. Although the focus of this text is on nutrition, the nurse takes a holistic view of the patient with his or her many needs; nutritional needs are one of the many facets of care.

The assessment phase involves data gathering. The nurse uses the patient history and laboratory reports, as well as physical assessment, to gain information about the patient's needs and problems. The patient history may provide clues as to physical impairments, such as stroke or illness, that may alter the intake or digestion of foods. Physical assessment may provide information about body functioning that may necessitate dietary alterations. Visual evidence of edema would lead the nurse to monitor the laboratory reports to note the levels of serum sodium. The nurse may then be involved in teaching the patient the importance of adhering to the diet prescription.

The diagnosis phase is analytical in nature. Nursing diagnoses are derived from the informa-tion obtained during the assessment. Examples of possible nursing diagnoses are included in subsequent chapters to serve as a guide in identifying specific nursing interventions for patients suffering from various disorders that require possible nutrition alterations.

Once the nursing diagnoses are identified, planning is required to reduce or eliminate the problems and promote health. The plan includes setting priorities, establishing goals or outcomes, prescribing nursing interventions, and documenting the nursing care (44). The implementation component involves putting the plan into action; nursing interventions are carried out and then tested. Any action that is implemented must be evaluated so that the nurse can assess the client's progress in attaining the goals. If the goals were not achieved, changes must be made in the nursing-care plan. Benefits of the nursing process include continuity of care; dynamic, ongoing assessment and evaluation of care; flexibility; and efficiency, since the health alterations of patients can be described in clear and concise terms (44).

TOPIC OF INTEREST

The Food and Drug Administration (FDA) has always taken an interest in the nutritional well-being of the American public. The FDA has, among other duties, responsibility for assuring that information on food labels (with the exception of meat products, which are governed by the USDA) is accurate. The FDA issues regulations that food processors must follow when labeling the nutritional content of foods, and has stipulated the types of claims that can be made on labels. In the past, the FDA has allowed implicit health claims such as "low calorie," "reduced calorie," "sodium free," "very low sodium," "low sodium," and "reduced sodium." Due to the increased public interest in the relationship between nutrition and health, the FDA is considering allowing explicit health-related or disease-prevention claims on food labels. This is a very new area for FDA, which historically has prohibited such claims (45).

In 1987, the FDA issued a proposal for public comment that detailed the procedures companies would need to follow in order to make label claims (46). There were numerous responses to the proposal, both positive and negative. Currently, the final regulation is in the Office of Management and Budget (OMB) for approval. The final rule would permit claims in five areas: calcium and osteoporosis; sodium and hypertension; lipids and heart disease; lipids and cancer; and fiber and cancer. Food manufacturers would be able to use model statements prescribed by the FDA that pertain to these five areas. Thus, a food product that is low in sodium could conceivably have a label with a printed statement regarding the usefulness of low sodium products in the prevention of hypertension.

Another program for which the FDA is drafting regulations is an in-store shelf-labeling program (47). The regulation would standardize definitions for "low fat," "excellent fiber source," and "good" sources of nutrients, for example. The terms would be used on the grocery shelves to help consumers quickly identify foods with the attributes they desire. These programs illustrate the commitment of the FDA to deliver truthful, accurate information to consumers that may help to forge the dietary changes that are currently being recommended by the government.

SPOTLIGHT ON LEARNING

Ms. Marks is a lacto-vegetarian. She recently had radiation therapy on her neck and finds it painful to swallow. You notice that she has been returning most of the food on her meal trays untouched. Her evening snack, a meat sandwich, is never eaten. The last time you weighed Ms. Marks, you noticed a drop in weight of three pounds.

1. What can you do to optimize the nutritional care of Ms. Marks?
2. What foods would be appropriate to offer?

REVIEW QUESTIONS

1. The overconsumption of which of the following dietary components is targeted as the primary priority for change according to the Surgeon General's Report on Nutrition and Health?
   a. sugar
   b. complex carbohydrates
   c. fat
   d. sodium

2. Vegans abstain from which of the following?
   a. all animal products
   b. all animal products except milk products
   c. all animal products except milk products and eggs
   d. all animal products except milk products, eggs, and poultry

3. Which of the following is not an essential amino acid?
   a. glutamine
   b. tryptophan
   c. phenylalanine
   d. lysine

4. Animal sources are weak in which amino acid?
   a. lysine
   b. isoleucine
   c. tryptophan
   d. none

5. The Asian diet is most likely to lack which of the following?
   a. iron
   b. vitamin B_{12}
   c. vitamin C
   d. calcium

6. Which of the following can prevent malnutrition in the hospital from occurring?
   a. offering clear liquids to patients
   b. screening patients on admission
   c. shortening hospital stays
   d. scheduling surgery

7. Bacteria generally do not need which of the following to cause food-borne illness?
   a. moisture
   b. warmth
   c. carbon dioxide
   d. time

8. Which of the following populations is not more vulnerable to some bacteria?
   a. the elderly
   b. pregnant women
   c. teenagers
   d. AIDS patients

9. Which member of the health-care team has responsibility for coordination of all of the patient's therapies?
   a. registered dietitian
   b. pharmacist
   c. nurse
   d. occupational therapist

10. Which of the following is not part of the nursing process?
   a. diagnosis
   b. assessment
   c. evaluation
   d. objectives

ACTIVITIES

1. Keep a record of dietary intake for one day. Does your intake include foods from the basic food groups? If not, how could you better balance your intake? Using a food composition table, total the amount of kilocalories and grams of fat, calculate the percentage of kilocalories from fat, and compare it with the National Academy of Sciences' recommendation to reduce total fat intake to 30% or less of kilocalories. What was the result? What foods in your diet contributed most heavily to total fat intake?

2. Investigate the dietary customs of a religious or ethnic group not covered in this chapter. Prepare a short report on the topic.

3. Take a trip to the grocery store and investigate the produce area. What Hispanic or Asian fruits and vegetables did you see? What other items in the grocery store could you find that appeal to a particular religious or ethnic group?

4. Imagine that you are going on a picnic. What precautions would you need to take to ensure that the food you pack does not turn into a breeding ground for bacteria? What would you do if there were leftovers?

5. Invite a member of the health-care team to class to discuss the interaction that member has with the nursing staff.

REFERENCES

1. Guthrie, H.A. *Introductory nutrition.* 5th ed. St. Louis: C.V. Mosby Company, 1983.
2. Committee on Dietary Allowances, Food and Nutrition Board, National Research Council. *Recommended dietary allowances.* 8th rev. ed. Washington, D.C.: National Academy of Sciences, 1974.
3. Senate Select Committee on Nutrition and Human Needs. *Dietary goals for the United States.* 2d ed. Washington, D.C., 1977.
4. Committee on Diet, Nutrition and Cancer, Assembly of Life Sciences, National Research Council. *Diet, nutrition and cancer.* Washington, D.C.: National Academy Press, 1982.
5. American Heart Association, Nutrition Committee Position Statement. *Dietary guidelines for healthy American adults.* Dallas: American Heart Association, 1986.
6. National Institutes of Health. Consensus Development Conference Statement. Osteoporosis. *Journal of the American Medical Association* 252 (1984):799–802.
7. U.S. Department of Health and Human Services, Public Health Service. *The surgeon general's report on nutrition and health: Summary and recommendations 1988.* Publication No. 88-50211.
8. Nestle, M. The surgeon general's report on nutrition and health: New federal dietary guidance policy, *Journal of Nutrition Education* 20 (1988):252–54.

9. Committee on Diet and Health, Food and Nutrition Board, Commission on Life Sciences, National Research Council, *Diet and health: Implications for reducing chronic disease risk.* Washington, D.C.: National Academy Press, 1989.

10. Senauer, B. Economics and nutrition. In *What is America eating?* Food and Nutrition Board, Commission on Life Sciences, National Research Council, 46–57. Washington, D.C.: National Academy Press, 1986.

11. U.S. Department of Agriculture. Human Nutrition Information Service, Nutrition Monitoring Division. *Nationwide food consumption survey. Continuing survey of food intakes by individuals. Women 19–50 years and their children 1–5 years, 4 days, 1985.* Report No. 85-4. Issued August 1987.

12. U.S. Department of Agriculture. Human Nutrition Information Service, Nutrition Monitoring Division. *Nationwide food consumption survey. Continuing survey of food intakes by individuals. Women 19–50 years and their children 1–5 years, 4 days, 1986.* Report No. 86-3. Issued September 1988.

13. U.S. Department of Agriculture. Human Nutrition Information Service, Nutrition Monitoring Division. *Nationwide food consumption survey. Continuing survey of food intakes by individuals. Men 19–50 years, 1 day, 1985.* Report No. 85-3. Issued November 1986.

14. Greenwood, M.R.C., and V.A. Pittman-Waller. Weight control: A complex, various and controversial problem. In *Obesity and weight control: The health professional's guide to understanding and treatment,* edited by R.T. Frankle and M. Yang, 3–15. Rockville: Aspen Publishers, Inc., 1988.

15. National Dairy Council. Nutrition and modern lifestyles. *Dairy Council Digest* 59, no. 5 (September–October, 1988).

16. ———. Consumers: Price is nice, but time is prime. *Progressive Grocer* (January 1987):47–52.

17. Regenstein, J.M, and C.E. Regenstein. The kosher dietary laws and their implementation in the food industry. *Food Technology* 42 (1988):86–94.

18. Nelson, M.S., and L.J. Jovanovic. Pregnancy, diabetes and Jewish dietary law: The challenge for the pregnant diabetic woman who keeps kosher. *Journal of the American Dietetic Association* 87 (1987):1054–57.

19. Twaigery, S., and D. Spillman. An introduction to Moslem dietary laws. *Food Technology* 43 (1989):88–90.

20. American Dietetic Association. Position of the American Dietetic Association: Vegetarian diets. *Journal of the American Dietetic Association* 88 (1988):351–55.

21. Herbert, V. Vitamin B$_{12}$: Plant sources, requirements and assay. *American Journal of Clinical Nutrition* 48 (1988):852–58.

22. National Dairy Council. Diet and nutrition-related concerns of Blacks and other ethnic minorities. *Dairy Council Digest* 59 (November–December 1988):31–36.

23. Sills-Levy, E. U.S. food trends leading to the year 2000. *Food Technology* 43 (1989):128–32.

24. Community Nutrition Institute. Hispanic population grows; Faces special food needs. *Nutrition Week*, November 14, 1985.

25. Aaron, J., and G.S. Salom. *The art of Mexican cooking.* Garden City: Doubleday and Company, Inc., 1965.

26. Ziegler, V.S., K.P. Sucher, and N.J. Downes. Southeast Asian renal exchange

list. *Journal of the American Dietetic Association* 89 (1989):85–92.

27. Ngo, B., and G. Zimmerman. The classic cuisine of Vietnam. Woodbury: Barron's Educational Series, Inc., 1979.

28. Samagalski, A., and M. Buckley. China: A travel survival kit. Victoria, Australia: Lonely Planet Publications, 1984.

29. Teitelman, R. Skeletons in the closet. *Forbes,* April 9, 1984.

30. Butterworth, C.E. Skeleton in the hospital closet. *Nutrition Today* 9 (1974):4–8.

31. Gilbride, J., C. Cowell, and M.D. Simko. The process of nutrition assessment. In *Nutrition assessment: A comprehensive guide for planning intervention*, 1–12. Rockville: Aspen Systems Corporation, 1984.

32. Shils, M.E. Nutrition assessment in support of the malnourished patient. In *Nutrition assessment: A comprehensive guide for planning intervention*, edited by M.D. Simko, C. Cowell, and J. Gilbride, 237–39. Rockville: Aspen Systems Corporation, 1984.

33. Heymsfield, S.B., and P.J. Williams. Nutritional assessment by clinical and biochemical methods. In *Modern nutrition in health and disease*, 7th ed., edited by M.E. Shils and V.R. Young, 817–60. Philadelphia: Lea & Febiger, 1988.

34. Glassman, R.G. Nutrition assessment: A critical review. *Topics in Clinical Nutrition* 1 (1986):16–27.

35. Hedberg, A., et al. Nutritional risk screening: Development of a standardized protocol using dietetic technicians. *Journal of the American Dietetic Association* 88 (1988):1553–56.

36. Archer, D.L. The true impact of foodborne infections. *Food Technology* 42 (1988):53–58.

37. Institute of Food Technologists' Expert Panel on Food Safety and Nutrition. Bacteria associated with foodborne illness. Scientific status summary. *Food Technology* 42 (1988):181–82 and 200.

38. Columbia University Institute of Human Nutrition. *Nutrition and Health* 3, no. 4 (1981).

39. Miller, R.W. Mother nature's regulations on food safety. DHHS Publication No. (FDA) 88-2223.

40. Marth, E.H. Disease characteristics of Listeria monocytogenes. *Food Technology* 42 (1988):165–68.

41. Zottola, E.A. Foodborne disease I. *Contemporary Nutrition* 2, no. 9 (1977).

42. U.S. Department of Agriculture. *Food-borne bacterial poisoning.* Food Safety and Inspection Service. Washington, D.C.: U.S. Government Printing Office, 1985.

43. Barbrow, E., and I. Laquatra. *Diet therapy and nutrition care in disease.* University Park: The Pennsylvania State University, 1983.

44. Alfaro, R. *Application of nursing process. A step-by-step guide.* Philadelphia: J.B. Lippincott Company, 1986.

45. National Dairy Council. Nutrition labeling and health claims. *Dairy Council Digest* 57, no. 6 (November–December 1986).

46. Food and Drug Administration. Food labeling; public health messages on food labels and labeling. 21 CFR Part 101. Federal Register 52 (1987):28843–49.

47. ———. Definitions for use in shelf label programs outlined by FDA. *Food Chemical News* (December 12, 1988), 32–34.

CHAPTER
2

AN OVERVIEW OF NUTRITION PRINCIPLES

Objectives

After studying this chapter, you will be able to
- describe the process of digestion.
- explain the metabolism of protein, carbohydrate, and fat.
- describe the metabolism of alcohol.
- discuss the functions of vitamins and minerals.
- list food sources of vitamins and minerals.
- explain symptoms of toxicity from ingesting high levels of specific vitamin supplements.

Overview

The purpose of food is to provide energy for body processes, including for example, energy for growth, activity, regulation of body temperature, and storage. The energy value of foods is measured in kilocalories. A kilocalorie is the amount of heat required to raise the temperature of one kilogram of water by 1° C. In most texts, the terms calorie and kilocalorie are used interchangeably, although such usage is technically incorrect, since a calorie is the amount of heat required to raise the temperature of one *gram* of water by 1° C.

Carbohydrate, protein, fat, and alcohol are the sole sources of kilocalories in the diet. The caloric value of these substances to the body is known as the physiological fuel value, which is the portion of the energy provided by carbohydrate, protein, fat, and alcohol that is available for transformation in the body, taking into account any loss of energy as a result of digestion. The physiological fuel value of carbohydrate and protein is four kilocalories per gram; for fat, nine kilocalories per gram; and for alcohol, seven kilocalories per gram. Vitamins and minerals, although not providing kilocalories themselves, play a critical role in the metabolism of the energy-yielding substances. This chapter provides an overview of the digestion of food and the metabolism of the six classes of nutrients: carbohydrate, protein, fat, vitamins, minerals, and water. Alcohol, because it is not needed for growth or maintenance of body tissues, is not considered a nutrient; however, because its use is so prevalent in our society, a brief review of its metabolism is included.

REVIEW OF THE GASTROINTESTINAL TRACT

The gastrointestinal tract (G-I tract) (see Figure 2-1) performs four functions: (1) moves digestive contents from one portion of the tract to another; (2) breaks down food into usable forms; (3) allows the absorption of nutrients into the bloodstream; and (4) excretes waste products. Each day, only 10% of all liquids and solids ingested and digestive juices secreted into the gastrointestinal tract are excreted (1). Food passing from the stomach to the ileum takes approximately 30–90 minutes, how-

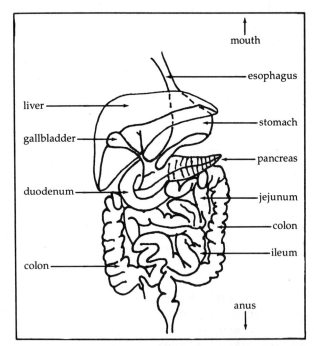

Figure 2-1 The gastrointestinal tract.

ever, passage through the colon can take from one to seven days. The cells of the G-I tract are completely renewed every three to seven days. Both voluntary and involuntary functions are controlled by the central nervous system and the hormones. Each section of the G-I tract is responsible for specific activities, which are briefly reviewed in the following paragraphs.

The Mouth

The mouth breaks down the cellulose walls of carbohydrates, decreases the size of food particles, and increases the surface area of foods. The last function mentioned is significant because digestive juices act only on the surface of food particles.

In the mouth, food is mixed with saliva, a slightly acid digestive juice secreted by the salivary glands. Saliva is 99% water and 1% enzymes, urea, glucose, mucus, and electrolytes and acts as a lubricant, moistening food and reducing it to a semisolid mass. The enzymes in saliva include salivary amylase (ptyalin) and lingual lipase.

The Stomach

The functions of the stomach are to mix the food with gastric juice to form chyme and store the chyme until it can be handled by the intestine. (The secretions of the cells in the stomach lining (see Figure 2-2) form the gastric juice. The surface epithelium of the stomach secretes mucus, which acts as a protection against the highly acidic environment of the stomach. The parietal cells produce hydrochloric acid and intrinsic factor (discussed later in the chapter), and the chief cells release an

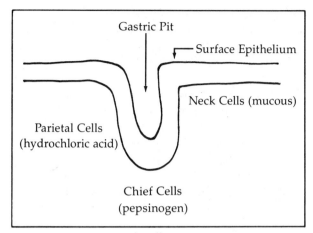

Figure 2-2. The stomach cells.

inactive precursor of pepsin known as pepsinogen. The total composition of gastric juice is hydrochloric acid (.2%–.5%), pepsin, rennin, lipase, and inorganic salts and water (97%–99%), with a pH of 1.0. The hydrochloric acid is critical for the conversion of pepsinogen to pepsin, an enzyme that partially digests protein and functions best at a pH of 1.0 to 3.0.

Digestion in the stomach begins with the release of the hormone gastrin. Stimulation of the vagus nerve through tasting, smelling, and chewing food promotes the release of gastrin, as does the distention of the stomach caused by the presence of food. Gastrin is the most potent activator of gastric acid secretion, because it stimulates the parietal cells to release hydrochloric acid. Gastrin can also decrease the rate of stomach emptying into the duodenum. High levels of gastric acid serve to inhibit gastrin release through a feedback loop.

The Exocrine Pancreas

Chyme enters the duodenum via the pyloric sphincter of the stomach. The presence of hydrochloric acid, fat, protein, and carbohydrate stimulates the release of the hormones secretin and cholecystokinin-pancreozymin (CCK-PZ) from the duodenal and jejunal mucosa. Secretin is a powerful stimulant of water and bicarbonate secretion of the pancreas, and it inhibits gastric acid secretion. Cholecystokinin-pancreozymin stimu-

lates the production of fluid from the pancreas, which is high in enzyme content and controls contraction of the gallbladder. The resultant pancreatic juice that enters the intestine is similar to saliva in water content. It is alkaline (as a result of its bicarbonate content), with a pH of 7.5–8.0 or higher. Some of the enzymes in pancreatic juice include trypsin, chymotrypsin, carboxypeptidases, alpha-amylase, lipase, and cholesterol ester hydrolase. Some of the enzymes are released as inactive precursors (zymogens), which become activated on contact with the intestinal mucosa.

The Small Intestine

The small intestine includes the duodenum, the jejunum, and the ileum and is approximately 15 ft in length. The major part of digestion and absorption occurs in the duodenum and jejunum. Chyme in the small intestine is mixed with intestinal juice secreted by the glands of Brunner and Lieberkuhn. Intestinal juice is high in enzyme content, containing peptidases, disaccharidases, phosphatase, and nucleotidases. The small intestine is uniquely structured to encourage absorption through its extremely large surface area. The mucosal area of the small intestine is 1.9–2.7 sq m. The presence of villi and microvilli forming the brush border increase the area further, making the total absorptive area of the small intestine 200–500 sq m (2).

The Liver and Gallbladder

The liver produces bile, which contains bile acids (also called bile salts), lecithin, cholesterol, and bile pigments. Bile is stored in the gallbladder, where it becomes more concentrated. During digestion, cholecystokinin-pancreozymin causes contraction of the gallbladder, causing release of bile into the intestine via the common bile duct. Once in the intestine, bile emulsifies fat and neutralizes the acidity of the chyme. Approximately 90% of the bile acids secreted in the bile are reabsorbed almost exclusively in the ileum and returned to the liver. The recycling of the bile acids occurs 6–10 times each day, and thus only a small fraction of the bile acids actually reaches the colon for excretion. The recycling system is known as the enterohepatic circulation.

The Large Intestine

As stated previously, most nutrients are absorbed in the small intestine. The chyme reaching the large intestine contains undigested food residues, water, desquamated cells (cells shed from epithelial lining), enzyme secretions of the digestive tract, mucus, and electrolytes. Considerable water is absorbed in the last third of the large intestine. Also, some of the residue (dietary fiber and a small amount of dietary protein) is attacked by bacteria. The action of bacteria on dietary fiber is known as fermentation. Short-chain fatty acids, the by-products of bacterial fermentation, are then absorbed from the colon and may be used for energy (3). The lower third of the large intestine functions as a reservoir for the stool. Intestinal bacteria account for approximately 10% of the dry weight of the stool.

THE ENERGY-YIELDING SUBSTRATES

Carbohydrate

Food sources of carbohydrate include sugar, starch, and dietary fiber. As a group, carbohydrates are classified according to the number of saccharide units contained in the molecule. *Monosaccharides* are carbohydrates that cannot be hydrolyzed into a simpler form, and include pentoses (e.g., ribose), hexoses (e.g., glucose), and trioses (e.g., glycerose). *Oligosaccharides* yield 2 to as many as 10 monosaccharides when hydrolyzed (4). The most prevalent oligosaccharides in nature are the disaccharides, which yield two monosaccharides when hydrolyzed. Examples of disaccharides are sucrose, lactose, and maltose. *Polysaccharides* are the most complex of the carbohydrates, and yield more than 10 monosaccharides when hydrolyzed. The most common polysaccharide is starch, which may be linear (amylose) or branched (amylopectin).

Digestion. Digestion of carbohydrate begins in the mouth, where ptyalin attacks the linear linked starch (alpha 1,4 links). Ptyalin acts for only a short time, because it is inactivated by the acid environment of the stomach. The next major area for carbohydrate digestion is in the duodenum, where pancreatic alpha amylase acts on the alpha 1,4 links of amylopectin and amylose, resulting in the formation of disaccharides and oligosaccharides. The final hydrolysis to monosaccharides occurs as a result of enzyme action at the glycocalyx (brush border) in the jejunum. The monosaccharides are absorbed into the intestinal cell, pass through the portal vein, and enter the liver. The monosaccharides, fructose and galactose, are converted to glucose in the liver.

Metabolism. Glucose is transported from the liver to all body tissues, and, depending on the state of the body, can be stored (as glycogen), converted to fat, or oxidized to provide energy. Glycolysis is the initial stage of the metabolism of glucose for energy. The process takes place in the cell cytoplasm and produces pyruvate from glucose and energy in the form of adenosine triphosphate (ATP).

When oxygen is in short supply, the pyruvate is reduced to lactate, and glycolysis continues. Under aerobic conditions, pyruvate is further oxidized in the mitochondria of the cell through the citric-acid cycle (also known and the Kreb's cycle and the tricarboxylic-acid cycle). The net result from the citric-acid cycle is carbon dioxide, water, heat, and ATP. The generation of ATP from the citric-acid cycle is much higher than that produced by glycolysis.

The pentose phosphate shunt is an alternate path for glucose oxidation. The major purpose of the shunt is not to provide energy, but to provide substrates for the synthesis of fatty acids, steroids, amino acids, and nucleic acids.

Protein

The fundamental unit of protein is the amino acid. On the average, approximately 20 amino acids are contained in most proteins (4). All amino acids contain nitrogen, carbon, hydrogen, and oxygen. Protein plays several roles in the body. It is essential for the growth and maintenance of tissue, and the formation of hormones, enzymes, antibodies, hemoglobin, and neurotransmitters. Protein also helps to maintain body neutrality by acting as a buffer, reacting with acids and bases. Finally, protein aids in the transport of nutrients. For example, transferrin protein (containing iron) and lipoproteins are lipid-protein complexes that are essential for the transport of lipids in the body.

Amino acids are classified as essential and nonessential. Essential amino acids are those with carbon skeletons that are not produced by the body at a rate sufficient to meet growth and maintenance needs. The essential amino acids are phenylalanine, valine, threonine, tryptophan, isoleucine, methionine, leucine, lysine, and histidine (for children). The protein quality of a food is assessed by evaluating the patterns of essential amino acids.

An ideal amino acid pattern, considered a standard, was developed by the Food and Agricultural Organization/World Health Organization and is based on the needs of a school-age child (5). High-quality protein sources are those foods that come closest to the standard and include meat, fish, poultry, eggs, and dairy products. Other sources of protein (grains, seeds, legumes) are considered to be of lower quality due to their amino-acid patterns that may be lacking in one or more essential amino acids. It is possible to mix foods of vegetable origin to obtain an appropriate amino-acid pattern, thus increasing their biological value (see Chapter 1 for a discussion of complementing protein sources).

Digestion. Protein in foods must be hydrolyzed to amino acids to be absorbed and used by the body. Protein digestion begins in the stomach through the action of the enzyme pepsin. The results of stomach digestion are the intermediates—polypeptides and peptones. Gastric digestion of protein is not essential, since individuals with achlorhydria (absence of hydrochloric acid) or those who have undergone total gastrectomies have no difficulty digesting protein (4). It is in the small intestine where the major digestion of protein occurs. Enzymes in the pancreatic juice (trypsin, chymotrypsin, carboxypeptidase, aminopeptidase, dipeptidase) and in the intestine itself (aminopeptidase, dipeptidase) hydrolyze peptide linkages. The end result of hydrolysis is the creation of amino acids that are absorbed into the portal vein and transported to the liver.

Metabolism. After reaching the liver, amino acids may be transported to other tissues and may be incorporated into tissue protein (anabolism) that is used in the synthesis of other nitrogen-containing compounds, such as purines, or broken down (catabolized) to produce energy. The dynamic process of synthesis and breakdown is known as protein turnover.

For synthesis of protein to occur, all essential amino acids must be present in the cell simultaneously. If all the essential amino acids are not available, the cell will release the amino acids or use them for energy. The pattern for protein synthesis is encoded in cellular DNA. The pattern is transferred to the ribosomes in the cell via messenger RNA. The ribosomes pick up the required amino acids in the proper order from transfer RNA. The amino acids are then incorporated in the protein molecule. The muscle is the primary site for branched-chain amino-acid (leucine, valine, and isoleucine) uptake and metabolism. The liver is the primary site for nonbranched-chain amino-acid uptake and metabolism.

Because amino acids are not excreted in the urine in significant quantities, breakdown (catabolism) must occur. When amino acids are catabolized, a carbon skeleton and nitrogen are the products. The energy state of the body determines the use of the carbon skeleton. It may be used to form glycogen or fat for storage, or it can enter the citric-acid cycle for the production of ATP. The major pathway of nitrogen excretion in humans is as urea synthesized in the liver, released into the blood, and cleared by the kidneys.

Fat

Currently, dietary fat accounts for approximately 37% of the total energy intake of Americans, well above the level of 30% of total kilocalories recommended by health organizations (6). The major sources of fat in the American diet are meat, poultry, fish, dairy products, fats, and oils. A complete discussion of the types of fat in the diet is included in Chapter 9.

Digestion. Fat in food is in the form of triglycerides (three fatty acids attached to a glycerol backbone). Through the process of digestion, the triglycerides are hydrolyzed to monoglycerides and fatty acids. The release of fat from the stomach is slow, accounting for its high satiety value. Only a small amount of fat is digested in the stomach, with the major portion of fat digestion occurring in the small intestine.

Fat in the small intestine stimulates the release of cholecystokinin-pancreozymin, which in turn causes the gallbladder to contract and release bile into the intestine. The bile acids in the bile work to emulsify the fat; that is, they break up the fat into smaller fat droplets to increase the surface area to accommodate hydrolysis by digestive enzymes. Pancreatic lipase then attacks the triglyceride molecules resulting in the formation of glycerol; short-, medium-, and long-chain fatty acids; and monoglycerides. Short- and medium-chain fatty acids, containing less than 10 or 12 carbon atoms, are directly absorbed into the portal vein and transported to the liver. The long-chain fatty acids (monoglycerides, phospholipids, cholesterol, fat-soluble vitamins, and bile acids) are grouped in the small intestine into water-soluble molecules known as micelles. The micelles deliver all of their contents, except the bile acids, to the mucosal cells. The bile acids continue to the ileum, where they are recycled via the enterohepatic circulation.

Once in the mucosal cell, triglycerides are resynthesized from fatty acids and monoglycerides. The cholesterol, triglyceride, phospholipid, and fat-soluble vitamins are then packaged into chylomicrons, molecules with a lipid core and protein coat. Chylomicrons are released from the intestinal cell into the lymphatic system and delivered to bloodstream for metabolism. Chylomicrons in the bloodstream bombard the adipose tissue cell. Lipoprotein lipase on the surface of the adipose tissue cell hydrolyzes the chylomicron triglyceride to monoglycerides and fatty acids. These components are then absorbed by the adipose cell and reesterified (rejoined) to form triglycerides, the most concentrated form in which energy can be stored. The liver shows a special affinity for chylomicron remnants, which are rich in cholesterol and fat-soluble vitamins. Once in the hepatocyte, chylomicron remnants are completely hydrolyzed.

Metabolism. Fatty acids are catabolized for energy through the process of beta-oxidation. Beta-oxidation, which occurs in the mitochondria (powerhouse of the cell), is a series of reactions by which two-carbon fragments are removed from the fatty acid molecule at a time. The two-carbon fragments, acetyl-CoAs, enter the citric-acid cycle with the resultant production of ATP. Beta-oxidation is important during aerobic exercise and between meals, when the body relies on fat catabolism for energy.

Although humans have the capability for synthesizing some fatty acids, other fatty acids, which are known as "essential fatty acids," cannot be produced by the body. The essential fatty acids, found in vegetable oils, are linoleic, linolenic, and arachidonic acids. Essential fatty acids are needed for the proper functioning of all tissues and are precursors of prostaglandins, compounds that are important in the regulation of blood pressure and blood aggregation and that are intermediates in pain sensation. Human essential-fatty-acid deficiency used to be regarded as a rare disease. However, with the use of more sensitive criteria in recent years, the existence of essential-fatty-acid deficiency has been demonstrated in elderly patients with peripheral vascular disease, in fat malabsorption after major intestinal resection, and in patients after serious accidents and burns (7). Symptoms of deficiency include growth retardation, scaliness of the skin, and male and female infertility. Kidney abnormalities, fatty liver, increased fragility of erythrocytes, and increased susceptibility to infections have also been noted.

Alcohol

Alcohol, although not considered a nutrient, is a source of kilocalories in the diet. The use of alcohol is quite common in the United States, and alcoholic beverages are regularly consumed by many individuals (8).

Digestion. Alcohol (ethanol) needs no digestion. It is both water soluble and lipid soluble, readily permeating membranes. Absorption occurs from the stomach, duodenum, and jejunum.

Metabolism. Because ethanol is not stored in the body, and very little is excreted from the lungs and kidney, it must be oxidized. The liver is the main site of the metabolism of ethanol. The capacity of the liver for oxidation of ethanol is 10 ml per hour. The major system in the liver for the oxidation of ethanol is the alcohol dehydrogenase system, in which ethanol is oxidized to acetyl-CoA. Other routes of ethanol oxidation include the microsomal ethanol oxidizing system (MEOS) and catalase, an enzyme that converts ethanol to acetaldehyde. The MEOS and catalase routes are responsible for only 10%–20% of ethanol oxidation (8).

The body does not use ethanol efficiently; that is, the seven kilocalories per gram are not useful kilocalories. Unlike the results of carbohydrate, fat, and protein oxidation, the energy formed from oxidation of ethanol is not conserved as ATP but is given off as heat.

Ethanol oxidation affects carbohydrate, protein, and lipid metabolism. It inhibits gluconeogenesis and depletes glycogen, increasing the chance of hypoglycemia. Ethanol also inhibits albumin synthesis and increases triglyceride accumulation in the liver and in the circulatory system. Even with an adequate diet, ethanol is toxic. It inflames the stomach (gastritis), may affect the structure and metabolism of the intestinal mucosa, causing an induced disaccharidase deficiency, may result in pancreatitis, and may damage the liver (cirrhosis).

VITAMINS

Vitamins are organic substances in the diet that are required in minute amounts for metabolic ac-
tions in the cell. The vitamins are normally classified into fat-soluble and water-soluble groups. The fat-soluble vitamins include vitamins A, D, E, and K. Water-soluble vitamins are vitamin C, thiamin, riboflavin, niacin, folate, vitamin B_{12}, vitamin B_6, biotin, and pantothenic acid.

Fat-Soluble Vitamins

Vitamin A. Vitamin A is actually several biologically active compounds. These include retinol (the alcohol), retinal (the aldehyde), and retinoic acid. Not all forms of vitamin A are active in the same body functions. For example, while retinol, retinal, and retinoic acid are all active participants in growth and maintenance of epithelial tissue and bone, only retinol and retinal have an active role in vision and reproduction. Precursors of vitamin A are the carotenes, which are converted to retinol in the body with varying efficiency. Beta carotene is the most important of the vitamin A precursors.

Vitamin A is found in animal and plant sources (see Table 2-1). Vitamin A from animal sources is preformed and well absorbed. The plant sources of vitamin A contain the precursors or carotenes. The liver is the major storage depot for vitamin A, and utilization and absorption are dependent on the amount of fat in the diet.

When vitamin A is needed by the tissue, retinyl ester (inorganic salt) is converted by a liver enzyme to retinol and bound to a protein. The bound retinol travels in the circulatory system to various body tissues. In the eye, vitamin A is involved in vision in dim light as well as acute perception. Vitamin A is also essential for growth, cellular differentiation, reproduction, and the integrity of the immune system (9).

The RDA for vitamin A is listed in Appendix B. Deficiency of vitamin A results in night blindness and drying of the conjunctiva (mucous membrane that lines the eyelids). If vitamin-A deficiency progresses, the cornea dries, then softens, and finally perforates, allowing the lens to pop out of the perforation and causing permanent blindness. Although rare in the United States, acute vitamin-A

Table 2-1. MAJOR FOOD SOURCES OF VITAMIN A

ANIMAL SOURCES	PLANT SOURCES

Fish-liver oils
Liver
Kidney
Whole milk
Eggs
Dairy products
	Dark, leafy green vegetables:
	  beet, dandelion, mustard, and turnip greens; collards; endive;
	  escarole; green leaf lettuce; kale; spinach; swiss chard.
	
	Other vegetables:
	  tomatoes, broccoli
	
	Deep-orange-yellow vegetables and fruits:
	  carrots, sweet potatoes, winter squash, apricots, cantaloupe,
	  mango, oranges, papaya, peaches, pumpkin.

deficiency is a major problem in less-developed countries, accounting for approximately 250,000 cases of blindness in children each year (9).

Toxicity of vitamin A occurs when 10 times the RDA is ingested as preformed vitamin A for long periods (10). Most cases of toxicity are the result of overuse of vitamin supplements rather than ingestion of food sources of preformed vitamin A. The reported incidences of vitamin-A toxicity have averaged less than 10 cases per year from 1976–1987 (11). Symptoms of vitamin-A toxicity include anemia, bone or joint pain, dryness of mucous membranes, fatigue, headache, insomnia, irregular menses, liver abnormalities, loss of body hair, and vomiting.

Excess consumption of carotene does not convert to vitamin A rapidly enough to be toxic. The only side effect from excess carotene consumption is yellow discoloration of the skin.

Vitamin D. Vitamin D is considered both a vitamin and a hormone. Like a vitamin, it functions as a micronutrient and must be supplied through the diet for most urban populations. However, some individuals do not need dietary vitamin D due to an adequate supply from activation of a vitamin D precursor in the skin through exposure to the ultraviolet rays in sunshine. The activated vitamin D then exhibits its effects on various target tissues.

Dietary sources of vitamin D supply differing forms of the vitamin. Animal sources supply vitamin D_3 (calciol), while plant sources supply vitamin D_2 (ercalciol). There are not many food sources of vitamin D. High amounts of vitamin D are found in cod-liver and tuna-liver oils. Minimal amounts are found in egg yolk, butter, and cheese. Milk, although not a naturally good source of vitamin D, is usually fortified with the vitamin. Absorption of dietary vitamin D occurs in the small intestine, and the vitamin is transported to the liver via chylomicrons. Most vitamin-D needs (approximately 80%) are satisfied by the conversion of 7-dehydrocholesterol in the skin to calciol through the action of ultraviolet light.

Vitamin D is intimately involved in calcium homeostasis. In order for vitamin D to carry out its functions in the body, it must first be activated. The initial step in the activation of vitamin D occurs in the liver, where it is hydroxylated to form calcidiol.

Calcidiol remains in circulation until a decrease in serum calcium triggers the release of parathyroid hormone from the parathyroid gland. The hormone stimulates the conversion in the kidney of calcidiol to calcitriol, the most potent form of vitamin D. Calcitriol is then released into the blood to travel to the target tissues: the intestine, the bone, and the kidney. In the intestine, calcitriol stimulates calcium and phosphorus absorption. Along with parathyroid hormone, calcitriol improves renal reabsorption of calcium and phosphorus. In the bone, calcitriol, along with parathyroid hormone, stimulates mobilization of calcium.

The net result of these activities is an increase in serum calcium. The increase in serum calcium suppresses parathyroid hormone release and therefore conversion of calcidiol to calcitriol in the kidney. Excretion of vitamin-D metabolites occurs through the bile.

The RDA for vitamin D is given in Appendix B. As previously noted, dietary sources of vitamin D are not necessary if individuals are exposed to adequate ultraviolet light (sunlight). Urban populations seem to need a dietary supply due to lack of exposure. Ultraviolet light cannot penetrate fog, smog, smoke, regular window glass, and clothing.

Vitamin-D deficiency results in rickets in children and osteomalacia in adults. Inadequate deposition of calcium and phosphorus in the bone matrix occurs in rickets. The bones become soft and pliable, and deformities result: bowing of the legs, knock knees, pigeon breast, and beading of the ribs. Other characteristics of rickets include retarded growth and problems with the teeth, such as later eruption, poor formation, and greater susceptibility to decay. Osteomalacia is also a defect in bone formation, resulting in softening and distortion of the bone.

The toxic level of vitamin D varies. Intakes beyond five times the RDA are inadvisable. Symptoms of toxicity are appetite loss, nausea, weight loss, failure to thrive, and renal and heart damage.

Vitamin E. There are eight naturally occurring vitamin-E compounds, with the most active form in foods known as alpha-tocopherol. The major sources of vitamin E are vegetable oils. Vitamin E is absorbed from the intestine unchanged, and like other fat-soluble vitamins, it is packaged in chylomicrons. Under normal conditions, approximately one-half of the vitamin E taken in is absorbed, and the more vitamin E ingested, the less absorbed. Storage sites for vitamin E include the adipose tissue, muscle, liver, heart, uterus, testes, and adrenals. Excretion is through urine or bile.

In the body, vitamin E functions as an antioxidant. It stabilizes the cell membrane and protects it against oxidative destruction. Vitamin E is also involved in cellular respiration and the synthesis of heme. The RDA for vitamin E is quite low, as illustrated in the table in Appendix B. The RDA is related to the polyunsaturated fatty-acid content of the cellular membranes, which in turn is dependent on the polyunsaturated fatty-acid level in the diet. Sources of polyunsaturated fat in the diet are also vitamin E sources.

In animals, vitamin-E deficiency causes abberations in the muscle, nervous, reproductive, and vascular systems. In adult humans, vitamin-E deficiency is extremely rare. Infants delivered prematurely show evidence of vitamin-E deficiency manifested by hemolytic anemia due to limited tissue storage, intestinal malabsorption, and rapid growth rates (13). These infants require vitamin-E supplementation.

Vitamin E appears to be the least toxic of the fat-soluble vitamins. Still, caution is necessary, since continuous storage of vitamin E can occur in the adipose tissue. Many individuals take vitamin-E supplements to treat numerous ailments, despite the lack of evidence that such supplementation is beneficial. Vitamin-E supplementation has no effect on the aging process or virility. Some favorable results have been obtained in the treatment of intermittent claudication when 300 mg per day of vitamin E are administered.

Vitamin K. Two forms of vitamin K are found in animal (including human) tissues. These are phylloquinone and menaquinone. The source of phylloquinone is plants, particularly green leafy vegetables. Menaquinone is vitamin K produced by bacterial biosynthesis in the jejunum and ileum. As is the case with all fat-soluble vitamins, absorption of vitamin K from the intestine requires bile. Vitamin K is packaged in chylomicrons for transport to the liver, which is the primary storage site.

Vitamin K is essential for the synthesis of blood-clotting factors in the liver (see Appendix B for the RDA for vitamin K). Primary deficiency is uncommon in adult humans due to the bacterial biosynthesis in the gastrointestinal tract even when dietary sources are not ingested. Secondary deficiencies of vitamin K can occur in instances of injury, renal insufficiency, and chronic treatment with antibiotics, which sterilize the gut (14). These

Table 2-2. DIETARY SOURCES OF VITAMIN C

FRUITS	VEGETABLES
Guava, oranges, papaya, strawberries	Beet greens, broccoli, brussels sprouts, cabbage, cauliflower, chives, collards, kale, kohlrabi, mustard greens, parsley, potatoes, spinach, sweet peppers, tomatoes, turnip greens

conditions are marked by a decrease in plasma prothrombin (normal range is 80–120 mcg/ml). The toxicity of vitamin K is very low, even when large amounts are taken over an extended period of time.

Water-Soluble Vitamins

Vitamin C. Vitamin C, or L-ascorbic acid, is a six-carbon compound related to monosaccharides. Humans do not synthesize vitamin C; therefore, the vitamin must be acquired through food sources.

Plants are the best sources of vitamin C (see Table 2-2). Note that many of the sources of vitamin C are also good sources of the vitamin A precursor, beta carotene. Vitamin C is very labile (easily decomposed), and large losses can occur as a result of storage and preparation techniques. Refrigeration decreases vitamin-C loss; however, prolonged storage will result in lower vitamin-C levels. Cooking losses can be minimized if the foods are cooked in a minimum amount of water for the shortest time possible. Steaming and microwaving foods retain more vitamin C than boiling.

Vitamin C is absorbed in the upper intestine by active transport. Efficiency of absorption declines as intake increases: at doses of 4–64 mg, absorption efficiency can be as high as 98%; at doses of 1000 mg, absorption declines to 75%; and at levels of 6000 mg, absorption is 26% (15). Vitamin C is widely distributed in body tissues, with the highest concentrations in the adrenal gland, pituitary gland, and retina. Vitamin C and its metabolites are excreted in the urine. Oxalate is the major urinary excretion product, unless large doses of

vitamin C are ingested. At large doses, most of the vitamin C excreted in the urine is unmetabolized.

Vitamin C is involved in collagen formation (tissue healing) and neurotransmitter metabolism. It also facilitates iron absorption and storage and activates folic acid. The RDA for vitamin C is listed in Appendix B. For reasons that are unclear, smokers seem to need more vitamin C than nonsmokers to maintain an appropriate body pool. In addition, factors such as extremes in temperature, stress, and strenuous physical activity may increase the need for vitamin C (15).

Vitamin-C deficiency, or scurvy, occurs in two to three months when a vitamin-C-deficient diet is ingested. Scurvy is characterized by small pinpoint hemorrhages, swollen and bleeding gums, loss of hair, loosening of the teeth, fatigue, weakness, and death, if untreated. Marginal vitamin-C deficiency, that is, reduced biochemical functions of vitamin C without the appearance of overt clinical symptoms, has been observed in patients suffering from liver disease, rheumatoid arthritis, and cancer (16). The impact of marginal vitamin-C deficiency on health is unknown.

Approximately 21% of the adult population ingests supplements of vitamin C providing 300 mg or more of vitamin C daily (15), which is well above the RDA. Doses of vitamin C in the range of one or more grams daily have been claimed to aid in the treatment of colds and atherosclerosis. Well-controlled studies have not supported the claims. What is the effect of taking such large doses? Acute ingestion of large amounts of vitamin C can cause stomach cramps, nausea, and diarrhea, with no long-lasting adverse effects. Chronic consumption of large doses (one gram or more daily) has been

Table 2-3. DIETARY SOURCES OF FOLATE

MEATS	GRAINS	FRUITS	VEGETABLES	OTHER
Kidney, liver	Wheat germ	Bananas, cantaloupe, oranges, strawberries	Asparagus, broccoli, lima beans, mushrooms, spinach	Yeast

associated with uricosuria (increased uric acid secretion in the urine), reduced bactericidal activity of leukocytes, enhanced mobilization of bone calcium, impaired blood-coagulation time, and lowered plasma vitamin-B_{12} levels (15).

Folate. Folate (folic acid) is present in numerous foods (see Table 2-3). Because folate is sensitive to heat, a diet composed exclusively of thoroughly cooked foods is usually low in folate (17). The jejunum is the major site of folate absorption, although it can be absorbed along the entire length of the small intestine. The liver is the main storage site of folate in the body.

Folate functions as an intermediary in one-carbon transfers from one compound to another. One-carbon transfers are essential for the synthesis of nucleic acids (and therefore DNA) and for the conversion of the amino acids, serine, histidine, and homocysteine to glycine, glutamic acid, and methionine respectively. The RDA for healthy individuals is listed in Appendix B. When the basal-metabolic rate is increased, as in the case of infection, or when cell turnover increases, as in the case of tumors, folate requirements are higher.

A deficiency of folate leads to impaired cell division and to alterations in protein synthesis, making the effects of deficiency most notable in rapidly growing tissues such as the bone marrow. The red blood cells fail to mature and lose their nuclei, resulting in megaloblastic anemia characterized by large, immature nucleated red blood cells. Folic-acid deficiency is the most common cause of megaloblastic anemia in infants and children (17).

For the majority of individuals, folate is nontoxic at several hundred times the RDA, and excesses are excreted in the urine. In persons with epilepsy who are in continuous control by phenytoin, very large doses of folate (100 times the RDA) may precipitate convulsions because folic acid and phenytoin inhibit each other's uptake. Supplements for pregnancy containing 350 mcg folate significantly reduce zinc absorption and may cause maternal zinc depletion with an ultimate effect of intrauterine growth retardation (17).

Vitamin B_{12}. When discussing the adequacy of vegetarian diets, the topic of vitamin B_{12} (also known as cobalamin) inevitably emerges. All vitamin B_{12} in nature is made by microorganisms (18). Dietary sources of the vitamin include all animal products, which contain the vitamin as a result of the animal's ingestion of the vitamin-producing microorganisms (see Table 2-4). The vitamin is not found in plant products, unless they have been contaminated by the bacteria. The bacteria may be located on the root nodules of legumes or may result from fecal contamination of the plant, since microorganisms in the colon produce large amounts of the vitamin.

In food, vitamin B_{12} is linked to a polypeptide and must be released prior to absorption. This release is effected through the action of gastric acid and enzymes. Once freed, the vitamin is attached to a substance called "R binder" (19). The pancreatic proteases digest the R binder in the slightly alkaline environment of the upper small intestine. The vitamin is then able to combine with intrinsic factor (IF). The vitamin-B_{12}-IF complex is transported to the ileum, and in the presence of calcium and a pH greater than 6.0, the complex attaches to the brush border and is absorbed. Vitamin B_{12} can also be absorbed passively over the entire intestine; however, only a very small percentage is

Table 2-4. DIETARY SOURCES OF VITAMIN B$_{12}$

RICH SOURCES (>10 mcg/100 g):	MODERATELY RICH SOURCES (3–10 mcg/100 g):	MODERATE SOURCES (1–3 mcg/100 g):	FAIR SOURCES (<1 mcg/100 g):

Organ meats:
  beef liver
  kidney
  heart
Bivalves:
  oysters
  clams
	Nonfat dry milk
	Seafood:
	  crab
	  salmon
	  sardines
	Egg yolks
		Meats:
		  beef
		  lamb
		  pork
		  poultry
		Seafood:
		  flounder
		  haddock
		  lobster
		  scallops
		  swordfish
		  tuna
		Cheeses:
		  camembert
		  limburger
			Milk
			Cheeses:
			  cheddar
			  cottage cheese

Source: V. Herbert, "Vitamin B$_{12}$," In R.E. Olson, et al. *Nutrition Reviews' Present Knowledge in Nutrition*, 5th ed. (Washington, D.C.: The Nutrition Foundation, Inc., 1984).

absorbed in this manner, and then only at very high levels of vitamin-B$_{12}$ intake. Once absorbed, the vitamin is complexed with protein and transported to the liver. The vitamin is transported throughout the body attached to a protein, and receptors for the protein are located in the liver, bone marrow cells, reticulocytes, lymphoblasts, and fibroblasts. The major storage site in the body is the liver, and the amount of stored vitamin B$_{12}$ increases with age due to a very efficient recycling system: The vitamin is excreted in the bile, and then most is reabsorbed through the enterohepatic circulation.

Vitamin B$_{12}$ is critical in the transport and storage of folic acid, plays a role in hydrogen transfers, and is actively involved in the enzymes of carbohydrate, fat, and protein metabolism. The RDA for vitamin B$_{12}$ is listed in Appendix B. Due to the conservation of the vitamin through the enterohepatic circulation and the amount stored, a long time (up to two decades) can pass before deficiency

symptoms occur in adults consuming a deficient diet.

Deficiency of vitamin B$_{12}$ occurs as a result of inadequate intake or absorption. Strict vegetarians (vegans) are at particular risk due to their complete avoidance of animal products. Individuals who cannot absorb the vitamin must receive injections of the vitamin to avoid deficiency symptoms. Pernicious anemia (discussed in Chapter 10) is the disease caused by vitamin-B$_{12}$ deficiency, and it is characterized by megaloblastic anemia and neurological damage. The megaloblastic anemia results from the aberration that occurs in folate metabolism. As shown in Figure 2-3, lack of vitamin B$_{12}$ results in the trapping of folate in a form that is metabolically useless. Folate therefore cannot participate in the production of DNA, and the effect is seen most readily in cells with a rapid turnover, the red blood cells. Administration of folic acid can cure the megaloblastic anemia but not the associated neurological damage. The neurological dam-

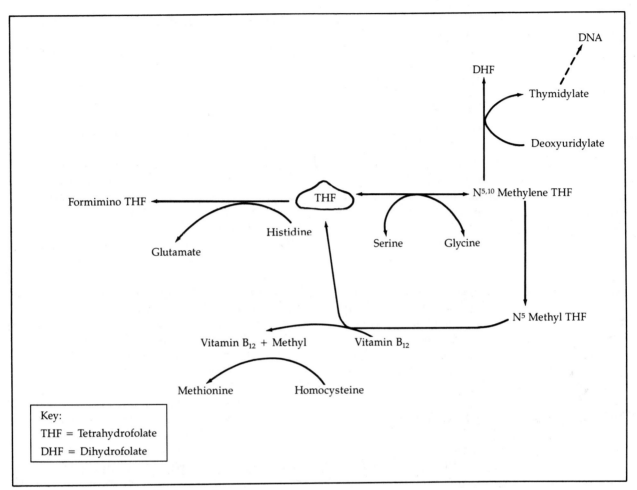

Figure 2-3. Folate-vitamin-B_{12} interaction.

age is a result of inadequate myelin synthesis and deterioration of the axon. Clinical symptoms include paresthesia, poor muscular coordination, mental slowness, confusion, depression, hallucinations, and psychosis. Left untreated, pernicious anemia can be fatal. No toxic reactions have been noted when vitamin B_{12} is taken in megadoses; however, there is no evidence that high doses of the vitamin are beneficial in the treatment of any disease other than pernicious anemia.

Thiamin (Vitamin B_1). The richest sources of thiamin in the diet are pork and pork products. Other sources include legumes, whole-grain breads and cereals, enriched breads and cereals, dried brewer's yeast, and wheat germ. Absorption of thiamin, which occurs in the duodenum, can be active or passive, depending on thiamin intake. At low intakes, absorption is active, and at large intakes, passive absorption occurs. Thiamin is absorbed into the mucosal cell, reacts with phosphate to become thiamin pyrophosphate, and is then transported to the liver.

Thiamin is required in carbohydrate metabolism: It is essential in the conversion of pyruvate to acetyl-CoA; it is important in the Kreb's cycle, in the conversion of alpha ketoglutarate to succinyl-

CoA; and it is required in the activation of transketolase, an enzyme in the pentose phosphate pathway. Because thiamin is required for the production of energy, the dietary recommendation has been usually based on energy intake. The RDA for thiamin is listed in Appendix B.

Diets low in thiamin will lead to the disease beriberi. Clinical signs of thiamin deficiency involve the nervous and cardiovascular systems: mental confusion, muscular weakness, edema (wet beriberi), muscle wasting (dry beriberi), anorexia, loss of tonus of the lower gastrointestinal tract resulting in constipation, and cardiac enlargement. Untreated, beriberi results in death. Alcoholics are at increased risk for developing thiamin deficiency due to decreased absorption (as a result of alcohol-induced changes in the intestinal wall), inadequate consumption, and increased requirement. Other at-risk individuals are renal patients on long-term dialysis treatment, patients fed intravenously for long periods, and patients with chronic febrile infections (10). Oral intake of thiamin, well in excess of the RDA, has not been associated with toxicity. Excess thiamin is excreted in the urine.

Riboflavin (Vitamin B₂). Riboflavin is widely distributed in animal and plant foods, but the best sources are eggs, lean meats, poultry, milk, and enriched breads and cereals. Ultraviolet light (sunlight) destroys riboflavin, and although the vitamin is heat stable, a portion can be lost through leaching when foods are cooked in large quantities of water.

Riboflavin is absorbed from the upper portion of the gastrointestinal tract. Absorption is regulated by a transport system. Once in the intestinal cell, a large portion of the riboflavin is linked with phosphate to form flavin mononucleotide (FMN). Riboflavin and FMN are transported in the blood linked to albumin as well as other proteins and released to all tissues, especially the liver. In the tissues, riboflavin and FMN can be converted to flavin-adenine dinucleotide (FAD).

Riboflavin is part of several enzymes and coenzymes and contributes to their capacity to accept and transfer hydrogen atoms. It participates in energy production in the respiratory chain, it activates vitamin B₆, and then facilitates the conversion of tryptophan to niacin. It converts folate to active forms, and it is important in the production of corticosteroids, red blood cells, glycogen synthesis, fatty-acid metabolism and thyroid activity. Clinical signs of riboflavin deficiency include personality changes, cheilosis (cracks at mouth corners and lip inflammation), glossitis (smooth, purplish-red tongue), growth retardation, decreased reproductive capacity, congenital malformations, alopecia (hair loss), and corneal vascularization. There have been no reports of toxicity when excessive amounts of riboflavin are ingested.

Niacin. Niacin refers to nicotinic acid and niacinamide. The richest sources of niacin in the diet are liver, meat, poultry, peanut butter, and legumes. Milk and eggs, although low in niacin, are high in tryptophan. Since tryptophan can be converted to niacin in the body, some of the requirement for niacin can be met with these foods. Enriched grains and cereals are also reliable sources of this B vitamin. Niacin is stable in foods and can withstand some heat.

Niacin is part of the coenzymes, nicotinamide adenine dinucleotide (NAD), and nicotinamide adenine dinucleotide phosphate (NADP). These coenzymes play vital roles in carbohydrate, protein and fat metabolism. Niacin (nicotinic acid) at pharmacologic levels has also been promoted for the lowering of serum cholesterol; however, due to the side effects of large doses of nicotinic acid, individuals should consult their physician before self-medicating with this vitamin.

The RDA for niacin is listed in Appendix B. The units are listed as "niacin equivalents" to account for the conversion of tryptophan to niacin in the body. A deficiency of niacin results in the disease pellagra. Pellagra is characterized by dermatitis, which occurs especially in areas of the skin exposed to sunlight; diarrhea, caused by inflammation of the mucous linings of the gastrointestinal tract; depression, characterized by irritability and sleeplessness initially and then severe mental symptoms as the disease progresses; and death, if untreated.

Unlike thiamin and riboflavin, large doses of niacin (as nicotinic acid) can be toxic. Massive doses produce flushing of the skin, gastrointestinal distress, unusual nervousness, recurring ulcers, increased uric acid secretion, and glucose intolerance. Due to the side effects of large doses of nicotinic acid, individuals should consult their physician before self-medicating to lower their serum cholesterol.

Vitamin B$_6$. The three natural forms of vitamin B$_6$ are pyridoxamine, pyridoxal, and pyridoxine. The vitamin is widely distributed in foods, and the richest sources are chicken and fish, liver, whole-grain cereals and egg yolks. Approximately one-half of the daily needs of Americans are met from meats, fish, poultry, and eggs. Pyridoxamine and pyridoxal are the most prevalent forms of the vitamin in animal sources, and their bioavailability is very high. Pyridoxine is the form of vitamin B$_6$ in plants. The absorption of the vitamin from plant foods is lower due to the presence of fiber and a less available form of pyridoxine (20). Substantial losses of the vitamin occur during cooking.

The dietary requirement for vitamin B$_6$ varies with the protein content of the diet—the more protein in the diet, the higher the need for the vitamin. A ratio of .02 mg vitamin B$_6$ per gram of protein has been suggested (21). See Appendix B for a listing of the RDA for vitamin B$_6$ for the various age groups. Vitamin B$_6$ is important in the synthesis and catabolism of all amino acids; it is necessary in transaminations, deaminations, and decarboxylations. It is also a factor in hemoglobin synthesis, the conversion of tryptophan to niacin, antibody production, and lipid and glycogen metabolism. Although uncommon, vitamin-B$_6$ deficiency can occur through inadequate intake, or it can be induced by antagonists such as isoniazid. Lack of vitamin B$_6$ in infants results in convulsions. In adults, symptoms such as weakness, irritability, nervousness, insomnia, and difficulty in walking have been observed. Toxicity is low, because virtually no storage of the vitamin in the body occurs. However, intakes in the range of 2000–6000 mg per day for several months has been associated with neurological damage.

Biotin. Biotin is widely available in foods, and sources include liver, kidney, egg yolk, milk, fish, and nuts. In addition, intestinal microflora make a significant contribution to the body pool of biotin. Absorption of biotin from the small intestine is through active transport. Once absorbed into the body, biotin plays an important role in the metabolism of fat and carbohydrate: it functions as a coenzyme in fatty-acid synthesis, fatty-acid catabolism, and gluconeogenesis. Biotin is also required in the catabolism of some amino acids. Due to the production of biotin by intestinal flora, the dietary requirement is unclear. The estimated safe and adequate intake is listed in Appendix C.

Deficiency of biotin as a result of inadequate intake in healthy individuals is rare; however, it can be produced if parenteral solutions do not contain the vitamin, if large amounts of raw egg white are ingested, or when certain medications are used. Raw egg whites contain the glycoprotein avidin, which renders biotin unavailable. The anticonvulsants, carbamazepine (tegretol) and primidone (mysoline), appear to be competitive inhibitors of biotin in the intestine, thereby interfering with absorption (22). Symptoms of biotin deficiency include anorexia, nausea, vomiting, glossitis, pallor, mental depression, and dry, scaly dermatitis. There have been no reports of toxicity of biotin when large amounts are ingested.

Pantothenic Acid. Pantothenic acid is widely distributed in foods and particularly good sources include meat and poultry, whole-grain cereals, and legumes. Other sources of the vitamin are milk, vegetables, and fruits. After absorption from the small intestine, pantothenic acid plays its critical role as a component of coenzyme A. Coenzyme A is required in the metabolism of fats and carbohydrates, in gluconeogenesis, and in the synthesis of compounds such as steroid hormones, porphyrins, and acetylcholine. Estimated adequate intake of pantothenic acid is listed in Appendix C.

Isolated dietary deficiencies of pantothenic acid are uncommon due to its wide distribution in foods; however, marginal deficiencies can exist in malnourished individuals. In animals, induced deficiency resulted in symptoms such as infertility, abortion, retarded growth rate, abnormalities of the skin and hair, neuromuscular disorders, gastrointestinal malfunction, adrenal cortical failure, and sudden death. In humans, pantothenic-acid deficiency caused symptoms such as postural hypotension, rapid heart rate on exertion, anorexia, constipation, numbness and tingling of the hands and feet, and hyperactive deep tendon reflexes (23). No evidence exists regarding toxicity of the vitamin when large doses are ingested.

MINERALS

Calcium

Approximately 1.5%–2.0% of total body weight is calcium. Most (99%) of the calcium present in the body resides in the bones and teeth, and the remainder is widely distributed throughout the body. The blood levels of calcium are tightly controlled in the 9–11 mg/dl range through a variety of mechanisms. When blood calcium falls below 7 mg/dl, parathyroid hormone is released, resulting in renal reabsorption of the mineral (occurs within minutes), bone resorption (occurs within hours), and increased absorption from the gastrointestinal tract (occurs within days). When calcium levels in the blood rise, the hormone calcitonin is released, stimulating bone mineralization and renal and intestinal excretion.

Sources of calcium in the diet are the dairy foods, milk and milk products, including cheeses. Leafy greens low in oxalic acid such as broccoli and turnip greens, fish with edible bones (sardines), and calcium-containing tofu are also good sources of the mineral. Calcium is usually complexed in foods and must be freed prior to absorption in the upper small intestine. It is incompletely absorbed, and normal absorption rates are 20%–30% of intake. Factors that favor calcium absorption are vitamin D, acid conditions that increase the solubility of calcium, lactose (milk sugar), and possibly the ratio of calcium to phosphorus in the diet and body needs. The importance of the calcium to phosphorus ratio is controversial. Although animal studies are quite clear and indicate an opti-

mum calcium to phosphorus ratio of 2:1, human studies are less definitive (10). It appears that humans can tolerate a much wider calcium to phosphorus ratio, and in cases of adequate calcium intake, the ratio may have no bearing on absorption at all. The Food and Nutrition Board has recommended a one-to-one ratio of calcium to phosphorus in the diet (10). With increased body needs, more calcium is absorbed, so that growing children absorb more calcium than do adults. Adaptation to low-calcium intake occurs, and individuals consuming low intakes of calcium are very efficient in their absorption. Still, despite increased efficiency of calcium absorption when intakes are low, the total calcium absorbed may not be adequate to meet body needs. Further, the ability to adapt to low intakes declines with age.

Certain factors inhibit the absorption of calcium from the gastrointestinal tract and/or increase its excretion from the body. These factors include the presence of oxalic acid and phytic acid (found in whole grains) in foods, stress, immobilization, alcohol intake, gender, and age. Oxalic acid and phytic acid in foods can complex with calcium to form an insoluble unabsorbable compound. This reaction is no longer considered important if the amount of calcium consumed is liberal (10). With liberal intakes, enough calcium will be absorbed despite the losses that occur when some of the calcium is complexed. Stress appears to decrease absorption and increase excretion of calcium due to the decreased activation of vitamin D caused by glucocorticoids. Immobilization results in calcium loss from the bone and the body. The cause is uncertain but may be linked to lack of weight on the bones or decreased vascularity resulting in less stimulus for bone formation. Alcohol has a direct effect on the mucosal cells, causing less calcium to be absorbed. Males are more efficient at absorbing calcium than women, and absorption of the mineral declines with age.

Calcium is excreted through the fecal and urinary routes. Fecal excretion represents unabsorbed calcium and endogenous calcium released into the gastrointestinal tract. Urinary excretion is quite low, since most calcium is reabsorbed. Calcium has numerous roles in the body. Most people are familiar with its role in bone formation and remodeling. Calcium is part of the hydroxyapatite crystal in the solid phase of bone. Bone undergoes constant remodeling and turnover; therefore, bone calcium is resorbed and replaced constantly. During the third or fourth decade, bone resorption is greater than bone replacement and skeletal mass begins to decrease. Men have a greater skeletal mass than women, and blacks have greater skeletal mass than Caucasians. Menopause accelerates bone loss in some females, so that the effects of bone loss (skeletal fracture) are seen most frequently in white, postmenopausal females.

Calcium is also involved in tooth formation. The hydroxyapatite that forms the dentin and enamel is more dense, with less water content than that in bones. Unlike the calcium in bones, the calcium in teeth is not available to the blood for the maintenance of calcium levels. Calcium plays a role in blood clotting by participating in the conversion of prothrombin to thrombin. It is a catalyst for biological reactions, including absorption of vitamin B_{12}, activation of pancreatic lipase, participation in carbohydrate, fat and protein metabolism, release of insulin from the pancreas, and the formation and breakdown of acetylcholine. Calcium is involved in the maintenance and function of the cell membranes and is critical for muscular contraction and nerve impulse transmission.

The RDA for calcium is listed in Appendix B. In 1984, the National Institutes of Health recommended an intake of 1000–1500 mg calcium per day to prevent osteoporosis in males and postmenopausal females (24). Numerous studies have been conducted on calcium and its role in osteoporosis, and it is clear that osteoporosis is not a calcium deficiency disease, but has multiple causes, including inadequate calcium intake, declining estrogen levels, decreased plasma levels of the active form of vitamin D, smoking, and lack of physical activity. It is currently recommended that calcium intake be encouraged throughout the lifespan, especially during the bone-growth period. Unfortunately, beginning in their teenage years, women usually fail to ingest the RDA for calcium,

often because of the exclusion of milk in their diets. If oral calcium supplementation is prescribed, it is important to realize that the supplements differ in the amount of elemental calcium they contain: calcium gluconate contains 9% calcium; calcium lactate contains 13% calcium, and calcium carbonate contains 40% calcium (25). High intakes of supplemental calcium in the range of 1000–2500 mg per day have not been associated with harmful effects. Hypercalcemia is encountered not by an increased dietary intake of calcium, but by vitamin-D toxicity.

Phosphorus

Like calcium, most phosphorus in the body resides in the skeleton. Sources of phosphorus are numerous, with milk, poultry, fish, and meat providing the highest amounts. Soft drinks also contain substantial phosphorus and most likely contribute to dietary intake of the mineral due to the high consumption of soft drinks in the United States. Approximately 60%–70% of dietary phosphorus is absorbed, and absorption is increased with lower intakes. Excretion routes are the feces and urine. The kidney is very efficient at reabsorbing phosphorus, depending on body needs.

Phosphorus, like calcium, is part of hydroxyapatite and is therefore required for bone formation and maintenance. It is also involved in protein, fat, and carbohydrate metabolism as a cofactor in enzyme systems. It is integral to energy-transfer systems in the body in the form of adenosine diphosphate (ADP), adenosine triphosphate (ATP), nicotinamide adenine dinucleotide phosphate (NADP), and dihydronicotinamide adenine dinucleotide phosphate (NADPH). Deficiency is extremely rare. Phosphorus depletion can occur as a result of prolonged and excessive intake of antacids. Symptoms of phosphorus depletion are weakness, anorexia, malaise, and pain in the bones (10). Toxicity has not been reported.

Magnesium

Most of the magnesium in the body is located in the bone. Only a small amount (less than 1%)

occurs in the plasma, and next to potassium, it is the predominant cation (positively charged ion) in cells. Dietary sources include vegetables, especially leafy green vegetables such as spinach, collards, dandelion greens, lettuce, and mustard greens. Legumes, seafood, nuts, whole-grain breads and cereals, and dairy products are also good sources. Absorption of magnesium from the small intestine is not efficient. As with other minerals, efficiency of magnesium absorption is higher when intake is low. Excretion is regulated through the kidney.

Magnesium performs numerous functions in the body. It is a cofactor for many enzymes, including those involved in carbohydrate, fat, protein, and nucleic-acid metabolism. The mineral is also required for normal cell-membrane permeability and normal calcium metabolism. Calcium and magnesium interact throughout the body. In the muscle, calcium is the stimulator, and magnesium is the relaxant; in the presynaptic neuron, calcium binding results in acetycholine release, and magnesium binding inhibits release (26). Magnesium is also essential for calcium mobilization from the bone.

The RDA for magnesium is given in Appendix B. Due to its involvement in many reactions throughout the body, clinical symptoms of magnesium deficiency are varied. On a severely deficient diet, the body's control over contraction and relaxation of the muscle is lost, with uncontrolled neuromuscular activity resulting. In the early stages, this is manifested as tremors; in later stages, seizures occur. Hypocalcemia and hypokalemia also occur. Chronic deficiency of magnesium results in elevated parathyroid hormone concentration and decreased bone responsiveness to the hormone, resulting in low serum calcium levels. As magnesium deficiency becomes more severe, the parathyroid gland is unable to secrete parathyroid hormone (27). Low levels of serum magnesium are related to higher membrane permeability, allowing potassium and magnesium to flow out of the cell and sodium and calcium to flow into the cell. The cellular shift of potassium and calcium can result in cardiac arrhythmias (27).

Some hospitalized patients have an increased risk for developing magnesium deficiency. Alcoholic patients, patients receiving diuretics for congestive heart failure or hypertension (especially loop diuretics, which increase urinary magnesium loss), patients with chronic obstructive pulmonary disease, those on total parenteral nutrition therapy without adequate magnesium, and those who suffer from vomiting and diarrhea seem to develop magnesium deficiency frequently (28). Toxicity of magnesium has not been reported in individuals with normal kidney function.

TRACE ELEMENTS

Trace elements are minerals that are required in very small quantities but that are involved in critical body processes in humans. The following is a description of iron, zinc, and copper. Other trace elements about which less is known are summarized in Table 2-5.

Iron

In the body, iron exists in either a functional or storage form. Approximately 70% of iron is in functional forms: hemoglobin, myoglobin, and tissue enzymes (cytochrome oxidase and catalase). Thirty percent is storage iron and includes ferritin, hemosiderin, and transferrin. Iron is stored in the liver, spleen, and bone marrow.

Food iron is classified as heme or nonheme iron. Heme iron is found in meat, fish, and poultry, and depending on individual needs, approximately 15%–35% of heme iron is absorbed. Iron in all other foods (grains, vegetables, fruits, nuts, eggs, and dairy products) and 60% of the iron in meat, fish, and poultry is the nonheme form, which has a lower absorption rate of 2%–20% (29). Absorption of both iron forms occurs in the duodenum and is dependent on body stores—the higher the need, the greater the absorption. In addition to needs, nonheme-iron absorption is affected by meal composition. Tannins (found in tea and coffee) bind nonheme iron and make it unavailable for absorption. Phytate in bran also exhibits an inhibitory effect. Factors that increase nonheme absorption include ascorbic acid and meat, fish, and poultry (29). Very little iron is excreted; therefore, the major regulation of iron balance in the body is absorption from the gastrointestinal tract.

Iron functions as a carrier of oxygen and carbon dioxide to body tissues. It is involved in the formation of red blood cells as a component of hemoglobin. Iron is also involved in the conversion of beta carotene to vitamin A, the synthesis of purines,

collagen synthesis, antibody production, and the detoxification of drugs in the liver.

The RDA for iron is listed in Appendix B. Needs are determined by losses and growth. Only a small amount of iron is lost in the urine, perspiration, and desquamated cells. In addition to these small losses, females lose 16–32 mg of iron monthly through menstruation. Growth is accompanied by an increase in blood volume, and the more hemoglobin produced, the more iron that is needed.

Table 2-5. TRACE ELEMENTS

TRACE ELEMENTS	DIETARY SOURCES	FUNCTIONS	DEFICIENCY SYMPTOMS	TOXICITY SYMPTOMS
Iodine	Iodized table salt, seafood, milk (if iodine-based cleaning agents used)	Integral part of thyroid hormones	Goiter	Thyrotoxicosis (thyroid disorders)
Fluoride	Water supply, ubiquitous	Part of hydroxyapatite in bones and teeth; increases caries resistance in teeth	Not observed	Mottling of teeth
Manganese	Nuts, whole-grain breads, cereals	Part of enzyme systems in protein and energy metabolism	Not observed in humans	Toxicity is known only in workers exposed to high levels of manganese dust in air; affects CNS
Selenium	Seafood, kidney, liver, meat	Part of the enzyme glutathione peroxidase (protects against oxidative damage of cell)	Keshan disease (cardiomyopathy)[1]	In animals: liver cirrhosis, growth depression, splenomegaly

Continued

Table 2-5. TRACE ELEMENTS (*continued*)

TRACE ELEMENTS	DIETARY SOURCES	FUNCTIONS	DEFICIENCY SYMPTOMS	TOXICITY SYMPTOMS
Chromium	Brewer's yeast, meat products, cheeses, whole grains	Maintenance of normal glucose and lipid metabolism	Glucose intolerance; neuropathy, encephalopathy in patients on TPN	Unknown
Molybdenum	Meat, grains, legumes	Part of enzymes for uric acid production; oxidation of aldehydes	Not observed	Gout-like syndrome; significant urinary copper loss

Sources:

Committee on Dietary Allowances, Food and Nutrition Board, Division of Biological Sciences, Assembly of Life Sciences, National Research Council, *Recommended Dietary Allowances*, 9th rev. ed. (Washington, D.C.: National Academy of Sciences, 1980).

M.E. Shils and V.R. Young (eds.), *Modern Nutrition in Health and Disease*, 7th ed. (Philadelphia: Lea and Febiger, 1988).

[1]Note that selenium deficiency alone may not cause the disease. A virus may also be necessary.

Iron deficiency occurs when total body iron is reduced. There are three stages of iron deficiency (30) (Table 2-6). The first stage is iron depletion, reflected by a drop in plasma ferritin (storage iron) to less than 12 mcg per liter. The second stage is normocytic iron-deficient erythropoiesis. Hemoglobin level is normal, but red-cell protoporphyrin (hemoglobin precursor) is elevated and transferrin (transport iron) saturation is reduced. The third stage is iron-deficiency anemia. The red blood cells are microcytic (small) and hypochromic (pale), and hemoglobin levels are below normal. Symptoms of iron-deficiency anemia include reduced exercise performance, weakness, altered behavior, pale color, and alterations in cellular immunity.

Iron toxicity from foods (other than long-term intake of beverages made in iron stills) has not been reported in people without genetic defects (30). Iron poisoning can occur from ingestion of excessive iron supplements. The genetic disease associated with iron toxicity is hemochromatosis, and it affects 0.1% of the population. In hemochromatosis, absorption of iron is not regulated. Iron is stored in tissues that are not normally storage depots. Symptoms of hemochromatosis are cirrhosis, diabetes mellitus, hyperpigmentation of the skin, and cardiac failure.

Zinc

Approximately 70% of body zinc is located in the skeleton, but these stores do not appear to be involved in maintaining equilibrium. The body pool of biologically available zinc is small and has a rapid turnover (10). Meat, liver, eggs, and seafood (especially oysters) are good sources of zinc. The zinc in whole-grain products is less available, since phytic acid interferes with the absorption of zinc.

Table 2-6. STAGES OF IRON-DEFICIENCY ANEMIA

	CHARACTERISTICS	NORMAL VALUES
Stage 1: Iron depletion	Serum ferritin: < 12 mcg/liter	Serum ferritin: 90 mcg/liter (males), 30 mcg/liter (females)
Stage 2: Normocytic iron-deficient erythropoiesis	Low serum ferritin plus RBC protoporphyrin: > 100 mcg/dl	RBC protoporphyrin: 60–100 mcg/dl
Stage 3: Iron-deficiency anemia	Low serum ferritin, elevated RBC protoporphyrin plus hemoglobin: <13 g/dl (males), <12 g/dl (females)	Hemoglobin: 13–16 g/dl (males), 12–16 g/dl (females)

Source: V. Herbert, "Recommended Dietary Intakes (RDI) of Iron in Humans," *American Journal of Clinical Nutrition* 45 (1987):679–86.

Calcium and nonheme iron also interfere with zinc absorption. Zinc is absorbed from the upper intestine and excretion is primarily through the feces.

On a biochemical level, zinc is an essential component. It is important in the functioning of enzymes involved in major metabolic pathways, including, for example, carbonic anhydrase, DNA polymerase, RNA polymerase, and carboxypeptidases. It also plays a role in reproduction, wound healing, taste and smell, and growth. The RDA for zinc is given in Appendix B.

Primary zinc deficiency is rare; however, zinc deficiency can occur as a result of other diseases such as uremia, alcoholic cirrhosis, inflammatory bowel diseases, hemolytic anemias, and viral hepatitis. Clinical signs of zinc deficiency are diverse: Growth retardation, delayed sexual maturation, alopecia, skin lesions, immune deficiencies, hypogeusia (impaired sense of taste), hyposmia (impaired sense of smell), and impaired wound healing have been observed in humans (31). Zinc toxicity has been observed when intakes of two grams or more are ingested. Large amounts of zinc cause gastrointestinal irritation and vomiting. In addition, excessive intakes of zinc can aggravate marginal copper deficiency.

Copper

Although copper is essential in human nutrition, all facets of copper's metabolism are as yet unknown. Food sources of copper include oysters, nuts, liver, kidney, corn oil margarine, and dried legumes. Once absorbed, copper is stored in the liver or transported to tissues in the form of ceruloplasmin. Copper is a component of many enzymes, including those involved in mitochondrial energy production, cross-linking of collagen, protection from oxidants, iron oxidation, catecholamine synthesis, and melanin synthesis (32). The major route of excretion of copper is the bile.

An estimated range of safe intake for copper is included in Appendix C. Under normal conditions, copper deficiency in humans has not been observed; however, patients on long-term total parenteral nutrition without added copper have shown signs of copper deficiency. Symptoms of deficiency include hypochromic anemia not responsive to iron, decreased pigmentation of the skin, depigmented hair, vascular abnormalities, and neurological abnormalities. Copper is toxic, and at levels of 10–15 mg can cause vomiting and diarrhea. Higher intakes can be fatal (32).

WATER AND ELECTROLYTES

Water

Humans can live for weeks without the intake of food, but they can survive only a few days without water. Approximately 60% of total body weight is water. Most of the body water is located in muscle, followed by adipose tissue, the teeth, bone, and cartilage. Water serves as a solvent for nutrients and waste products such as carbon dioxide and ammonia. It is also a transporter of nutrients to the cells; is incorporated in glycogen, fat, and muscle; acts as a catalyst in many reactions; functions as a lubricant between joints; and serves as a temperature regulator. The evaporation of water from the skin rids the body of extra heat produced by the metabolism of protein, fat, and carbohydrate. Water also conducts heat and distributes it throughout the body. The requirement of water is two liters daily from liquids and food sources. Water is lost through respiration, the skin, the stool, and the urine. Regulation of water balance is accomplished through stimulation of the thirst mechanism and by the antidiuretic hormone, which increases water reabsorption at the site of the kidney distal tubules and collecting ducts.

Sodium

Sodium has acquired a negative reputation, primarily because in the United States, consumption far outpaces needs. Although the major emphasis today is to decrease dietary intake of sodium, it should be recognized that sodium does play a critical role in the body.

Sodium is available from animal sources and plant sources, from food processing, and as table salt (sodium chloride). Absorption of sodium is virtually 100%. Sodium balance is maintained by the hormone aldosterone, which promotes reabsorption of sodium in the kidney.

Sodium is the major cation in the extracellular fluid. In conjunction with chloride and bicarbonate, it plays an important role in the maintenance of the acid-base balance in the body. Sodium is also critical for the maintenance of osmotic pressure of body fluid and preserves normal muscle irritability and cellular permeability (33). The estimated minimum requirement for sodium is listed in Appendix C. Sodium deficiency has not been noted in healthy humans; hypertension in sensitive individuals is believed by some to be a symptom of toxicity. Hypertension is discussed in detail in Chapter 9.

Potassium

Potassium is the major cation in the intracellular fluid. Meat, milk, and fruits are good sources of the mineral. In the body, potassium functions as a catalyst, maintains osmotic pressure in the cell, plays a role in the release of insulin, and is involved in the transmission of nerve impulses. The estimated minimum requirement for potassium is listed in Appendix C. Deficiencies of potassium have been noted in patients on diuretics that do not spare potassium, such as chlorothiazide. Potassium deficiency can also be caused by diarrhea and vomiting. Some liquid-protein diets have been associated with potassium deficiency. Symptoms of potassium deficiency are disordered smooth-muscle functioning, arrhythmias, weakness, and lethargy. Excessive intakes of potassium result in arrhythmias and cardiac arrest. The relationship between potassium and hypertension is discussed in Chapter 9.

SUPPLEMENTS AND FORTIFIED FOODS

Despite recent recommendations from the National Academy of Sciences discouraging the use of nutrient supplements and encouraging the intake of a variety of foods to meet nutrient needs, approximately 35%–40% of the American population regularly uses nutrient supplements (34, 35). While it is true that certain subgroups may require additional amounts of some nutrients (e.g., pregnant women, hospitalized patients suffering from various diseases), the likelihood that 40% of the population needs supplementation is remote. Individuals take supplements for a variety of reasons: as insurance against dietary deficiencies, to give extra energy or strength, to protect against stress, and to prevent or cure chronic disease (35).

There is little scientific evidence supporting the benefits of ingesting nutrients beyond the RDA. The RDA for nutrients are set to *exceed* the requirements of most healthy individuals, and eating a variety of foods ensures adequate intake of nutrients. A single daily dose of a multivitamin or multimineral supplement containing 100% of the RDA is not known to be harmful or beneficial; however, vitamin-mineral supplements that exceed the RDA or single supplements of specific vitamins or minerals have no known health benefits and can have harmful effects on the general population (34). As described in "TOPIC OF INTEREST" in this chapter, nutrients interact with each other, and imbalances can occur.

At present, the FDA, with few exceptions, cannot limit the potency of vitamin and mineral supplements; however, the agency has begun to track reports of toxic reactions from supplement use. The information should provide the substantiation necessary for setting maximum limits for supplement potency (35).

Fortified food products have also become "hot buttons" during a time when individuals are concerned about health. The FDA has a fortification policy that outlines when nutrients should be added to foods. The FDA does not encourage indiscriminate addition of nutrients to foods, nor does it encourage the addition of nutrients to fresh produce, meat, poultry, fish, sugars, or snack foods (36). Some nutrients added to foods have reduced the prevalence of nutrition-related diseases; for example, iodine added to salt to prevent goiter, vitamin D added to milk to prevent rickets, and B vitamins added to cereals and grains to replace those lost in processing. Unfortunately, in recent years, single nutrients have been added to foods without complete attention to bioavailability or interaction with other nutrients. Examples are the addition of calcium and beta carotene to everything from breakfast cereals to soft drinks. While it is unlikely that serious health problems to the general public will occur as a result of such fortification, the real question of benefit remains.

TOPIC OF INTEREST

As knowledge about nutrients increases, more interactions among nutrients are being discovered. In some cases, the interactions are beneficial; however, in other instances, nutrients may exert negative interactive effects. Some interactions (positive and negative) have been discussed in this chapter. For example, vitamin D increases intestinal absorption of calcium; vitamin C activates folate and enhances the absorption of nonheme iron; riboflavin is involved in the activation of vitamin B_6; vitamin B_{12} is critical in the transport and storage of folate; vitamin B_6 is required for the conversion of tryptophan to niacin; and excess zinc interferes with copper metabolism. Numerous other interactions exist. Additional beneficial interactions that have been noted include the following:

- Adequate vitamin E improves the body's use of vitamin A (37);
- Vitamin E and selenium act together as antioxidants in the cell (37); and
- Copper is important for the mobilization of iron (32).

Negative consequences of nutrient interactions include the following:
- Large doses of zinc can reduce intestinal absorption of calcium (35);
- Zinc absorption may be reduced by iron supplements (35);
- High doses of vitamin A reduce tissue storage of vitamin C (11); and
- Riboflavin deficiency may reduce iron absorption and increase iron loss (38).

As nutrient metabolism becomes increasingly understood, it is likely that more interactions among nutrients will be noted. Future dietary recommendations will take into account nutrient-nutrient interactions.

SPOTLIGHT ON LEARNING

Ms. Durns, age 35, currently takes a vitamin-E supplement to protect her against the effects of pollution; a vitamin-C supplement to prevent the possibility of catching a cold; and a B-complex vitamin (thiamin, riboflavin, niacin, vitamin B_6, pantothenic acid) to help her deal with stresses in her life. Fearful of developing osteoporosis, she just began taking a calcium supplement.

1. What information do you need to know to assess whether or not Ms. Durns needs vitamin and/or mineral supplementation?
2. What information do you need to assess whether or not Ms. Durns may have an adverse reaction to the supplements?
3. Suppose Ms. Durns needs the calcium supplement. How can you judge whether it is a good one for the money she is paying?

REVIEW QUESTIONS

1. One gram of fat yields how many kilocalories?
   a. 4
   b. 7
   c. 9
   d. 10

2. Which of the following is not an essential amino acid?
   a. phenylalanine
   b. arginine
   c. isoleucine
   d. lysine

3. Alcohol is metabolized primarily in which of the following?
   a. liver
   b. kidney
   c. brain
   d. pancreas

4. Which of the following is not a food source of Vitamin A?
   a. carrots
   b. liver
   c. spinach
   d. whole grain cereal

5. Vitamin D is essential for the absorption of which of the following?
   a. calcium
   b. iron
   c. vitamin B_6
   d. riboflavin

6. Which is the least toxic of the fat-soluble vitamins?
   a. vitamin A
   b. vitamin D
   c. vitamin E
   d. vitamin K

7. The megaloblastic anemia observed in vitamin B_{12} deficiency is a result of the trapping of which of the following?
   a. niacin
   b. iron
   c. vitamin C
   d. folate

8. Nonheme iron absorption is enhanced if which of the following is consumed at the same time?
   a. meat
   b. phytate
   c. tea
   d. biotin

9. Which of the following is a major extracellular cation?
   a. potassium
   b. sodium
   c. magnesium
   d. fluoride

10. Which of the following is a major intracellular cation?
    a. potassium
    b. sodium
    c. magnesium
    d. fluoride

ACTIVITIES

1. Visit a grocery store or drug store and randomly select three bottles of nutrient supplements. Record the RDA of the vitamins and/or minerals in the supplements. For whom might the supplements be necessary? What are the possible harmful effects (if any) of the supplements chosen?

2. Look through some magazines on body building. What claims (if any) are made for supplements? What is your estimation of the validity of the claims?

3. Visit a grocery store and locate food items that have been fortified. List the food items, the nutrients added, and the amount of the nutrients added. What benefits can you list for the fortification? What fortification seems unnecessary?

4. Interview five people about their use of supplements. Obtain answers to the following:
   a. Do you use supplements? If yes,
      What supplements do you use?
      What are your reasons for using the supplements?
   b. If no, What are your reasons for not using supplements?

REFERENCES

1. Wilson, P.C., and H.L. Greene. The gastrointestinal tract: Portal to nutrient utilization. In *Modern nutrition in health and disease,* 7th ed., edited by M.E. Shils and V.R. Young. Philadelphia: Lea and Febiger, 1988.
2. Davenport, H.W. *Physiology of the digestive tract.* 4th ed. Chicago: Year Book Medical Publishers, Inc., 1977.
3. Cummings, J.H. Consequences of the metabolism of fiber in the human large intestine. In *Dietary fiber in health and disease,* edited by G.V. Vahouny and D. Kritchevsky. New York: Plenum Press, 1982.
4. Pike, R.L., and M.L. Browne. *Nutrition: An integrated approach.* 3rd ed. New York: John Wiley & Sons, 1984.
5. Food and Agricultural Organization/World Health Organization. *Energy and protein requirements. Report of a joint FAO/WHO ad hoc expert committee on energy and protein requirements.* WHO Technical Report Series, No. 522: Geneva; FAO Nutrition Meeting Report Series, No. 52: Rome, 1973.
6. U.S. Department of Health and Human Services, Public Health Service. *The Surgeon General's report on nutrition and health. Summary and recommendations.* DHHS (PHS) Publication No. 88-50211. Washington, D.C.: Superintendent of Documents, GPO, 1988.
7. Linscheer, W.G., and A.J. Vergroesen. Lipids. In *Modern nutrition in health and disease,* 7th ed., edited by M.E. Shils and V.R. Young. Philadelphia: Lea and Febiger, 1988.

8. Eisenstein, A.B. Nutritional and metabolic effects of alcohol. *Journal of the American Dietetic Association* 81 (1982):247–51.

9. Olson, J.A. Recommended dietary intakes (RDI) of vitamin A in humans. *American Journal of Clinical Nutrition* 45 (1987): 704–16.

10. Committee on Dietary Allowances, Food and Nutrition Board, Division of Biological Sciences, Assembly of Life Sciences, National Research Council. *Recommended dietary allowances.* 9th rev. ed. Washington, D.C.: National Academy of Sciences, 1980.

11. Bendich, A., and L. Langseth. Safety of vitamin A. *American Journal of Clinical Nutrition* 49 (1989):358–71.

12. DeLuca, H.F. Vitamin D and its metabolites. In *Modern Nutrition in Health and Disease,* 7th ed., edited by M.E. Shils and V.R. Young. Philadelphia: Lea and Febiger, 1988.

13. Farrell, P.M. Vitamin E. In *Modern Nutrition in Health and Disease,* 7th ed., edited by M.E. Shils and V.R. Young. Philadelphia: Lea and Febiger, 1988.

14. Olson, J.A. Recommended dietary intakes (RDI) of vitamin K in humans. *American Journal of Clinical Nutrition* 45 (1987): 687–92.

15. Olson, J.A., and R.E. Hodges. Recommended dietary intakes (RDI) of vitamin C in humans. *American Journal of Clinical Nutrition* 45 (1987):693–703.

16. Hornig, D.H., U. Moser, and B.E. Glatthaar. Ascorbic acid. In *Modern Nutrition in Health and Disease,* 7th ed., edited by M.E. Shils and V.R. Young. Philadelphia: Lea and Febiger, 1988.

17. Herbert, V. Recommended dietary intakes (RDI) of folate in humans. *American Journal of Clinical Nutrition* 45 (1987):661–70.

18. Herbert, V. Vitamin B$_{12}$. In *Nutrition reviews' present knowledge in nutrition,* 5th ed., edited by R.E. Olson, et al. Washington, D.C.: The Nutrition Foundation, Inc., 1984.

19. Herbert, V. Vitamin B-12: plant sources, requirements, and assay. *American Journal of Clinical Nutrition* 48 (1988):852–58.

20. Reynolds, R.D. Bioavailability of vitamin B-6 from plant foods. *American Journal of Clinical Nutrition* 48 (1988):863–67.

21. McCormick, D.B. Vitamin B$_6$. In *Modern nutrition in health and disease,* 7th ed., edited by M.E. Shils and V.R. Young. Philadelphia: Lea and Febiger, 1988.

22. Said, H.M., R. Redha, and W. Nyalander. Biotin transport in the human intestine: Inhibition by anticonvulsant drugs. *American Journal of Clinical Nutrition* 49 (1989):127–31.

23. McCormick, D.B. Pantothenic acid. In *Modern nutrition in health and disease,* 7th ed., edited by M.E. Shils and V.R. Young. Philadelphia: Lea and Febiger, 1988.

24. National Institutes of Health. Consensus Development Conference Statement. Osteoporosis, 1984. *Journal of the American Medical Association* 252 (1984):799–802.

25. Avioli, L.V. Calcium and phosphorus. In *Modern nutrition in health and disease,* 7th ed., edited by M.E. Shils and V.R. Young. Philadelphia: Lea and Febiger, 1988.

26. Shils, M.E. Magnesium. In *Modern nutrition in health and disease,* 7th ed., edited by M.E. Shils and V.R. Young. Philadelphia: Lea and Febiger, 1988.

27. Franz, K.B. Magnesium in human nutrition. *Nutrition & the M.D.* 14 (1988):1–3.
28. ———. Hypomagnesemia in hospitals. *Nutrition & the M.D.* 14, no. 11 (1988):1.
29. Monsen, E.R. Iron nutrition and absorption: Dietary factors which impact iron availability. *Journal of the American Dietetic Association* 88 (1988):786–90.
30. Herbert, V. Recommended dietary intakes (RDI) of iron in humans. *American Journal of Clinical Nutrition* 45 (1987):679–86.
31. Solomons, N.W. Zinc and copper. In *Modern nutrition in health and disease,* 7th ed., edited by M.E. Shils and V.R. Young. Philadelphia: Lea and Febiger, 1988.
32. Turnlund, J.R. Copper nutriture, bioavailability, and the influence of dietary factors. *Journal of the American Dietetic Association* 88 (1988):303–8.
33. Tyler, D.D. Water and mineral metabolism. In *Review of physiological chemistry,* 17th ed., edited by H.A. Harper, V.W. Rodwell, and P.A. Mayes. Los Altos: Lange Medical Publications, 1979.
34. Committee on Diet and Health, Food and Nutrition Board, Commission on Life Sciences, National Research Council. *Diet and health: Implications for reducing chronic disease risk. Executive summary.* Washington, D.C.: National Academy Press, 1989.
35. ———. Food versus pills versus fortified foods. *Dairy Council Digest* 58 (March–April 1987):7–12.
36. Food and Drug Administration, HHS. 21 CFR Ch.1. Subpart B—*Fortification policy. 104.20 Statement of purpose.* Issued April 1, 1985.
37. ———. Vitamin interaction. Part I: How nutrients help one another and protect the body. *American Institute for Cancer Research Newsletter* Spring 1986.
38. ———. Possible effects of riboflavin deficiency on iron utilization. *Food and Nutrition News* 61 (1989):11.

CHAPTER
3

NUTRITION FOR PREGNANCY, FETAL DEVELOPMENT, AND LACTATION

Objectives

After studying this chapter, you will be able to

- explain the nutritional requirements of pregnant females that are different from the requirements for nonpregnant females of the same age.
- specify the unique nutritional needs of pregnant adolescents and the older primigravida and multipara.
- list appropriate nutrition interventions for common discomforts experienced during pregnancy;
- identify the nutritional adaptations for the commonly occurring problems associated with pregnancy.
- explain the differences in the nutritional requirements during pregnancy and lactation.
- translate the nutritional requirements to dietary recommendations.
- identify the Special Supplemental Food Program for Women, Infants and Children (WIC).

Overview

Pregnancy, described as a "metabolic tour de force" (or feat of strength), is an anabolic event accommodated by physiologic adaptations of the mother (1). The metabolic changes result in additional nutritional needs to support growth of the mother and fetus. The major goals of pregnancy are the birth of a full-term infant at optimal physical and mental development and the maintenance of the good health of the mother during and following pregnancy (2).

It is a well-accepted fact that good nutrition is important to the health of the mother and developing fetus. However, the specific effects of nutrition on pregnancy outcome are difficult to isolate due to the complex influences of heredity and social, economic, environmental, and lifestyle factors. Teaching nutritional principles to pregnant women should, therefore, emphasize optimal health as the goal. With adequate dietary intake in the absence of harmful influences, mothers can benefit themselves and their unborn children.

POSSIBLE NURSING DIAGNOSES

Knowledge deficit related to
- understanding of the relationship between good nutrition and normal fetal development and/or lactation.
- problems associated with teenage pregnancy.
- hazards of excess caffeine, drug, or alcohol intake.

Noncompliance related to
- lack of understanding of the role of adequate nutrition and normal maternal weight gain to normal fetal development and/or lactation.
- lack of money (including lack of refrigeration and/or cooking facilities or transportation).
- cultural differences between client and established system of care.

Alteration in comfort regarding
- heartburn related to pressure from enlarging uterus and hormonal changes.
- nausea or vomiting related to morning sickness;
- constipation related to hemorhoid formation.

Alteration in bowel elimination regarding constipation related to decreased intestinal movement, pressure from the enlarging uterus, and/or iron supplements.

Potential inadequate coping related to stress, leading to inhibition of lactation.

Potential for infection during lactation related to milk production or trauma during breast-feeding.

NUTRIENT NEEDS DURING PREGNANCY

The developing fetus is totally dependent on the mother for adequate nutrition. The actual provision of nutrients is accomplished through activities in the placenta. Here, the maternal and fetal circulation come in close contact, although they never directly interface. The placenta allows diffusion of nutrients from maternal to fetal blood and diffusion of excretory products from fetal to maternal blood. In addition, the mother undergoes anabolic changes to support the pregnant state.

The growth requirements of the mother and fetus result in an increased need for kilocalories as well as all nutrients (Table 3-1).

Energy Needs

The energy needs during pregnancy are influenced by maternal, fetal, and placental growth, as well as by maternal basal-metabolic rate and muscular activity. The growth in the mother includes an enlargement of the uterus and breasts. Fat reserves increase as a protection against catabolism and as a buffer against deprivation and to provide

Table 3-1. RECOMMENDED DIETARY ALLOWANCES FOR WOMEN (REVISED 1989)

Age (yr)	Weight (lb)	Height (in)	Kcals	Protein (g)	WATER-SOLUBLE VITAMINS Vitamin C (mg)	Thiamine (mg)	Riboflavin (mg)	Niacin (mg)	Vitamin B$_6$ (mg)	Folate (mcg)	Vitamin B$_{12}$ (mcg)
11–14	101	62	2200	46	50	1.1	1.3	15	1.4	150	2.0
15–18	120	64	2200	44	60	1.1	1.3	15	1.5	180	2.0
19–24	128	65	2200	46	60	1.1	1.3	15	1.6	180	2.0
25–50	138	64	2200	50	60	1.1	1.3	15	1.6	180	2.0
51+	143	63	1900	50	60	1.0	1.2	13	1.6	180	2.0
Pregnant 1st trimester			+0	60	70	1.5	1.6	17	2.2	400	2.2
2nd trimester			+300								
3rd trimester			+300								
Lactating 1st 6 mo.			+500	65	95	1.6	1.8	20	2.1	280	2.6
2nd 6 mo.			+500	62	90	1.6	1.7	20	2.1	260	2.6

Age (years)	Weight (pounds)	Height (inches)	FAT-SOLUBLE VITAMINS Vitamin A (mcg)	Vitamin D (mcg)	Vitamin E (mg)	MINERALS Calcium (mg)	Phosphorus (mg)	Magnesium (mg)	Iron (mg)	Zinc (mg)	Iodine (mcg)
11–14	101	62	800	10	8	1200	1200	280	15	12	150
15–18	120	64	800	10	8	1200	1200	300	15	12	150
19–24	128	65	800	7.5	8	1200	1200	280	15	12	150
25–50	138	64	800	5	8	800	800	280	15	12	150
51+	143	63	800	5	8	800	800	280	10	12	150
Pregnant			800	10	10	1200	1200	320	30	15	175
Lactating 1st 6 mo.			1300	10	12	1200	1200	355	15	19	200
2nd 6 mo.			1200	10	11	1200	1200	340	15	16	200

Source: Reprinted from the *Recommended Dietary Allowances*, 10th ed., © 1989 by the National Academy of Sciences, National Academy Press, Washington, D.C.

for lactation. Fat reserves are also used to satisfy the energy needs of the fetus, sparing protein for cellular growth. Fetal growth requires increased kilocalories, particularly during the third trimester of pregnancy. As the fetus grows, the placenta grows to accommodate the increased needs.

The basal-metabolic rate increases by about 15% during the latter half of pregnancy as a consequence of increased secretion of thyroxin, adrenal corticoid hormones, and the sex hormones. The increased basal-metabolic rate frequently results in the sensation of being overheated. In addition to an increased basal-metabolic rate, energy is required to carry the extra load of the fetus.

The RDA of an additional 300 kcal was calculated by estimating the total extra energy needs over the entire pregnancy (80000 kcal) and dividing by the number of days a normal pregnancy lasts following the first month (250 days) (3). Energy needs are smallest during the first trimester and increase as pregnancy progresses. A small, consistent increase in kilocalories is recommended by the Food and Nutrition Board of the National Research Council.

Weight Gain. Increased energy intake and growth of the fetus result in weight gain. The relationship between pounds of weight gained by a pregnant woman and the birth weight of her infant has been a focus of attention for several decades. In 1970 and 1981, the Committee on Maternal Nutrition of the National Research Council published reports that concluded that there is a relationship between maternal weight gain and mean birth weight; there is an inverse relationship between birth weight and perinatal morbidity and mortality; and the pattern and distribution of weight gain are just as important to consider as total weight gain during pregnancy (4).

Current research confirms the association between maternal weight gain and birth weight and supports the desirability of a range for a weight gain of 24–27 lb (11–12 kg) for the adult healthy woman of normal weight. Underweight women demonstrate more successful pregnancies when they gain approximately 28–36 lb, and obese women can support a successful pregnancy with a weight gain of 16–24 lb (5). However, pregnancy is not the time for an obese woman to diet; rather, a weight loss program should be followed prior to conception.

Inadequate weight gain increases the risk for the delivery of low birth weight (LBW) infants, defined as infants weighing less than 2500 g (approximately 5½ lb). Approximately two-thirds of LBW infants are the result of premature delivery (less than 37 weeks gestation). The remaining one-third are a result of intrauterine growth retardation producing smaller babies in relation to the gestational date, often due to malnutrition. Low birth weight infants are at greater risk of morbidity and mortality than infants of normal weight.

The weight gain during pregnancy is distributed as illustrated in Table 3-2. Although the figures listed are approximate, they clearly show the need for the range of weight gain recommended. Weight gained during pregnancy should be lost by six months after delivery. Approximately 9 lb (4 kg) are lost immediately after delivery, with the remainder lost in the ensuing months.

The pattern of weight gain during pregnancy is just as important a factor as total weight gain for a positive outcome of pregnancy. The suggested amount to gain during the first trimester is approximately 2–5 lb, with about 1 lb per week during the remainder of the pregnancy (5). After the 20th week, a sudden weight gain may be a sign of excess fluid retention. Although some fluid retention is normal, excess retention can result in serious consequences for the mother and infant. This condition, known as toxemia of pregnancy, is discussed later in this chapter.

Nutrient Needs

The need for all nutrients increases during pregnancy. For most nutrients, the needs are met through the physiological adaptations that occur in concert with an increased dietary intake. Some physiological changes enhance nutrient availability. For example, gastric movement and intestinal contraction decline during pregnancy, allowing for slower passage of digestive contents through the

Table 3-2. WEIGHT GAIN DURING PREGNANCY

	GRAMS	POUNDS
Fetus	3400	7.5
Placenta	650	1.4
Amniotic fluid	800	1.8
Uterus	1000	2.2
Breasts	400	.9
Blood Volume	1250	2.8
Interstitial fluid	1500	3.3
Maternal body stores	2000–3000	4.4–6.6
Total	11000–12000 (11–12 kg)	24.3–26.5 (24–27 lb)

Sources:

J.L. Duhring, "Nutrition in Pregnancy." In *Present Knowledge in Nutrition,* 5th ed., edited by R.E. Olson, et al. (Washington, D.C.: The Nutrition Foundation, Inc., 1984).

H.A. Guthrie, *Introductory Nutrition,* 5th ed. (St. Louis: C.V. Mosby Company, 1983).

gastrointestinal tract. Slower passage results in an increased opportunity for nutrient (particularly mineral) absorption.

Hormonal changes also influence absorption of nutrients. Increased levels of circulating parathyroid hormone during pregnancy result in an increase in calcium absorption. Elevated levels of aldosterone enhance the kidney's ability to reabsorb sodium from the kidney tubules.

Complementing the physiological changes, an increased intake of all nutrients is necessary to satisfy nutritional requirements. A pregnant woman must make wise choices in her dietary selections, since there is a large increase in nutrient needs compared with calorie needs. The calorie increase of 300 per day does not translate into "eating for two." In fact, an extra 300 kcal does not go far when obtained from a less nutrient-dense item such as pecan pie, which contains 490 kcal per slice with almost 50% of the calories coming from fat. The nurse may act as an adviser in providing resources, such as a food guide, to help pregnant women obtain the needed nutrients within the calorie recommendation. A food guide translates nutrient needs into recommendations for food intake. Table 3-3 is an example of a food guide showing the number of servings recommended for daily intake from the various food groups. Note the increases in intake required for pregnant adults compared with the intake for nonpregnant adults.

Even with the physiologic changes and increases in dietary intake, the demand for iron is so great that the requirements are difficult to achieve through the diet alone. Iron needs during pregnancy are influenced by an increased blood volume as well as fetal requirements. Total blood volume increases by almost one-third to accommodate the transport of nutrients to and waste products from the fetus. As blood volume increases, hemoglobin decreases, and the effect is hemodilution. The standards for measuring iron requirements are different in the pregnant versus the nonpregnant individual. Iron deficiency anemia in pregnancy is associated with a hemoglobin less than 11 g/dl (1).

Table 3-3. DAILY INTAKE FOOD GUIDE

FOOD GROUP	SERVING SIZE	SERVINGS FOR		
		NONPREGNANT ADULT	PREGNANT ADULT	LACTATING ADULT
Milk and milk products (whole, low-fat, and skim milk; powdered and canned milk; cheese; ice cream, puddings made with milk; yogurt; cottage cheese)	8 oz or equivalent	2	3	3
Meat, poultry, fish, and alternates (beef; pork; lamb; poultry; eggs; fish; dried beans, such as lentils and pinto beans, and peas; nuts; peanut butter)	approximately 3 oz	2–3 (5–7 oz lean)	2–3 5–7 oz lean)	2–3 (5–7 oz lean)
Fruits (including citrus fruits, such as oranges and grapefruits; avocados; pumpkin; melon; berries)	½ cup or equivalent	2–4	2–4	2–4
Vegetables (including dark leafy green vegetables, such as spinach and kale; deep-yellow vegetables, such as carrots, squash, and sweet potatoes; broccoli; chili peppers; bean sprouts; potatoes; snap beans; peas)	½ cup or equivalent	3–5	3–5	3–5
Breads, cereals, and other grain products (whole-grain breads and rolls; cornbread; ready-to-eat and cooked cereals; rice; oats; barley; wheat; grits; tortillas; crackers; macaroni products, including couscous and pasta)	½ cup or equivalent	6–11	6–11	6–11
Fats and sweets (avoid too many fats and sweets)				

Source: USDA Home and Garden Bulletin Number 232-1, April 1986.

For a nonpregnant individual, normal hemoglobin levels are 14–18 g/dl, and anemia corresponds to a hemoglobin of less than 12 g/dl (6). Towards the end of pregnancy, the bone marrow increases its activity, resulting in a closer-to-normal concentration of red blood cells.

In addition to accommodating the increase in blood volume, iron intake must be high enough to allow fetal accumulation of iron to last for the first three to four months of infancy. Despite the savings in iron resulting from the cessation of menstruation and increased absorption from the gastrointestinal tract, pregnant women cannot meet their iron needs through diet. A supplement of elemental iron is prescribed to meet the high demands of pregnancy (this is the current RDA recommendation).

Another nutrient, folic acid, may require supplementation as well. The increase in demand for folic acid is a result of the high rate of cellular growth, not only in maternal tissue but in fetal tissue as well. Some physicians routinely prescribe a supplement of 200–400 mcg of folacin, while others limit supplementation to individuals who are high risk, for folic-acid deficiency (7, 8).

LIFE-STYLE FACTORS AND PREGNANCY

Exercise

The physiological changes during pregnancy result in limitations on some types of exercise. The pregnancy-associated changes that have a direct impact on exercise are shortness of breath, weight gain, increased heart rate, light-headedness, and increased tendency towards injury due to softer connective tissue. Research has been conducted to address concerns such as uterine blood flow, temperature changes in the mother and fetus, fetal distress, and fetal outcome in exercise-conditioned pregnant women.

Depending on the intensity and duration of exercise, uterine blood flow can be affected twentyfold.

Research shows that even though exercise results in a decreased oxygen delivery to the fetus, a compensatory mechanism mitigates the negative effects. Body temperature is .5°C higher in the fetus than the mother, and little, if any, fetal distress has been found when the mother is exercising. Results from the studies on fetal outcome have been unclear because of poorly controlled experiments.

Benefits of exercise during pregnancy include fewer problems with bloating, constipation, morning sickness, and varicose veins. Exercise also helps to control excessive weight gain and aids in toning the body for labor and delivery. After weighing the benefits and risks of exercise, the American College of Obstetricians and Gynecologists recommends that regular exercise be encouraged during pregnancy. Brisk walking is considered to be especially good. Activities such as swimming, jogging, and tennis may be continued if the woman engaged in these activities regularly prior to becoming pregnant. Prolonged or strenuous aerobic exercise is not recommended (7).

Alcohol

Results of studies conducted on women who drank heavily during pregnancy have indicated that a significant number of infants were born with a pattern of physical, mental, and behavioral abnormalities referred to as FAS, or fetal alcohol syndrome (9). Alcohol passes rapidly through the placenta, and fetal blood alcohol reaches approximately the same concentration as maternal blood alcohol. In addition, fetal blood-alcohol concentration falls more slowly than the mother's because the fetus does not produce the enzyme (alcohol dehydrogenase) needed to metabolize alcohol. Consequently, the damaging effects have a longer period of activity in the fetus. Alcohol is toxic and results in changes in fetal acid-base balance, cerebral function, and metabolism (10). Features of FAS include prenatal and/or postnatal growth retardation, including height, weight, and/or head circumference measurements below the tenth percentile; retarded mental and motor abilities; and abnormal facial and eye features. When the full syndrome is not present, the abnormalities resulting from heavy or moderate alcohol use during pregnancy are referred to as FAE, or fetal alcohol effects (10).

Currently, no safe level for alcohol intake during pregnancy has been defined. An intake of two to three drinks daily (one to two ounces ethanol) has been associated with decreased weight, hyperactivity, and motor problems (11). Because FAS is totally preventable, the risks of alcohol consumption during pregnancy are so great, and no known safe level of alcohol consumption in pregnancy can be set, the Surgeon General advises pregnant women or those women planning a pregnancy to abstain from alcohol consumption (12).

Smoking

Smoking during pregnancy is associated with twice the incidence of LBW infants and an increase in fetal and neonatal mortality. Smoking has negative effects on the mother as well, increasing the risk for heart disease and cancer.

Medications, Drugs

Medications, including aspirin and laxatives should not be taken unless prescribed by the physician, particularly during the first 12 weeks of pregnancy. Additionally, amphetamines, barbitu-

rates, cocaine, crack, narcotics, marijuana, and hallucinogens can cross the placenta and affect the fetus. Infants have been born addicted to drugs and go through withdrawal, which can be serious and sometimes fatal (13).

Caffeine

Caffeine is a stimulant to the central nervous system that can cross the placenta. Concern about caffeine consumption during pregnancy was caused by research suggesting an association with birth defects. Results from a teratology study in pregnant rats that were force-fed large quantities of caffeine by stomach tube prompted the FDA in late 1980 to recommend that pregnant women avoid or decrease caffeine consumption (14). Since that time, more studies have been completed, and no human evidence exists to suggest that moderate caffeine intake causes birth defects (15). The FDA's concerns over human consumption have diminished; however, the agency is not prepared to rescind its original warning (14). A daily intake of 400 mg or less of caffeine has been suggested as a safe level (11).

Caffeine-containing foods include coffee, tea, cocoa, chocolate, and some soft drinks. Caffeine is also an ingredient in drugs, both prescription and over-the-counter. (See Table 3–4.)

Table 3-4. CAFFEINE CONTENT OF COMMON ITEMS

ITEM	AVERAGE CAFFEINE (mg)
Coffee (5-oz cup)	
brewed, drip	115
brewed, percolator	80
instant	65
decaffeinated, brewed	3
decaffeinated, instant	2

Continued

Table 3-4. CAFFEINE CONTENT OF COMMON ITEMS *(continued)*

ITEM	AVERAGE CAFFEINE (mg)
Tea (5-oz cup)	
brewed	40
instant	30
iced (12 oz)	70
Hot cocoa (5-oz cup)	4
Chocolate milk (8 oz)	5
Milk chocolate (1 oz)	6
Dark chocolate, semisweet (1 oz)	20
Chocolate syrup (1 oz)	4
Soft drinks (12 oz)	
cola	30–46
cola, decaffeinated	0–0.18
cola, diet	0.6
cola, diet decaffeinated	0–0.2
ginger ale	0
ginger ale, diet	0
lemon-lime	0
lemon-lime, diet	0
root beer	0
root beer, diet	0
seltzer	0
Prescription drugs	
Cafergot (1 tablet)	100
Norgesic	30
Fioricet	40
Darvon compound	32.4
Synalgos-DC	30
Over-the-counter drugs	
No Doz	100
Vivarin	200
Anacin, maximum strength	32
Excedrin	65
Midol	32.4
Aqua-Ban	100

Source: C.W. Lecos, "Caffeine Jitters: Some Safety Questions Remain." *FDA Consumer* 21, no. 10 (December 1987–January 1988):22–7.

COMMON DISCOMFORTS EXPERIENCED DURING PREGNANCY

Morning Sickness

Nausea and vomiting during pregnancy, or morning sickness, may occur at any time of the day and is common during early pregnancy. The problem appears to be the result of hormonal changes that occur initially in pregnancy. Some interventions with food intake are helpful for some women.

The goal is to alleviate the uncomfortable symptoms, avoid dehydration, and resume food intake. The following are some suggestions to reduce nausea and vomiting during pregnancy:

- Eat small frequent meals.
- Eat a dry carbohydrate food, such as crackers and dry toast before rising in the morning.
- Avoid drinking with meals; consume beverages between meals.
- Avoid coffee, tea, and spicy foods.
- Avoid foods that are high in fat, such as fried food and rich desserts.
- If possible, try to occasionally have someone else prepare meals. Often, the smell rather than the taste of food causes the upset.

Heartburn

Heartburn and indigestion result from increased pressure of the uterus on the stomach but also may be due to relaxation of the cardiac sphincter of the stomach due to hormonal changes. To reduce the chances of developing heartburn, small frequent meals are recommended. In addition, avoiding high-fat foods and spicy foods may be helpful. Maintaining an upright position for at least one hour following meals may also help to prevent gastric reflex (refer to Chapter 7). Self-medication with antacids should be discouraged, because there is a potential for alkalemia. Antacids can also bind with iron and predispose to anemia.

Constipation

The decline in gastric movement, decreased intestinal contraction, and pressure from the enlarging uterus are thought to cause constipation. Iron supplements may also be a factor. The following suggestions may help relieve this common problem:

- Increase consumption of fresh fruits and vegetables.
- Include whole-grain cereals, whole-wheat or cracked-wheat breads and rolls in the diet.
- Consume adequate fluids such as water, milk, and juices.
- Include regular exercise and adequate rest in the schedule.

(A complete discussion of constipation and its treatment is given in Chapter 7.)

Food Cravings and Aversions

Research on mechanisms involved in food cravings and aversions during pregnancy is scant. The studies that have been completed indicate a high incidence of cravings or aversions, occurring in one-half to two-thirds of pregnancies (16). The cravings or aversions appear most often in the first trimester. It is speculated that hormonal-metabolic changes in pregnancy are somehow related.

Aversions and cravings during pregnancy are normally not serious unless the aversions result in inadequate nutrient intake or the cravings are for nonfood items. Compulsive consumption of nonfood items, such as laundry starch or red clay, is known as *pica*. It should be noted that pica is not only restricted to pregnancy; it can occur in both sexes at any age and may be related to cultural and/or geographic factors.

Pica has been associated with iron deficiency; however, the relationship is far from clear, especially since the substances craved are rarely rich in iron and actually inhibit iron absorption. In addition, not all individuals with iron deficiency exhibit pica. It has therefore been theorized that pica is a result of the complex interrelationship among nutrient deficiency and cultural and psychological factors (17). Consumption of the nonfood item can be so high that intestinal obstruction, bowel perforation, and infection can result. Educational campaigns about the dangers of pica as well as dietary improvement have been successful in reducing the incidences of pica.

POSSIBLE COMPLICATIONS OF PREGNANCY

Toxemia

The causes of toxemia during pregnancy are unknown, but it is characterized by inflammation and spasm of the arterioles in many parts of the body, decreased renal blood flow, and decreased glomerular filtration rate. Clinically, this translates to a sudden, excessive weight gain after 20 weeks gestation, edema, and often elevation of blood pressure.

Severe toxemia during pregnancy is referred to as eclampsia, characterized by hypertension, headache, proteinuria, seizures, and possibly death. Milder degrees of eclampsia are referred to as preeclampsia.

A greater occurrence of eclampsia has been noted in individuals who are overweight when they conceive and gain excessive weight in the latter half of pregnancy. However, it is most severe in underweight women who fail to gain enough weight during pregnancy (11). Prevention requires adequate preparation before conception and close monitoring of the pregnancy by medical professionals.

Gestational Diabetes

Gestational diabetes is caused by the lack of pancreatic response to the increased requirements for insulin during pregnancy. Untreated, gestational diabetes can result in intrauterine or neonatal death or hypoglycemia, hypocalcemia, polycythemia, and hyperbilirubinemia in the infant.

Treatment of gestational diabetes involves efforts to maintain normal blood glucose levels. Diet therapy is the recommended first step. If diet alone proves inadequate to control blood glucose levels, insulin treatment may be necessary. Treatment with hypoglycemic agents is not advised.

Because pregnancy is normally accompanied by a degree of glucose intolerance, recommendations for diagnosing gestational diabetes have been issued. Current recommendations include screening pregnant women for glucose intolerance between the 24th and 28th week of pregnancy with an oral glucose load of 50g. A blood glucose value of greater than or equal to 140 mg/dl one hour after ingestion suggests a need for a full glucose tolerance test (18). (See Chapter 13 for a full description of diabetes diagnosis and treatment.)

With proper medical care, women with gestational diabetes can deliver healthy babies. Usually, glucose tolerance returns to normal after pregnancy although the mother is at an increased risk for developing diabetes later in life. In addition, the children of mothers who experience gestational diabetes have a greater risk for glucose intolerance.

SPECIAL CARE SITUATIONS

Adolescent Pregnancy

Adolescent pregnancy is a significant problem in the United States, with approximately 600,000 births per year reported for girls in their teens (19). Additionally, 19% of infants born to teenagers are classified as LBW (20). The outcomes of adolescent pregnancies are profoundly influenced by nutritional, environmental, and social conditions.

Adolescence is a time of growth and, therefore, increased energy and nutrient needs. When a young adolescent is pregnant, the energy and nutrient needs are compounded, because she must not only support her normal growth, but she must also support the growth required during pregnancy and the growth of the fetus. It has been reported that adolescents with a gynecologic age (chronologic age minus age at menarche) of two years or less have higher energy and nutrient needs than those of older pregnant adolescents (21). This is due to the higher needs for the teen's growth, which do not end until four to seven years after menarche. To these needs are added the requirements for pregnancy. (Refer to Table 3-1 for the calorie and nutrient needs of adolescents.)

An optimal weight gain in adolescent pregnancy is not known. Adolescents often gain less than 16 lb during pregnancy. Weight gain in the range of 26–35 lb has been found to lower the risk of LBW and decrease fetal mortality (20).

It is a challenge to encourage teenagers to follow food guidelines (Table 3-5), because they often have poor dietary habits. They are apt to skip meals, consume snacks of low nutrient density, and limit food intake for fear of gaining too much weight or to hide the pregnancy. In addition to the nutritional risks, pregnant teenagers often face disruptions in schooling and family life. Some high schools have special programs for pregnant teens that include classes on pregnancy and child care in the curriculum. These programs often offer a support system when one is lacking in the home.

Table 3-5. FOOD GUIDE FOR THE PREGNANT ADOLESCENT

GROUP	SERVING SIZE	AMOUNT	EXAMPLES
MILK AND MILK PRODUCTS	8 oz or equivalent	4 Servings	Cheese; ice cream; puddings made with milk; yogurt; milk (whole, low-fat, skim); cottage cheese; powdered and canned milk
MEAT, POULTRY, FISH, AND ALTERNATES	approximately 3 oz	2–3 Servings (total 5 to 7 oz lean)	Eggs; dried beans and peas such as lentils and pinto beans; nuts; peanut butter; poultry; fish; beef; pork; lamb
FRUITS	½ cup or equivalent	2–4 Servings	All fruits including citrus fruits such as oranges and grapefruits; avocados; pumpkin; melon; berries
VEGETABLES	½ cup or equivalent	3–5 Servings	All vegetables including dark, leafy green vegetables such as spinach and kale; deep-yellow vegetables such as carrots, squash, and sweet potatoes; broccoli; chili peppers; bean sprouts; potatoes; snap beans; peas
BREADS, CEREALS, AND OTHER GRAIN PRODUCTS	½ cup or equivalent	6–11 Servings	Rice; oats; barley; wheat; grits; cornbread; tortillas; crepes; whole-grain breads and rolls; crackers; macaroni products including couscous and pasta; cereals (ready-to-eat and cooked)
FATS AND SWEETS Avoid too many fats and sweets			

Source: USDA Home and Garden Bulletin Number 232-1, April 1986.

The Older *Primigravida* (a woman during her first pregnancy) and *Multipara* (a woman who has borne more than one offspring)

The number of women aged 35 and over having first pregnancies is on the increase. Reasons for delaying motherhood include later marriages as well as dual-career marriages. The main potential complication that has been reported in older pregnancy is hypertension (22).

Research on the nutritional needs of the older pregnant woman is lacking. Energy needs may be less due to the decrease in resting metabolism, which occurs with age. Despite lower calorie needs, nutrient requirements are similar. The older pregnant woman should therefore be guided towards more nutrient-dense foods.

Nutrition Implications During Labor

During early labor, clear carbohydrate liquids may be prescribed, because these will be more readily absorbed by the body. Foods containing protein and fat are avoided due to the longer time required to digest these substances. Solid foods are not given during labor because the movement of the stomach is greatly diminished. Foodstuffs could be retained; should vomiting occur, there would be a greater chance for aspiration.

When the woman enters the period of active labor, she is maintained NPO (nothing by mouth). Small quantities of ice chips and lollipops may be offered to alleviate thirst. A lollipop is preferable to hard candy since there is less chance of aspiration during forceful uterine contractions. If the labor process is prolonged, intravenous fluids will be prescribed.

LACTATION

Before World War II, almost three-fourths of infants were breast-fed. From this high level, a steady decline occurred in incidence and duration of breast-feeding during the 1950s and 1960s. The steady lengthy decline ended in the 1970s, and incidence has been on the increase ever since (23).

The Committee on Nutrition of the American Academy of Pediatrics has endorsed breast-feeding as the best means of feeding for the newborn (19). Also, the Committee on Nutrition of the Mother and Preschool Child of the National Research Council has suggested that any healthy mother with the least inclination toward breast-feeding her newborn should be encouraged to do so, and given all possible assistance from health professionals (9). Approaches that have been shown to promote breast-feeding include increased information and support to mothers, changes in hospital routines to accommodate breast-feeding, such as immediate skin-to-skin contact and rooming-in, and direct modeling of breast-feeding (24).

Breast-feeding has physiological and psychological advantages for both the infant and the mother. Among the major advantages to the infant are the transmission of maternal immunity through colostrum (early milk), the delivery of a food considered to be best suited for the infant's needs (25), and the development of strong bonding between the mother and infant. For the mother, lactation causes contraction of the uterus wall, facilitating its return to normal size and a faster return to prepregnancy weight.

The quantity and nutritional composition of breast milk can be affected by the mother's dietary intake in some cases. Poorly nourished mothers produce less milk than well-nourished mothers (19). The water-soluble vitamin profile of breast milk and, to a lesser extent, the mineral content, is influenced by maternal diet. However, the major constituents of breast milk are maintained at the expense of the mother (11).

As shown in Table 3-1, calorie and nutrient needs of lactating women are increased. Of special interest are energy and iron needs. Energy or calorie requirements for lactation are proportional to the quantity of milk produced (3). According to the *Recommended Dietary Allowances*, the additional 500 kcal needed each day by a lactating woman are based on the production of breast milk daily.

Iron needs during lactation are not greatly different from those during nonpregnancy.

The recommendation for fluid intake during lactation is two quarts daily (19). Variations in fluid intake will not affect the volume of milk; rather, the urine becomes more concentrated to accommodate the lower fluid intake.

The daily food guide illustrated in Table 3-3 is a translation of the dietary recommendations for lactation. Note the differences between the amounts of food recommended for lactation versus pregnancy.

In addition to recommendations on items to include in the diet, there are specific cautions for lactating women. Persons who test positive for human immunodeficiency virus (HIV) should be discouraged from breast-feeding. Excessive caffeine consumption should be avoided due to its stimulatory effects. Abstinence from alcohol is recommended until after weaning. A number of drugs are excreted in breast milk. Drugs that are thought to be contraindications to breast-feeding include those that suppress immune function, radioactive isotopes, some antithyroid drugs, some sulfonamides, bromocriptine (Parlodel), and chlorothiazide (Diuril). The latter two suppress lactation (19). Judgments about beginning or continuing breast-feeding while on medication are based on the drug, dose schedule, infant feeding patterns, infant age, and dietary intake (19).

GOVERNMENT PROGRAMS FOR PREGNANT AND LACTATING WOMEN

The Special Supplemental Food Program for Women, Infants and Children was first authorized in 1972. Through this program, pregnant, postpartum, and lactating women and infants and children up to five years of age at nutritional risk due to inadequate nutrition and income are provided with nutritious supplemental foods or vouchers for these foods, redeemable at local grocery stores. The supplemental foods contain the nutrients most often lacking in the diets of low-income populations: high-quality protein, iron, calcium, vitamin A, and vitamin C.

The program originates at the federal government level. Cash grants are distributed from the federal government to health departments in each state. The states oversee and fund the development of WIC programs to serve low-income populations at the local level. A unique aspect of WIC is the provision of nutrition education in addition to the food or vouchers. Research supports that WIC has a positive impact on participants (26).

NURSING INTERVENTIONS RELATED TO DIETARY MANAGEMENT

- Work closely with the dietitian or nutritionist and the physician as may be required to assist a woman in achieving optimum nutrition during pregnancy.
- Act as a resource person in providing information related to physiological demands of the pregnancy; conducting dietary assessments; referring a woman or her family to the appropriate community agencies for additional assistance (financial, medical, etc.).
- Dispel myths associated with pregnancy (e.g., a tooth is lost for every pregnancy).
- Monitor weight gains.
- Interpret the results of laboratory tests, blood-pressure readings, and weight gain as a reflection of dietary status.
- Assess for discomforts related to pregnancy (heartburn, constipation, and nausea or vomiting), offer suggestions that may help to control the problem.

Continued

NURSING INTERVENTIONS *(continued)*
- Stress the importance of good nutrition throughout the life span.
- Be alert for situations that may require special consideration, such as teenage pregnancy, the older primigravida, or alcohol- or drug-related problems.

- Encourage the new mother and family during the process of lactation (if appropriate).
- Refer the nursing mother to support groups such as La Leche League.

TOPIC OF INTEREST

Teen pregnancy programs have been shown to be effective in encouraging adolescents to gain weight and in reducing the incidence of LBW infants (27). In these programs, interdisciplinary teams deliver prenatal and postpartum medical care, social services, and health education. The value of such programs is easily measured, since the financial cost associated with LBW infants can be substantial: $13,616 per LBW infant for postpartum care in 1983 dollars (20).

SPOTLIGHT ON LEARNING

Ms. M. is three months pregnant, and she reports having problems with morning sickness. She also states that she simply cannot drink milk, although she knows she should. Her food intake over a 24-hour period is as follows:

Breakfast: 1 donut, 1 cup coffee with 1 tbls cream and 1 tsp sugar
Lunch: Roast beef sandwich (2 slices white bread, 2 oz roast beef, 1 oz cheddar cheese, 2 tsp mayonnaise), 1 orange, 2 chocolate chip cookies, 12 oz cola
Snack: 1-oz bag of potato chips
Dinner: 3 oz fried chicken, french fries, steamed carrots, tossed salad with 1 tbls Italian dressing, 1 piece coconut cream pie, 1 cup coffee with 1 tbls cream and 1 tsp sugar
Snack: 1 cup tea with lemon and 1 tsp honey, 1 container (6 oz) fruited yogurt

1. What guidance can you offer to help her deal with morning sickness?
2. What substitutions are appropriate for milk to satisfy her calcium requirements?
3. What strengths and weaknesses do you see with her diet?
4. Is follow-up guidance needed?
5. When and to whom would you send this woman?

REVIEW QUESTIONS

1. What is the recommended amount of weight gain during pregnancy for a woman of normal weight?
   a. 12–17 lb
   b. 20–25 lb
   c. 24–27 lb
   d. 30–35 lb

2. Select the letter that represents an adequate diet for a pregnant woman.
   a. 3 servings milk, 2–3 servings meat, 2–4 servings fruits, 3–5 servings vegetables, 6–11 servings breads and grains
   b. 4 servings milk, 2–3 servings meat, 2–3 servings fruits, 3 servings vegetables, 2 servings breads and grains
   c. 2 servings milk, 2 servings meat, 2–4 servings fruits, 3–5 servings vegetables, 6–11 servings breads and grains
   d. 5 servings milk, 4 servings meat, 2 servings fruits, 3 servings vegetables, 4 servings breads and grains

3. Which of the following is not recommended for relieving constipation during pregnancy?
   a. increase consumption of fresh fruits and vegetables
   b. include whole-grain cereals and breads in the diet
   c. consume adequate fluids
   d. increase the fat content of the diet

4. What is the recommendation regarding the consumption of alcohol during pregnancy?
   a. reduce intake to no more than 1–2 drinks per day
   b. abstain from alcohol
   c. moderate consumption
   d. limit intake to 1 drink per week

5. Which of the following is not a source of caffeine?
   a. colas
   b. chocolate
   c. tea
   d. lemonade

6. A patient with toxemia during pregnancy is asked to choose from the following list those foods that contain the least amount of sodium. Which choice is appropriate?
   a. hot dog with mustard
   b. grilled cheese on wheat bread
   c. sliced turkey breast and tomato wedges
   d. bacon, lettuce, and tomato on white toast

NUTRITION FOR PREGNANCY, FETAL DEVELOPMENT, AND LACTATION   71

7. What is gynecologic age?
   a. chronologic age
   b. age at menarche
   c. chronologic age minus age at first pregnancy
   d. chronologic age minus age at menarche

8. What is the most common complication of an older woman undergoing her first pregnancy?
   a. gestational diabetes
   b. inadequate weight gain
   c. premature labor
   d. hypertension

9. What are the additional 500 kcal recommended during lactation based on?
   a. activity of the mother
   b. weight of the infant
   c. quantity of milk produced
   d. age of the infant

10. The foods provided through the WIC program emphasize which of the following nutrients?
   a. vitamin A, vitamin C, thiamin, riboflavin, niacin
   b. protein, iron, calcium, vitamin A, vitamin C
   c. carbohydrate, fiber, zinc, copper
   d. phosphorus, fluoride, magnesium, pyridoxine

ACTIVITIES

1. Record your previous 24-hour food intake. Compare your intake with the daily food guide for a pregnant woman. How does it differ?

2. Interview a woman who has given birth in the last year. Ask what directions she was given concerning the amount of weight women should gain during pregnancy. Interview a woman who gave birth at least 15 years ago. Ask what directions she was given concerning weight gain. How does the advice compare?

3. Interview a woman who chose to breast-feed her child. What influenced her to do so?

4. Visit the grocery store and your library. Using food labels and food composition tables, identify the amount of iron per serving in the following foods:

Food	Amount
Chicken	3 oz
Beef	3 oz.
Fish	3 oz
Liver	3 oz
Milk	1 cup
Cheese	1 oz
Total cereal	½ cup
Kix cereal	½ cup
Cream of wheat	½ cup cooked
Saltines	6
Bread, wheat	1 slice
Macaroni	½ cup cooked
Orange juice	½ cup
Prune juice	½ cup
Lima beans	½ cup cooked
Lettuce	2 large leaves
Tomato	1 medium
Cola	12-oz can
Tea	6 oz
Chocolate cake	1 square

Which foods would you recommend for a pregnant woman to increase her dietary intake of iron?

5. Invite a nurse to class to speak about her experiences with adolescent pregnancy and first pregnancies of women aged 35 and older.

6. Spend one day at a local WIC clinic. Sit in on an interview of a client by a nutritionist. Examine pamphlets available for patient education. Inquire about the number of clients who keep their appointments and return to the nutritionist for follow-up.

REFERENCES

1. Duhring, J.L. Nutrition in Pregnancy. In *Present knowledge in nutrition,* 5th ed., edited by R.E. Olson, et al. Washington, D.C.: The Nutrition Foundation, Inc., 1984.

2. National Research Council, Committee on Nutrition of the Mother and Pre-school Child. *Nutrition services in perinatal care.* Washington, D.C.: National Academy of Sciences, 1981.

3. National Research Council, Committee on Dietary Allowances, Food and Nutrition Board. *Recommended Dietary Allowances.* 9th ed. Washington, D.C.: National Academy of Sciences, 1980.

4. Chez, R. Weight gain during pregnancy. *American Journal of Public Health* 76 (1986):1390–91.

5. Worthington-Roberts, B.S., J. Vermeersch, and S.R. Williams. *Nutrition in pregnancy and lactation.* St. Louis: Times Mirror/Mosby College Publishing, 1985.

6. Hallberg, L. Iron. In *Present knowledge in nutrition,* 5th ed., edited by R.E. Olson, et al. Washington, D.C.: The Nutrition Foundation, Inc., 1984.

7. American College of Obstetricians and Gynecologists. *Standards for obstetric-gynecologic services.* 6th ed. Washington, D.C.: The American College of Obstetricians and Gynecologists, 1985.

8. Huber, A.M., and L.L. Wallins. Folate nutriture in pregnancy. *Journal of the American Dietetic Association* 88 (1988):791–95.

9. National Research Council, Committee on Nutrition of the Mother and Pre-school Child. *Alternative dietary practices and nutritional abuses in pregnancy.* Washington, D.C.: National Academy of Sciences, 1982.

10. Ouellette, E.M. The fetal alcohol syndrome. *Contemporary Nutrition* 9 (no. 3) (1984) Minneapolis: General Mills, Inc.

11. Guthrie, H.A. *Introductory nutrition.* 5th ed. St. Louis: C.V. Mosby Company, 1983.

12. U.S. Department of Health and Human Services, National Institute on Alcohol Abuse and Alcoholism. *My baby strong and healthy.* Washington, D.C.: GPO, 1986.

13. U.S. Department of Health and Human Services, Public Health Service/Health Resources and Services Administration. Bureau of Health Care Delivery and Assistance. Division of Maternal Health. *Prenatal and Postnatal Care.* DHHS Publication No. (HRSA) 83-5070. Rockville: 1983.

14. Lecos, C.W. Caffeine jitters: Some safety questions remain. *FDA Consumer* 21, no. 10 (December 1987–January 1988):22–7.

15. Scientific Status Summary. Evaluation of caffeine safety. *Food Technology* 41 (1987):105–13.

16. Rozin, P. The selection of foods by rats, humans, and other animals. In *Advances in the study of behavior,* edited by S.S. Rosenblatt, et al. New York: Academic Press, 1976.

17. Zamula, E. The curious compulsion called pica. *FDA Consumer* 19, no. 10 (December 1985–January 1986):29–32.
18. Medical news. Gestational diabetes: Panelists set guidelines for detection, control. *Journal of the American Medical Association* 254, no. 4 (1985):465–70.
19. Committee on Nutrition, American Academy of Pediatrics. *Pediatric nutrition handbook*. Elk Grove Village: American Academy of Pediatrics, 1985.
20. Position of the American Dietetic Association. Nutrition management of adolescent pregnancy. *Journal of the American Dietetic Association* 89 (1989):104.
21. Story, M., and I. Alton. Nutrition issues and adolescent pregnancy. *Contemporary Nutrition* Volume 12, Number 1, (1987). Minneapolis: General Mills, Inc.
22. Weigley, E.S. Nutrition and the older primigravida. *Journal of the American Dietetic Association* 82 (1983):529–30.
23. Hendershot, G.E. Trends in breast-feeding. *Pediatrics Supplement* 74, no. 4 (1984):591–602.
24. Reiff, M.I., and S.M. Essock-Vitale. Hospital influences in early infant-feeding practices. *Pediatrics* 76 (1985):872–79.
25. U.S. Department of Health and Human Services, Bureau of Health Care Delivery and Assistance, Division of Maternal and Child Health. *Report of the Surgeon General's workshop on breast-feeding and human lactation*. DHHS: 1984.
26. Rush, D., Principal Investigator. The national WIC evaluation: Evaluation of the Special Supplemental Food Program for Women, Infants and Children. *American Journal of Clinical Nutrition Supplement* 48, no. 2 (1988): entire issue.
27. Nutrition management of adolescent pregnancy. Technical support paper. *Journal of the American Dietetic Association* 89 (1989):105–9.

CHAPTER
4

NUTRITION DURING INFANCY, CHILDHOOD, AND ADOLESCENCE

Objectives

After studying this chapter, you will be able to

- explain the differences among human milk, commercial infant formula, and cow's milk.
- identify the physiological changes of infancy related to the introduction of solid foods.
- describe the usual pattern for the introduction of solid foods.
- recognize those foods most likely to cause choking in the young child.
- describe possible solutions to typical childhood feeding problems.
- discuss the changes during adolescence that have an impact on nutritional status.
- identify nursing interventions related to dietary management during infancy, childhood, and adolescence.

Overview

Infancy, childhood, and adolescence are marked by periods of growth that strongly influence energy and nutrient needs. During infancy, tremendous growth occurs. On a body-weight basis, nutritional needs are higher in infancy than at any other time during life. In fact, if weight continued to increase at the same rate after infancy as it does during the first year of life, by five years of age, the child would weigh approximately 1800 pounds!

Childhood is marked by steady growth, although not at the rapid rate observed during infancy. The changes in needs are often reflected by variations in the child's appetite. Adolescence is characterized by the rapid increase in energy and nutrient needs associated with puberty. During each stage of life, from infancy to adolescence, intake is influenced not only by physiological needs but also by culture, family dietary and activity patterns, and peer pressure.

POSSIBLE NURSING DIAGNOSES

Growth and development—
  normal, related to
  - adequate parental knowledge of good nutrition and appropriate food choices for infant, child, and/or adolescent.
  - ability of infant to consume necessary nutrients.
  altered, related to
  - inadequate parental knowledge of principles of good nutrition.
  - poor nutritional intake due to lack of financial or other resources to provide adequate nutrition.

Knowledge deficit related to
  - understanding of the relationship between good nutrition and normal infant, child, or adolescent development.
  - use of community resources that may be available to supplement nutritional needs.
  - methods of food preparation.
  - availability of community resources to supplement nutritional needs.
Noncompliance related to
  - lack of understanding of the role of adequate nutrition to normal developmental patterns.
  - lack of resources (financial and transportational, etc.).

INFANCY

The goal for feeding during infancy is to provide kilocalories and nutrients that will contribute to a healthy childhood, aid in optimal physical and mental development, and establish patterns of food consumption that prevent future health problems (1). During the first year of life, the infant progresses through three overlapping stages of feeding: the nursing period, during which human milk or a commercial formula (along with necessary supplements) is the source of nutrients; the transitional period, characterized by the addition of solid foods to the diet of breast milk or formula; and the modified adult period, when the majority of foods come from the table (2). Progress through the three feeding periods is dependent on physiological changes in the infant.

The Nursing Period

The nursing period usually lasts for at least the first four to six months of life. During this time, breast milk or formula best suits the infant's capabilities and needs. The normal infant is physiologically equipped for breast or bottle feeding at birth. Strong rooting, sucking, and swallowing reflexes; the presence of fat pads in the cheeks; and the large size of the tongue compared with the lower jaw are examples of the neuromotor and physical characteristics that make breast- or bottle-feeding possible (3). The infant's gastrointestinal tract and kidneys are not mature enough to handle other types of foods at this time.

Human milk continues to be the feeding of choice for infants during the nursing period. Mothers who are not able to breast-feed because of medical problems or who choose not to breast-feed can find an adequate replacement in commercial infant formula. The task of mimicking human milk is formidable, however, and distinct differences exist between human milk and commercial infant formula.

Human Milk. There are three types of "milk" secreted during lactation: colostrum, transitional milk, and mature human milk. Colostrum is a yellowish, transparent fluid released during the first few days after birth. Human colostrum is higher in protein than mature human milk but lower in fat, carbohydrate, and kilocalories (3). It is valued for its content of antibodies and anti-infective factors that protect the infant against enteric infections. Transitional milk appears between the third and sixth day. The protein content of transitional milk is greater than that of mature human milk. Transitional milk changes to mature milk by about the 10th day of lactation. Besides the nutrient differences in kilocalorie content, the antibody content of mature human milk is less than in earlier milks (4).

The nutrient content of human milk is extremely variable. Composition varies from woman to woman, throughout lactation, and even from the beginning (foremilk) to the end (hindmilk) of each feed. Significant differences have been observed in the macronutrient (fat, protein, kilocalorie) content of the milk of different mothers. Additionally, the fat and kilocalorie content of milk increases and the nitrogen content decreases significantly in women as lactation progresses (5). In Table 4-1, the changes

Table 4-1. ENERGY AND MACRONUTRIENTS IN BREAST MILK DURING THE FIRST MONTH OF LACTATION

NUTRIENTS	DAYS OF LACTATION			
	3–5	8–11	15–18	26–28
Energy (kcal/dl)	48 ± 3	59 ± 2	62 ± 2*	62 ± 1
Lipid (g/dl)	1.85 ± .35	2.9 ± .23	3.06 ± .21	3.05 ± .07*
Protein (g/dl)	1.87 ± .05*	1.7 ± .06*	1.5 ± .05*	1.29 ± .04*
Lactose (g/dl)	5.14 ± .22	5.98 ± .23	6 ± .2*	6.51 ± .23

Source: G.H. Anderson, S.A. Atkinson, and M.H. Bryan, "Energy and Macronutrient Content of Human Milk During Early Lactation from Mothers Giving Birth Prematurely and at Term." *American Journal of Clinical Nutrition* 34 (1981):258–65.

*Values derived from graphs

in the macronutrient content of milk during lactation are shown.

Micronutrients are also affected. Vitamin-A, vitamin-E, and zinc concentrations in human milk decrease throughout lactation, and thiamine concentration increases (6). Also, hindmilk is higher in fat content than foremilk (7). It has therefore been quite difficult to exactly characterize human milk, and averages for nutrients (Table 4-2) have been described based on pooled samples.

Breast milk contains macronutrients in forms that are easily used by the newborn. The protein in breast milk is in the form of lactalbumin, which forms an easily digested curd in the infant's stomach. The protein in human milk supports growth without contributing an excessive renal solute load for the infant's immature kidneys. The amino acid content of the protein complements the enzyme systems of the infant. The primary carbohydrate in breast milk is lactose. Lactose provides a medium for the growth of the bacteria, lactobacillus, in the intestinal tract of the infant. Lactobacillus microorganisms produce an acidic environment in the gastrointestinal tract, thus interfering with the growth of pathogenic organisms. The fat of breast milk is easily digested because of the presence of lingual lipase in the infant and bile salts-stimulated lipase in human milk. The fatty-acid profile of human milk is responsive to maternal intakes. Unsaturated fatty acids, particularly linoleic acid, are affected. Linoleic acid is an essential fatty acid for growth (8).

A breast-fed infant is fed on demand, and during the first three months, normally averages an intake of 600–700 ml breast milk daily (9). The infant is considered adequately nourished if given at least six feedings daily during the first weeks of life (2). The number of wet diapers (at least six), number of stools, and weight gain are variables monitored to assure that breast-fed babies are doing well (2). According to the National Center for Health Statistics Standards, infants usually double their birth weight at about 4 months and triple their birth weight at approximately 12 months of age (10).

Nutrient supplementation for the breast-fed infant often includes vitamin K, vitamin D, fluoride, and iron (11–13). Vitamin K is given as a single, intramuscular dose of 0.5–1.0 mg or as an oral dose of 1–2 mg in newborns as prophylaxis against hemorrhagic disease (2). Administration of vitamin K to newborns is mandated in some states. The vitamin D content of human milk is very low, and if breast-fed infants are not exposed to sunlight, rickets can occur. Fluoride supplementation in the breast-fed infant is controversial. The Committee on Nutrition of the American Academy of Pediatrics recommends that a fluoride supplement be initiated shortly after birth in the breast-fed infant but acknowledges that it can be delayed until six months of age (2). Even though the iron content of human milk is low, it is very well absorbed. Neonatal iron stores formed before birth usually last for the first three months of infancy. Another source of iron is required in addition to that in breast milk by four to six months of age and can be obtained from an iron-fortified infant cereal.

Commercial Infant Formulas. If an infant is not breast-fed or if breast-feeding is stopped early, a commercially prepared infant formula is an acceptable alternative. Standards for the nutrient composition of commercial infant formulas were established by the Infant Formula Act of 1980 and are based on recommendations of the Committee on Nutrition, American Academy of Pediatrics. In 1985, the FDA published nutrient specifications for infant formulas (see Table 4-2). These standards provide commercial infant formula manufacturers with guidelines for formulas that reflect the nutrient composition of breast milk and meet infant needs as reflected by the RDA (see Appendices A, B, and C for the RDA for infancy).

Many different commercial infant formulas exist. The most timely information on the nutrient composition of specific brands of infant formulas is available in the Physician's Desk Reference (PDR) for the current year. Basically, infant formulas can be divided into three categories: cow-milk-based, soy-based, and specialized formulas (14). Cow-milk-based formulas are most often used for normal, healthy, full-term infants. In Table 4-3, the protein, fat, and carbohydrate sources for three major cow-milk-based formulas are listed.

Table 4-2. NUTRIENT CONTENT OF MATURE HUMAN MILK, INFANT FORMULA, AND COW'S MILK

NUTRIENT	MATURE HUMAN MILK[1]	FORMULA[2]	COW'S MILK[3]
		Per 100 Kcals Minimum/Maximum	
Fat (g)	5.4	3.3/6.0	5.7
Protein (g)	1.4	1.8/4.5	5.1
Carbohydrate (g)	10.0	None specified	7.2
Linoleic Acid (g)	.5	.3	.1
Fat-Soluble Vitamins			
Vitamin A (IU)	310	250/750	215
Vitamin D (IU)	3.0	40/100	63.9*
Vitamin E (mg)	.32	.7	—**
Vitamin K (mcg)	.29	4	—**
Water-Soluble Vitamins			
Ascorbic acid (mg)	5.6	8	2.3
Biotin (mcg)	.56	1.5	—**
Folic acid (mcg)	7.0	4	7.6
Niacin (mcg)	208	250	130
Pantothenic acid (mcg)	250	300	487
Pyridoxine (mcg)	28.5	35	65
Riboflavin (mcg)	48.6	60	250
Thiamin (mcg)	29.2	40	59.2
Vitamin B_{12} (mcg)	.07	.15	.55
Minerals			
Calcium (mg)	39	60	185
Chloride (mg)	58	55/150	—**
Copper (mg)	.03	.06	.06***
Fluoride (mcg)	2.2	None Specified	—**
Iodine (mcg)	15.3	5/75	84****
Iron (mg)	.04	.15/3.0	.08
Magnesium (mg)	4.9	6	21

Continued

Table 4-2. NUTRIENT CONTENT OF MATURE HUMAN MILK, INFANT FORMULA, AND COW'S MILK (continued)

NUTRIENT	MATURE HUMAN MILK[1]	FORMULA[2]	COW'S MILK[3]
	Per 100 Kcals Minimum/Maximum		
Manganese (mcg)	0.8	5	—**
Phosphorus (mg)	19.5	30	144
Potassium (mg)	73	80/200	234
Selenium (mcg)	2.8	None Specified	—**
Sodium (mg)	25	20/60	76
Zinc (mg)	.17	.5	.6
Other Nutrients			
Choline (mg)	12.5	7	—**

Sources:

[1]Committee on Nutrition, American Academy of Pediatrics. *Pediatric Nutrition Handbook,* 2nd ed. (Elk Grove Village: American Academy of Pediatrics, 1985).

[2]Food and Drug Administration. "Rules and Regulations. Infant Formula. Labeling Requirements." *Federal Register* 50 (1985):1833–41.

[3]USDA Handbook 8

*fortified

**not listed

***See J.T. Pennington and D.H. Calloway, "Copper Content of Foods," *Journal of the American Dietetic Association* 63 (1973):143–53.

****See F. Taylor, "Iodine: Going from Hypo to Hyper," *FDA Consumer,* April 1981.

Soy-protein formulas differ in their protein and carbohydrate sources. Soy-protein isolate is the protein source, corn syrup and/or sucrose provide the carbohydrate, and a blend of oils similar to the cow-milk-based formulas provides the fat. The American Academy of Pediatrics released specific recommendations for the use of soy-protein formulas. Use of soy-protein formulas is indicated (1) when animal protein is not desired because of religious or family beliefs; (2) in the management of galactosemia and lactase deficiency; and (3) in infants with a family history of allergies who have *not yet* shown clinical signs of allergy. Soy-protein formulas should not be used for (1) feeding premature or LBW infants; (2) in the dietary management of documented allergy to cow's milk or soy protein; or (3) in the routine management of colic (15).

Soy-protein formulas are contraindicated in the feeding of premature or LBW infants because studies have shown that the calcium content of soy-protein formulas (and standard formulas) cannot

Table 4-3. SOURCES OF MACRONUTRIENTS IN COMMERCIAL INFANT FORMULAS

MACRONUTRIENT	SIMILAC[1]	ENFAMIL[2]	SMA[3]
Protein	Nonfat cow milk	Reduced mineral whey and nonfat cow milk	Nonfat cow milk, demineralized whey
Fat	soy, coconut oils	coconut, soy oil	oleo, coconut, oleic, soy oils
Carbohydrate	lactose	lactose	lactose

Sources:

[1]Ross Laboratories, Columbus, Ohio

[2]Mead Johnson Laboratories, Indianapolis, Indiana

[3]Wyeth Laboratories, Philadelphia, Pennsylvania

meet the needs of the rapidly growing infant with a very low LBW. This is cited as a major cause of osteoporosis in these sick infants. In addition, hypophosphatemia associated with prolonged use of soy-protein formulas for infants with very low LBW accelerates the development of hypophosphatemic rickets.

After infants show clinical signs of allergy to cow's milk, they have an increased intestinal permeability and show an immunological response to other proteins. They may, therefore, show an allergic reaction to soy protein, which can be severe. It is, therefore, recommended that infants with documented allergy to cow's milk be placed on a less antigenic formula such as Nutramigen, a lactose-free formula containing hydrolyzed casein as the protein source, corn syrup solids and modified corn starch as the carbohydrate source, and corn oil as the fat source.

While the causes of colic are not known, some studies suggest that cow's milk may be a precipitating factor. Use of casein-hydrolysate formulas rather than soy-protein formulas relieved symptoms in these studies. Thus, the soy-protein formulas are believed to have limited value in colicky infants.

Specialized infant formulas have been developed to meet the needs of infants with disorders in digestion, absorption, and metabolism. The car-

bohydrate, protein, and fat sources vary, depending on the particular problem under treatment. Examples include Pregestimil and Portagen. Pregestimil is lactose free and contains hydrolyzed casein as the protein source, corn syrup solids and modified tapioca starch as the carbohydrate source, and a mixture of corn oil and medium-chain triglycerides as the fat source. Portagen, which is also lactose free, contains sodium caseinate as the primary protein source, corn syrup and sucrose as the carbohydrate source, and medium-chain triglycerides as the fat source.

Commercial infant formulas are available in three forms in the marketplace. These are the ready-to-feed form requiring no preparation (most expensive), concentrates prepared by mixing equal part of formula and water, and powder made by mixing two ounces of water with each level tablespoon of powder. Health professionals should be aware of price differences among forms of formula, and some thought should be given about the cost of the recommended formula in relation to available funds.

How much formula does a healthy infant need? The quantity depends on variables such as age, weight, and rate of growth. The amount of formula required can be calculated using the RDA for kilocalories for infants (see Appendix A). Infants from birth to 0.5 years require an average of 115 kcal per kilogram body weight. For infants who are 0.5–1 year of age, an average of 105 kcal per kilogram is required. Most commercial infant formulas contain 20 kcal per ounce when prepared according to directions. Therefore, a one-month-old healthy infant weighing 4 kg (8.8 lb) would require approximately 460 kcal daily (115 kcal/kg × 4 kg). The amount of formula needed to meet this calorie need would be about 23 oz (460 kcal ÷ 20 kcal/oz).

It is important to remember that the volume of milk required will vary from infant to infant. Surveys of healthy infants in the United States indicate that an average intake is about 3 oz of formula per pound in the first weeks of life to 1⅓ oz per pound in the later months of infancy. When infants receive formula beyond six months of life, the volume should be limited to about 30 oz daily to encourage the consumption of semisolid (pureed) foods and thus insure an adequate nutrient intake (16).

Formula is often heated prior to feeding, and it must be stressed to new parents to check the temperature by testing a couple drops of the heated formula on the wrist or forearm before giving it to their infants. The formula should feel warm, not hot. Burns caused by formula that is too hot are tragic and easily avoided. Using the microwave oven to heat formula is not recommended due to uneven heating causing "hot spots" in the formula. Also, since the external container does not absorb heat, it may feel cool to the touch; however, the liquid inside can be extremely hot.

Other than vitamin K given soon after birth, infants consuming adequate amounts of iron-fortified commercial formula do not need vitamin and mineral supplementation during the first six months of life (2). Although a commonly held belief is that iron-fortified formulas cause constipation and gastrointestinal distress, carefully controlled research does not support this belief (17). Supplements are not required during the second six months if the formula is continued in combination with solid foods. If the formula is not iron fortified, a source of iron in the diet is required by the time the infant is four to six months of age.

The iron needs are satisfied by the addition of iron-fortified infant cereal to the diet.

Cow's Milk. The nutrient profile of cow's milk is significantly different from breast milk and formula. Unlike breast milk and formula, cow's milk is low in linoleic acid and high in saturated fatty acids (18). The protein in whole cow's milk is more difficult to digest than that in breast milk, and the sodium content is much higher than breast milk or formula, contributing to an excessive renal solute load. Whole cow's milk is also a poor iron source. (See Table 4-2).

Controversy exists concerning the appropriate age at which whole cow's milk can be safely introduced. In young infants, whole cow's milk causes occult bleeding in the gastrointestinal tract. Also, due to its low concentration of iron, whole cow's milk feeding in young infants has been associated with iron deficiency anemia. The consequences of whole cow's milk in the diet of older infants (beyond six months of age) are not completely clear. Research indicates no compromise of iron status in infants after 140 days of age when iron and vitamin-C supplements were given in addition to the milk (19). On the other hand, studies conducted on the nutrient content of infant diets containing whole cow's milk versus formula during the second six months of life indicated that infants consuming milk receive greater amounts of solid foods; more table versus baby food; higher protein, sodium, chloride, and potassium; and less iron and linoleic acid than infants fed iron-fortified commercial formula. Additionally, the nutrient profile for infants consuming an iron-fortified formula attained an intake of nutrients during the second six months more closely aligned with the RDA (18, 20). The implications of the effects of these different dietary profiles are unknown.

Currently, the American Academy of Pediatrics' viewpoint is that no convincing evidence exists that feeding whole cow's milk after six months of age is harmful, if adequate supplementary feedings are given (21). The Academy's recommendations are (1) if breast-feeding or bottle-feeding has been discontinued and infants are consuming one-third of their kilocalories as supplemental foods, whole cow's milk may be introduced; (2) whole cow's milk intake should be limited to one liter daily; and (3) if a significant portion of kilocalories are not coming from supplemental foods (i.e., less than one-third of daily kilocalories), iron-fortified infant formula should be given. Reduced-fat-content milk, such as skim or 2% milk, is not recommended during infancy. Skim milk contains less kilocalories than whole milk and lacks the essential fatty acid, linoleic acid. Infants receiving skim milk during this period exhibited a decrease in their skinfold thickness, suggesting depletion of fat stores. Additionally, weight gain occurs at a slower rate than in infants fed formula or whole cow's milk.

The Transitional Period

The transitional period is marked by the introduction of solid foods to the infant. The solid foods do not replace but are given in addition to breast milk or formula. Physically, the infant is able to handle foods other than liquids when the extrusion reflex (tongue thrust) of early infancy disappears, usually around four to five months of age. Also, the infant should have good control of head and neck movements and the ability to sit upright with support. Once in better control, infants can indicate desire or disinterest in food and swallow properly.

The American Academy of Pediatrics suggests a time frame of four to six months for the introduction of solid foods, and notes no nutritional advantage to earlier introduction (2). Despite the Academy's recommendation, baby food is often introduced too early. Findings indicate that most infants in the United States are fed some baby foods by two months of age (22). Reasons given for early introduction of solids included competition among mothers, advice of family members, and desire for the baby to sleep through the night.

The feeding of solid foods is considered a milestone, and sometimes parents feel pressured to show that their infants are progressing well or are advanced. Usually, when infants are spoon-fed before the loss of the extrusion reflex, more food is wasted than eaten, because the infant's tongue reflexively juts out and pushes the food out of the mouth and onto the spoon, face, high chair, or floor. Recommendations for infant feeding have changed significantly over the years, making some feeding practices followed by older family members in the past obsolete. Contrary to popular opinion, controlled studies of infant sleeping patterns show that early feeding of solids does not influence infant sleep patterns. Sleeping during the night is related to the infant's neurological development (23).

Introduction of solid foods before four months has been suggested as a possible cause of allergies (24). The infant's digestive tract is quite permeable early in infancy. Substances normally of low antigenicity may cross the gastrointestinal barrier and cause allergic reactions.

The experience of eating solid foods is a new one for the infant. Consider that infants are familiar with only one food—breast milk or formula—and only one consistency—liquid. The feel of the spoon in the mouth is a new sensation, and the tastes are very different. What tastes do infants experience, and which do they prefer?

Infants begin to taste even before birth (25). The day-old infant responds positively to sweet substances, can differentiate among sugars, and can even detect differences in the concentration of individual sugars (25). All evidence points to an innate sweet tooth (26). In contrast, while newborns can detect the salt taste, they are indifferent to or reject salt solutions. The preference for salty tastes does not appear until approximately four to six months of age and coincides with a more mature kidney (25).

Introducing Solid Foods. Variations exist for the sequence in which new foods are introduced to the infant. An iron-fortified infant rice cereal mixed with breast milk or formula is the most common first semisolid food for an infant in the United States. Rice is chosen first due to its low allergenicity. The iron fortification is considered necessary for infants fed human milk or nonfortified formula, because of the depletion of iron stores by this age. First feedings of cereal are small, only one to two teaspoons, and the consistency should be thin. Once the infant is familiar with spoon-feeding, larger amounts of thicker consistency are appropriate.

After rice cereal, other single-grain infant cereals can be introduced, followed by the introduction of single-ingredient pureed fruits, vegetables, and meats. The order of introduction is not critical; however, it is important that only single-ingredient foods be offered first, and only one new food introduced each week so that any food sensitivities can be detected easily (2). Juices should be introduced when the infant can drink from a cup.

New parents often have questions about how much to feed an infant and need to be reassured that their infants know best. Infants appear to be quite sensitive to their caloric needs (27). Parents ought to be aware of signs of satiety to avoid overfeeding. Satiety signals in the infant include showing sustained interest in surroundings versus food; pushing the food away; turning the head away; pursing the lips; and shaking the head "no."

Parents have a choice about the type of pureed food they choose for their infants. Homemade baby food, commercial baby food, or a combination of both are options. About 10% of parents make their own baby food. Making baby food is easy, but it does require some planning. Basic principles of food preparation should be followed to assure a nutritious, wholesome product. High-quality foods should be chosen. Fresh plain meats or poultry and fresh, frozen, or canned fruits and vegetables *without* added sweeteners or salt are appropriate. Clean hands and utensils are essential, since the infant's defenses against infection are not yet mature. Foods should be prepared by methods that allow maximum nutrient retention. Ripe bananas can be pureed and served without cooking. For other fruits and vegetables, steam cookery is an excellent way to preserve vitamins. Roasting is an acceptable method for cooking meats. Scrupulous cleanliness in all aspects of home food preparation cannot be overemphasized.

Once cooked, foods can be pureed, using a baby-food grinder or food processor. The foods can be served immediately, refrigerated for use in one

to two days, or frozen in ice cube trays and then packaged for later meals. The short refrigeration time is due to the large surface area of pureed foods, allowing easier attack by microorganisms.

Salt should not be added to homemade baby food. The natural sodium content of the food is enough to meet infant needs. The impact of high sodium intakes during infancy is not clear. One sweetener in particular (honey) should not be used in foods for infants less than one year old. Many samples of honey on the market contain C. botulinum spores. While spores pose no threat to children over one year of age and adults, the infant's immature gastrointestinal tract and immune system allow the spores to cultivate in the intestine. The spores produce toxins that can cause weakness, paralysis, and death. This condition is known as infant botulism.

Certain home-prepared vegetables are not appropriate for infants under four months of age because they may contain a high level of nitrates. When nitrate concentration is high, ingestion of the vegetable can cause methemoglobinemia. In methemoglobinemia, hemoglobin iron is oxidized from the ferrous to the ferric state. The blood is a chocolate brown color and useless as an oxygen carrier. Vegetables that may contain high nitrate levels are spinach, beets, turnips, carrots, and collard greens (2). It should be noted that only very young infants have been affected by this condition. Feeding these vegetables after the infant is at least four months of age is not associated with the problem, making the case for delaying introduction of solid foods even stronger. Also, the commercially prepared versions of the above-mentioned vegetables have not been associated with methemoglobinemia because of the methods followed in commercial processing. Such processing involves blanching and pureeing the vegetables in fresh water, thereby reducing the nitrate content.

A wide variety of commercial infant foods is available. In order to make the most appropriate choices for their infants, parents need to know how to read a baby food label. (See Figure 4-1).

In 1977, the addition of salt to commercial strained (pureed) baby food was discontinued by baby food

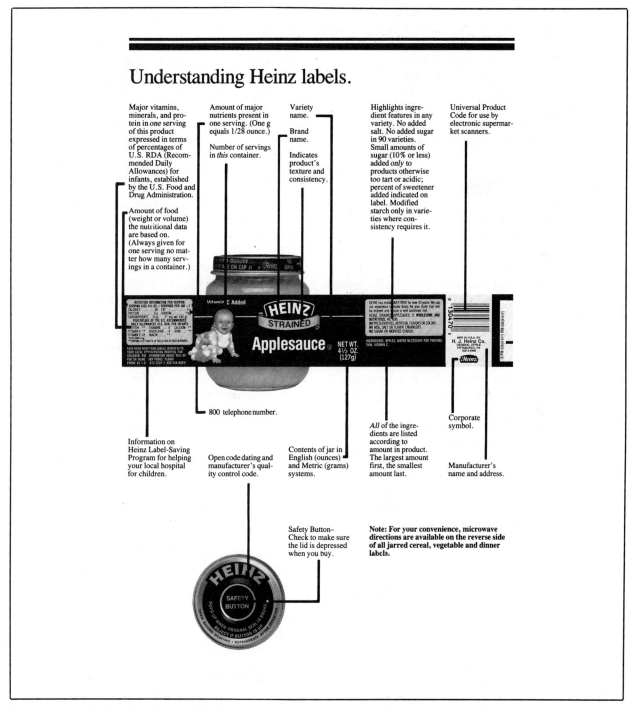

Figure 4-1. Analysis of a baby-food label.
(© Heinz USA, Division of the H.J. Heinz Company. Reprinted with permission.)

manufacturers (10). Sugar and corn syrup are added to some products; therefore, label reading is of utmost importance if parents want to limit their infants' intake of these carbohydrates. Modified food starch is a cross-linked, stabilized starch used in some varieties of baby food. Considered a safe ingredient suitable for use in infant foods, modified food starch maintains the uniformity in the texture of baby food as it travels through distribution channels (28). It also allows for uniform distribution of nutrients in baby food (29). No preservatives or artificial colors are added to any commercial baby foods.

Some commercial baby foods are fortified with nutrients. For example, most fruits and fruit juices are fortified with vitamin C. Iron is added to infant cereals and cereals with fruit. The ingredient list and the nutrient declarations on the label will indicate whether the food has been fortified with any nutrients.

Parents who choose to use commercial baby food should be aware of the following:

- A distinctive popping sound should occur when the jar is first opened. This is evidence that the seal was tight and intact, a sign of commercial sterility.
- Unless the infant can eat the entire jar, baby food should be spooned into a heating dish and the remainder recapped and refrigerated immediately. When the infant is fed directly from the jar, the saliva from the spoon mixes with the food. Enzymes in saliva will digest the food, making it watery and unappetizing.
- Once opened, jars of baby food should be refrigerated and used within two to three days to prevent microbiological contamination.
- If food has been heated, check the temperature of the food before feeding it to the infant. The food should be warm, not hot.
- Certain baby food should *never* be heated in a microwave oven. Strained meats and high-meat dinners heat unevenly and can explode.

At about six to eight months of age, rudimentary chewing movements begin, and the infant is ready for food with more texture. Soft, fork-mashed fruits and vegetables are often added to the infant's diet. It is believed to be critical to offer foods with more texture during this sensitive learning period to stimulate chewing. Infants may also start to finger-feed at this time. Popular finger foods are melba toast, rusks, and bread crusts. By about 9–12 months, the infant can handle finely cut-up fruits, vegetables, and meats from the table.

The Modified Adult Period

The onset of the modified adult period is less defined than the earlier periods, but it usually begins after one year of age (2). During this time, the infant obtains the majority of nutrients from table foods. Unfortunately, many of the table foods fed to infants are high in sodium, and the infant's sodium intake increases appreciably (30). Caretakers of infants should select foods lower in sodium and use a minimum, if any, salt in cooking food intended for the infant. Label reading is a must.

The table foods offered should be cut into small, easy-to-handle pieces so that the infant can self-feed and to minimize the hazards of choking. Specific types of foods have been implicated as choking hazards. Typical problem-food characteristics are (31):

- small, thin, and smooth or slick when wet
- hard, tough, and resistant to mastication
- round, cylindrical, and pliable
- highly viscous

Foods associated with childhood asphyxiation are hot dogs, round candies, peanuts and other nuts, grapes, raw carrots, popcorn, peanut butter, beans, berries, and chewing gum. In addition to the types of foods, environmental factors such as distractions during eating or poor parental supervision play a role in childhood choking.

Feeding during infancy and childhood should take place only while the child is seated and supervised. The child's balance and coordination are not advanced enough to allow eating while walking, and infants and young children do not yet have experience to determine the amount of food they can comfortably hold in their mouths.

Common Concerns and Problems During Infancy

Food Sensitivities. Food sensitivities are more common during infancy than at other life stages because the gastrointestinal tract is permeable to macromolecules and production of IgA (immunoglobulin gamma A) antibody is low prior to seven months of age (32). Approximately 4%–6% of infants experience true food allergies (33). The most common allergy during infancy is to cow's milk. Other problem foods include eggs (particularly egg whites), soy protein, nuts, fish, meats, chocolate, tomatoes, citrus fruits, and strawberries (34). Management of food allergy requires a detailed dietary history, elimination of the problem foods from the diet, and subsequent reintroduction of each food. Most of the time, the sensitivity to the food is transient, and the food can be reintroduced at a later age. Families with a history of allergies are encouraged to breast-feed, avoid foods that commonly cause problems, and introduce new foods slowly.

Diarrhea. Diarrhea in infancy may be acute or chronic and caused by specific foods or infections. Prevention of dehydration or rehydration can be accomplished with special oral hydration solutions administered under the supervision of the physician. In infants with acute diarrhea, it is recommended that the reintroduction of feeding not be delayed more than 24 hours (2). Breast milk can be reintroduced as such. Formula or milk feeding initially requires dilution. If an infant is on solid foods, suggestions for reintroduction to food include rice cereal, bananas, potatoes, and other lactose-free carbohydrate-rich foods (2). In chronic diarrhea, temporary or permanent (as in the case of celiac disease), removal of the offending food results in symptom improvement.

Obesity. The relationship between infant and adult obesity has challenged investigators for years. Although there is a risk that obese infants can grow into obese adults, most obese infants do not become obese adults and most adult obesity cannot be explained by obesity in infancy (35). There does seem to be an increased risk of obesity in adulthood, however, when obesity is present in late childhood and adolescence. Therefore, if an infant is in the high weight range and continues such a pattern into late childhood, then the risk for adult obesity is greatly increased (see Appendix D for growth charts).

Factors associated with obesity in infancy are not entirely clear. Heredity is considered an important determinant. When both parents are obese, the child has an 80% chance of becoming obese. When one parent is obese, the risk for the child is 40%. Feeding practices in infancy have not been good predictors of obesity. Neither early introduction of solids nor the use of formula instead of breast milk during infancy has been related to the prevalence of obesity in childhood (36).

Inordinate concern with obesity may cause some parents to restrict food intake of their infants with resultant problems in growth. Caloric restriction is contraindicated in infancy, and it is more important for parents to become aware of satiety cues of their infants to avoid overfeeding.

Nursing-Bottle Syndrome. Putting the infant to bed with a bottle filled with milk, juice, or sweetened water causes severe tooth decay once teeth erupt. Called nursing-bottle syndrome, it usually occurs in one- to four-year-olds; however, the pattern of feeding is often established during the first year. The carbohydrate (lactose in milk, natural sugar in fruit juice, and sugar added to water) comes into contact with the teeth and is not washed away or neutralized due to the reduced saliva production during sleep. The carbohydrate is a substrate for bacteria that produce an acid that destroys tooth enamel. The upper incisors are the most severely affected. Lower teeth are protected because the tongue covers them. Decay in the primary teeth can adversely affect dietary intake and the resultant pain can disrupt sleeping patterns. Premature loss of the primary teeth due to tooth decay can affect speech development and cause faulty alignment of the permanent teeth (34).

Nursing-bottle syndrome is easily prevented if plain water only (if anything) is given in a bottle at bedtime; pacifiers are not dipped in sugar or other sweeteners; and juices are served when the infant can drink from a cup (9–12 months).

Dietary Modifications. Due to the increased evidence that clearly links dietary patterns with disorders such as cardiovascular disease, recommendations have been issued for the adult population. Limiting fat and cholesterol intake has been advanced as a preventive measure to reduce the risk of heart disease. Reducing the cholesterol and fat content of the infant's diet is not appropriate and can have negative effects on growth and development. In addition, strong evidence is lacking that links feeding practices during infancy with subsequent serum lipid levels (37). Therefore, dietary modification is not recommended until after the age of two in children who show elevated cholesterol levels (37).

Colic. Colic is defined as excessive and uncontrollable crying of unknown origin in normal infants less than three months of age (38). Some evidence suggests that colic is caused by cow's milk protein. The protein can be passed to the infant via formula or passed from the mother to the infant in breast milk (39). Other causes that have not been substantiated are disturbed maternal-child relations, maternal anxiety, hypertonicity of babies, and trapped intestinal gas (40).

No cure exists for colic. Remedies such as medications, car rides, massaging the infant's abdomen, altering the diet to avoid cow's milk, and warm baths have been suggested; however, not all seem effective in all infants. Colic ends at about three to four months of age.

Special Care Situations

Low-Birth-Weight Infants. The nutritional needs of premature infants is an intense area of study, and providing adequate nutrition to LBW (less than 2500 g) and very low LBW (less than 1500 g) infants is an immense challenge. The American Academy of Pediatrics has stated that although the goal of nutrition for these infants is not known with certainty, a logical approach is to work to achieve postnatal growth that approximates growth in utero of the normal fetus at the same postconception age (2). Premature infants require increased kilocalories and amounts of certain nutrients (zinc, iron) due to lack of fat and nutrient storage that normally occurs during the last trimester of pregnancy (41). Four feeding approaches are currently used for providing nutrient needs: (1) human milk, (2) special commercial formulas, (3) enteral feeding, and (4) parenteral feeding.

Preterm infants fare better when fed preterm milk rather than pooled human milk from mothers of term infants. Milk from mothers of preterm infants contains more kilocalories, higher concentrations of fat, protein, and sodium, but lower concentrations of lactose, calcium, and phosphorus than milk from mothers of term infants (2, 42). Although it is not the perfect food, of present choices, preterm milk is considered the best due to its antiinfective properties and easier digestibility (43).

Special commercial formulas have been designed to meet the needs of preterm infants. Common features of the formulas include the use of whey as the major source of protein, carbohydrate mixtures of lactose and glucose polymers, and fat sources containing medium-chain triglycerides and unsaturated long-chain triglycerides (2). Examples of these formulas include Enfamil (Mead Johnson), SMA "Premie" (Wyeth), and Similac Special Care (Ross Laboratories).

Infants who cannot suck are given enteral feeding or parenteral feeds. Enteral feeding involves the use of the gastrointestinal tract. Bolus feedings into the stomach by gavage tube or nipple every two to three hours is the goal of feeding (2). Finally, parenteral nutrition, in which the gastrointestinal tract is completely bypassed and nutrients are infused directly into the bloodstream, has become a common practice, particularly in infants weighing less than 1000 g at birth (41). Positive results have been reported for total parenteral nutrition as well as for a combination of enteral and parenteral nutrition. Investigations on the nutritional requirements of this vulnerable population will no doubt continue, given the numbers of infants being kept alive by medical advances.

CHILDHOOD

Preschool Years (Ages 1–5 Years)

During the preschool years, the infant develops more coordination and gradually assumes more responsibility for self-feeding. Although chewing is more mature, choking is still a serious concern in this age group because the grinding action of the teeth is not very effective. Physical growth is not as rapid during this period of the child's life as it was during the first year; therefore, there is a gradual decline in caloric need relative to body weight. The energy and nutrient needs (RDA) of preschool children are listed in Appendices A, B, and C. The energy and nutrient needs can be met through offering a variety of foods according to the guidelines in Table 4-4. Note that the serving sizes are small. Children in this age group are easily overwhelmed, and the smaller serving sizes are easier for them to accept and handle. Young children best meet their nutrient needs when fed three meals and two snacks daily (2).

There is little reliable data on foods preferred by this age group, although certain food characteristics are commonly thought to be accepted by young children (Table 4-5). However, there are many exceptions, especially in different cultural groups.

The most common nutrition-related problems in this age group are iron-deficiency anemia and dental caries. Iron-deficiency anemia occurs between

Table 4-4. GUIDELINES FOR DIETARY INTAKE FOR THE PRESCHOOL YEARS (AGE 1–5 YEARS)

FOOD GROUP	SERVINGS
Milk	2 ¾–1 cup is one serving. Use only whole milk under 2 years of age.
Protein	2 1–1½ ounces is one serving.
Grain	4 Serving sizes: 1 slice bread, ½–¾ cup cereal, ½ cup macaroni or rice.
Fruit/Vegetable	4 Include fruits and vegetables rich in vitamin A and C. Vitamin A sources: dark, leafy green vegetables and deep yellow-orange fruits and vegetables. Vitamin C sources: citrus fruits, strawberries, broccoli. Serving size: ½ cup.
Other: Fats/Sweets	Moderate intake according to caloric needs. These foods should not replace food from other groups.

Sources:

USDA, National School Lunch Program

E. Satter, *How to Get Your Kid to Eat . . . But Not Too Much* (Palo Alto: Bull Publishing Company, 1987).

Note: Younger children may not be able to eat a full portion and should not be forced to do so.

Table 4-5. CHARACTERISTICS OF FOOD COMMONLY ACCEPTED BY PRESCHOOLERS

CHARACTERISTIC	COMMONLY ACCEPTED
Form	Single food rather than combination dishes
Color	Bright colors, high contrast
Flavor	Mild
Texture	Tender and moist
Temperature	No extremes

six months and three years and is a result of the child's increased growth and the high intake of milk, which is a poor iron source (2). In the preschooler, greater opportunities for improved iron intake occur through the use of a variety of foods, especially from the meat group. Meats contain heme iron, which is well absorbed. Better absorption of nonheme iron, which is found in fruits, vegetables, and grains, can be achieved when meat is included in the meal or when a source of ascorbic acid is included. Sources of vitamin C include citrus fruits and juices, broccoli, green peppers, and strawberries.

The frequency and number of dental caries can be held in check by effective teeth cleaning, water fluoridation, supervision of between-meal snacks, and substitution of less cariogenic foods (2). High cariogenic foods are high in sugar and sticky in consistency (raisins, hard candies, caramels, taffy, pastries). Foods that are considered to be protective are rich in protein and fat, and include cheeses. Professional dental care should begin by the time the child is three years old. Many dentists prefer to see the child at age two or even younger.

Common Feeding Problems in the Preschool Child

Both the parents and the children have responsibilities during feeding. The parent is responsible for providing a variety of foods in a healthy physical and emotional setting. The child is responsible for what and how much is eaten (44). During the preschool years, certain problems in feeding often occur. Rejection of new foods, rejection of certain foods, small appetite, and food jags are examples of feeding problems.

Rejection of New Foods. Research has shown that experience plays a major role in a child's food-acceptance patterns (45). Children often reject novel foods, but the negative reaction can be reduced by increasing exposure to that food. Even if the child does not taste the food at first, just seeing it will decrease its novelty and therefore reduce rejection on future trials. A small portion of the food should be placed on the plate and removed if the child will not eat it. This should be repeated until the food is tasted.

Rejection of Certain Foods. Receiving a food reward should not be contingent on eating foods the child rejects. For example, when children are told to eat their vegetables and then they can have dessert, they actually decrease their liking of the target vegetable. In addition, they show an increased preference for the reward food, which is the dessert (45). Ironically, the parents hope to encourage the exact opposite behavior. If children will not eat a certain food, it is best to remove the food without a fuss, but continue to offer the food. Sometimes, the rejected food will be accepted if it is prepared in a different manner. Also, alternate foods can be substituted to ensure adequate intake when a

Table 4-6. FOOD SUBSTITUTIONS

FOOD DISLIKED	FOOD SUBSTITUTIONS
Fluid milk	Cheese, cottage cheese, cream soups, yogurt
Carrots, spinach	Apricots, cantaloupe, sweet potatoes
Cooked vegetables	Raw vegetables cut into different shapes served with a yogurt-based dip, vegetable salads
Meat	Beans, fish, poultry

child dislikes or will not eat certain foods (Table 4-6).

Lack of Appetite. If the child's snacks are not interfering with meals and, therefore, are not the source of the problem, the lack of appetite is associated with the decreased growth rate during this period. Children can regulate their food intake based on internal, physiological cues and should never be forced to "clean the plate" (45). Offering smaller portions helps the child feel less overwhelmed, and regularly scheduled snacks ensure adequate nutritional intake. If the child does not eat at mealtime, the food should be removed without a fuss; however, the child must recognize that eating is over until the scheduled snack time. Snack foods should be of high nutrient density and include such items as small sandwiches, fresh fruits, yogurt, and cheese and crackers rather than cookies, cakes, or salted snack chips. Suggestions for dealing with small appetites include the following:

- Offer a variety of food in appropriate amounts in easy-to-eat form at regular intervals.
- Allow for a well-selected snack.
- Allow some choice in food selection.
- Provide a meal environment free of distractions.
- Allow for a premeal rest.
- Set a reasonable time for eating. If food is not eaten, casually remove it.
- Allow the child to help with food preparation.

Food Jags. It is not uncommon for a preschooler to eat the same food over an extended period. This type of behavior is known as a food jag. The less focus placed on the food jag, the more quickly it will pass. Other foods should continue to be offered, so that change is more easily facilitated.

The School-Aged Child (6–10 Years)

The school-aged child faces a period of slow, steady growth accompanied by increases in energy and nutritional needs. Appendices A, B, and C include a listing of the RDAs for these ages. Maintaining adequate nutritional status for the school-aged child has a direct effect on health. Infectious diseases are readily transmitted among this age group, and a well-nourished child is more likely to have a milder degree of illness and faster recovery. During this period, feeding provides the opportunity for improved eating skills, greater food acceptance, and socialization (44). Parents have less control over intake during this period than during the preschool years because of the influence of the child's peers, television, and after-school activities. Still, parents need to establish ground rules and set limits.

A major public health problem in the United States is childhood obesity. Risk factors include heredity and dietary and exercise patterns. The influence of heredity has already been mentioned. Eating beyond physiological needs contributes to weight gain. Children who are forced to eat even when they are not hungry begin a pattern of failing to respond to internal cues. In addition, the passive activity of watching television has been associated with childhood obesity. The average child aged 6–11 years spends 25 hours per week watching television, which is a significant amount of time not devoted to more energy expending activities (46). Overweight children should not be put on a diet. Instead, an evaluation of the dietary intake can be made and substitution of more nutrient-dense snacks can replace high-sugar, high-fat foods. Weight maintenance rather than weight loss is the goal so that the child can "grow into" his or her weight. Exercise is encouraged and is most successful when done as a family recreational activity.

ADOLESCENCE

Adolescence is a time marked by a dramatic increase in growth and changes in body composition. Increased growth rates occur in girls between 10 and 12 years of age and in boys approximately 2 years later (2). In females, body fat increases during this time, and in males, lean body mass and blood volume increases. In order to support the rapid growth, higher intakes of energy and nutrients are required. In Appendices A, B, and C, the RDA for energy and nutrients for all ages, including adolescence, are listed. (See Table 4-7 for a dietary guide for adolescents.)

Despite increased needs, adolescence is a time marked by irregular dietary patterns. Adolescents tend to skip meals, especially breakfast and lunch, snack heavily, and eat many of their meals away from home (47). In addition, some adolescents are subject to high-risk nutrition conditions, such as athletics, eating disorders, alcohol and drug abuse, and pregnancy (48).

Teens involved in athletics often follow bizarre dietary regimens in the hope of improving performance. Obesity in adolescence is increasing in prevalence as are anorexia nervosa and bulimia. Anorectic and bulimic teenagers experience abnormalities in their cardiovascular, endocrine, renal, hematologic, thermoregulatory, gastrointestinal, and electrolyte systems (49). (Eating disorders are

Table 4-7. DAILY FOOD GUIDE FOR ADOLESCENTS

FOOD GROUP	SUGGESTED DAILY SERVINGS
Bread, cereals, and other grain products	6 to 11 Include whole-grain products.
Fruits	2 to 4 Include citrus fruits.
Vegetables	3 to 5 Include dark green, leafy and yellow-orange vegetables several times each week.
Meat, poultry, fish, and alternates	2 to 3 (Total 5–7 ounces lean) Eggs, dry beans and peas, nuts, and seeds are alternates.
Milk, cheese, and yogurt	3 (4 for pregnant or breast-feeding teens)
Fats, sweets	Avoid too many fats and sweets.

Source: USDA, *Home and Garden Bulletin*, No. 232-1, April 1986.

discussed in detail in Chapter 15.) Alcohol and drug abuse during this period is a significant public health problem. The effect on nutritional status is not clear. Teen pregnancy can impose significant increases in nutrient requirements (see Chapter 3).

Despite their eating habits, the nutritional status of most adolescents is satisfactory (47). In addition, although adolescents have more freedom in food selection, they continue to benefit from reasonable and supportive limits from their parents. The need for nutrition education directed to adolescents is becoming increasingly apparent. Today's teens have taken more responsibility for grocery shopping and meal preparation than in past years. The trend is attributed to the influence of four factors: working mothers, single-parent households, dual-income households, and smaller families (50). The trend of increased responsibility of teenagers in food matters will most likely continue.

GOVERNMENT FEEDING PROGRAMS FOR INFANCY THROUGH ADOLESCENCE

The USDA administers the WIC program (see Chapter 3). The USDA also administers the National School Lunch Program. Through the program, the USDA provides cash reimbursement and supplemental foods to feeding programs that comply with federal regulations. The federal regulations require that the school lunches be offered free or at reduced cost to low-income families. Also, the meals must meet specific guidelines.

The nutritional goal of the school lunch program is to provide approximately one-third of the RDAs for children in the various age groups. Foods that must be served include one item from the meat/meat alternate group; two items from the vegetable/fruit group; and one item each from the bread/bread alternate and milk groups. (See Table 4-8.)

In the senior high school, an "offer-versus-serve" provision is required. At lower grades, it is discretionary. In the offer-versus-serve option, students must be offered all five food items in the pattern but may choose at least three for their lunch to be reimbursable. In additon to the School Lunch Program, the USDA administers a School Breakfast Program, a Special Milk Program, and a Child-Care Food Program, which also have regulations with regard to cost, type of food, and amount of food served.

Table 4-8. SCHOOL LUNCH PATTERNS FOR VARIOUS AGE/GRADE GROUPS

U.S. Department of Agriculture, National School Lunch Program—USDA recommends, but does not require, that you adjust portions by age/grade group to better meet the food and nutritional needs of children according to their ages, if you adjust portions. Groups I–IV are minimum requirements for the age/grade groups specified. If you do not adjust portions, the Group IV portions are the portions to serve all children.

COMPONENTS		Preschool ages 1–2 (Group I)	ages 3–4 (Group II)	Grades K-3 ages 5–8 (Group III)	Grades 4-12[1] age 9 & over (Group IV)	Grades 7-12 age 12 & over (Group V)	Specific Requirements
		MINIMUM QUANTITIES				RECOMMENDED QUANTITIES[2]	
Meat or Meat Alternate	A serving of one of the following or a combination to give an equivalent quantity:						• Must be served in the main dish or the main dish and one other menu item.
	Lean meat, poultry, or fish (edible portion as served)	1 oz	1½ oz	1½ oz	2 oz	3 oz	• Vegetables protein products, cheese alternate products, and enriched macaroni with fortified protein may be used to meet part of the meat/meat alternate requirement. Fact sheets on each of these alternate foods give detailed instructions for use.
	Cheese	1 oz	1½ oz	1½ oz	2 oz	3 oz	
	Large egg(s)	½	¾	¾	1	1½	
	Cooked dry beans or peas	¼ cup	⅜ cup	⅜ cup	½ cup	¾ cup	
	Peanut butter	2 Tbsp	3 Tbsp	3 Tbsp	4 Tbsp	6 Tbsp	

Continued

Table 4-8. SCHOOL LUNCH PATTERNS FOR VARIOUS AGE/GRADE GROUPS *(continued)*

U.S. Department of Agriculture, National School Lunch Program—USDA recommends, but does not require, that you adjust portions by age/grade group to better meet the food and nutritional needs of children according to their ages, if you adjust portions. Groups I–IV are minimum requirements for the age/grade groups specified. If you do not adjust portions, the Group IV portions are the portions to serve all children.

COMPONENTS		MINIMUM QUANTITIES Preschool ages 1–2 (Group I)	ages 3–4 (Group II)	Grades K-3 ages 5–8 (Group III)	Grades 4-12[1] age 9 & over (Group IV)	RECOMMENDED QUANTITIES[2] Grades 7-12 age 12 & over (Group V)	Specific Requirements
Vegetable and/or Fruit	Two or more servings of vegetable or fruit or both to total	½ cup	½ cup	½ cup	¾ cup	¾ cup	• No more than one-half of the total requirement may be met with full-strength fruit or vegetable juice. • Cooked dry beans or peas may be used as a meat alternate or as a vegetable but not as both in the same meal.
Bread or Bread Alternate	Servings of bread or bread alternate A serving is • 1 slice of whole-grain or enriched bread • A whole-grain or enriched biscuit, roll, muffin, etc. • ½ cup of cooked whole-grain or enriched rice, macaroni, noodles, whole-grain or enriched pasta products, or other cereal grains such as bulgur or corn grits. • A combination of any of the above.	5 per week	8 per week	8 per week	8 per week	10 per week	• At least ½ serving of bread or an equivalent quantity of bread alternate for Group I, and 1 serving for Groups II–V, must be served daily. • Enriched macaroni with fortified protein may be used as a meat alternate or as a bread alternate but not as both in the same meal. NOTE: *Food Buying Guide for Child Nutrition Programs,* PA-1331 (1983) provides the information for the minimum weight of a serving.
Milk	A serving of fluid milk	¾ cup (6 fl oz)	¾ cup (6 fl oz)	½ pint (8 fl oz)	½ pint (8 fl oz)	½ pint (8 fl oz)	At least one of the following forms of milk must be offered: • Unflavored lowfat milk • Unflavored skim milk • Unflavored buttermilk NOTE: This requirement does not prohibit offering other milks, such as whole milk or flavored milk, along with one or more of the above.

Source: U.S. Department of Agriculture. *National School Lunch Program Food Buying Guide,* 1984, page 3.

[1]Group IV is highlighted because it is the one meal pattern that will satisfy all requirements if no portion size adjustments are made.

[2]Group V specifies recommended, not required, quantities for students 12 years and older. These students may request smaller portions, but not smaller than those specified in Group IV.

NURSING INTERVENTIONS RELATED TO DIETARY MANAGEMENT

- Work closely with the dietitian or nutritionist and the physician, as may be required, to assist families in achieving optimum nutrition for the growing child.
- Act as a resource person in providing information related to the physiological demands of the varied age groups and the role of adequate nutrition; conducting dietary assessments; referring families to the appropriate community agencies for additional assistance (financial, nutritional, etc.); working with teachers, coaches, school administrators, etc., in providing nutritional information to children of all ages and their parents.
- Teach parents of infants which foods to initially offer an infant, to encourage the infant to eat, and to avoid.
- Teach hospitalized teenagers how to achieve a well-balanced diet.
- Assess for potential nutritional problems associated with children of all ages in the varied settings in which the nurse works (hospital, school, clinic, office, community, etc.).

TOPIC OF INTEREST

Numerous inborn errors of metabolism exist. Two that involve faulty metabolism of essential amino acids are phenylketonuria (PKU) and maple-syrup urine disease. In hereditary disorders involving essential amino acids, the intake of the offending essential amino acid must be restricted without interfering with normal growth and development. The metabolic defect in PKU is the lack of phenylalanine hydroxylase, a liver enzyme responsible for converting the essential amino acid phenylalanine to tyrosine. The lack of the converting enzyme alters the fate of ingested phenylalanine resulting in diversion of the amino acid to other metabolic pathways. These alternate pathways produce catabolites that are believed to cause brain damage in infants with PKU. The presence of the phenylalanine derivative, phenylacetic acid, in the urine and sweat causes a mousy body odor. Successful treatment of the disorder is achieved through strict adherence to a low phenylalanine diet instituted within the first eight weeks of life. Special commercial formulas (such as Analog XP, Ross Laboratories) must be used for feeding the infant. The low phenylalanine diet is continued throughout childhood. The age at which the diet can be discontinued with no adverse effects is highly controversial. Females with PKU who become pregnant must follow a phenylalanine restricted diet to avoid fetal abnormalities and complications during pregnancy.

Maple-syrup urine disease is characterized by defective metabolism of the essential amino acids leucine, isoleucine, and valine. Clinical manifestations of maple-syrup urine disease include lethargy, vomiting, spasticity, maple-syrup odor to the urine, and elevated levels of leucine, isoleucine, and valine. Untreated, maple-syrup urine disease results in severe mental retardation and death. A synthetic diet low in the offending amino acids is used to treat the disorder.

SPOTLIGHT ON LEARNING

Ms. M's three-year-old daughter, Missy, has two major feeding problems: She says she hates vegetables even though she may have never seen or tasted the vegetable before, and sometimes she eats, but at other times, she says she is not hungry.

1. Are the behaviors of Missy normal or abnormal for her age?
2. What suggestions could help Ms. M overcome the feeding difficulties?

REVIEW QUESTIONS

1. Cow's milk is inappropriate to feed during the first six months of life because it is too low in which of the following?
   a. iron
   b. sodium
   c. saturated fat
   d. protein

2. How long does the nursing period usually last?
   a. 6 weeks
   b. 2–3 months
   c. 4–6 months
   d. 7 days

3. Soy-protein formulas are frequently prescribed for which infants?
   a. premature or LBW infants
   b. colicky infants
   c. infants who cannot be breast-fed
   d. infants who have galactosemia and lactase deficiency

4. When or why are solid foods introduced to infants?
   a. to help them sleep through the night
   b. at about 4–6 months of age
   c. as soon as possible, preferably at 2 months
   d. when their taste buds mature

5. Which is the first solid food commonly fed to infants in the United States?
   a. meat
   b. mixed vegetables
   c. iron-fortified rice cereal
   d. honey-sweetened fruit

6. Which of the following include satiety cues in infancy?
   a. crying and fussiness
   b. grabbing the spoon
   c. showing sustained interest in surroundings versus food
   d. grabbing for the food

7. Which of the following foods is not associated with choking in the young child?
   a. hot dogs
   b. round candies
   c. toast
   d. nuts

8. When a child refuses to eat a food on his or her plate, what should the parent do?
   a. demand that the food be eaten
   b. remove the food after a specific time without a fuss
   c. offer a dessert if the child will eat the food
   d. send the child to his or her room without eating

9. Which are the most common nutrition-related problems in U.S. preschoolers?
   a. dental caries and iron-deficiency anemia
   b. obesity and hyperactivity
   c. iron-deficiency anemia and hypercholesterolemia
   d. hypertension and diabetes mellitus

10. What are the reasons for increased nutrient needs during adolescence?
    a. skipped meals
    b. growth rate increases
    c. anorexia
    d. snacking behaviors

ACTIVITIES

1. Visit a store that sells commercial infant formula. List the forms available and the cost of each. Compare the nutritional profile and ingredient listings for two competing brands. What differences did you note?

2. Take a trip to a grocery store and compare two brands of baby food. Compare the cost, nutritional declarations, and ingredients in one fruit, one vegetable, and one meat variety of each brand.

3. Plan a one-day menu for a healthy four-year-old. Be sure to take into account nutritional needs and dietary preferences at this age.

4. Analyze the school lunches in a nearby school district using the USDA guidelines (Table 4-8) and a food composition table. Do the lunches meet the USDA guidelines? Does the average composition over a one-week period meet one-third of the RDA for school-aged children?

5. Invite a dietitian into class to discuss nutrition and the high school athlete.

REFERENCES

1. Barness, L.A. History of infant feeding practices. *American Journal of Clinical Nutrition* 46 (1987):168–70.
2. Committee on Nutrition, American Academy of Pediatrics. *Pediatric nutrition handbook.* 2d ed. Elk Grove Village: American Academy of Pediatrics, 1985.
3. Pipes, P.L. *Nutrition in infancy and childhood.* St. Louis: Times Mirror/Mosby College Publishing, 1985.
4. Anderson, G.H. Human milk feeding. *The Pediatric Clinics of North America* 32 (1985):336.
5. Ferris, A.M., et al. Macronutrients in human milk at 2, 12, and 16 weeks postpartum. *Journal of the American Dietetic Association* 88 (1988):694–97.
6. Committee on Nutrition, American Academy of Pediatrics. Nutrition and lactation. *Pediatrics* 68 (1981):435–43.
7. Guthrie, H.A. *Introductory nutrition.* St. Louis: The C.V. Mosby Company, 1983.
8. Dudek, S. *Nutrition handbook for nursing practice.* Philadelphia: Lippincott, 1987.
9. Matheny, R., and M.F. Picciano. Feeding and growth characteristics of human milk-fed infants. *Journal of the American Dietetic Association* 86 (1986):327–31.
10. Jung, E., and D.M. Czajka-Narins. Birth weight doubling and tripling times: An updated look at the effects of birth weight, sex, race, and type of feeding. *American Journal of Clinical Nutrition* 42 (1985):182–89.
11. Fomon, S.J. Reflections on infant feeding in the 1970s and 1980s. *American Journal of Clinical Nutrition* 46 (1987):172–73.
12. Fomon, S.J. Breast-feeding and evolution. *Journal of the American Dietetic Association* 86 (1986):317–18.
13. Specker, B., and R. Tsang. Cyclical serum 25-hydroxyvitamin D concentrations paralleling sunshine exposure in exclusively breast-fed infants. *The Journal of Pediatrics* 110 (1987):744–47.
14. Krug-Wispe, S. *Formulas used in infant feeding.* The University of Iowa Hospitals and Clinics, Dietary Department, 1983.

15. Committee on Nutrition, American Academy of Pediatrics. Soy-protein formulas: Recommendations for use in infant feeding. *Pediatrics* 72 (1983):359–63.

16. Fomon, S.J., et al. Recommendations for feeding normal infants. *Pediatrics* 63 (1979):52–59.

17. Oski, F. Iron-fortified formulas and gastrointestinal symptoms in infants: A controlled study. *Pediatrics* 66 (1980):168–70.

18. Martinez, G.A., A.S. Ryan, and D.J. Malec. Nutrient intakes of American infants and children fed cow's milk or infant formula. *American Journal of Diseases of Children* 139 (1985):1010–18.

19. Fomon, S.J., et al. Milk feeding in infancy: Gastrointestinal blood loss and iron nutritional status. *Journal of Pediatrics* 98 (1981):540–45.

20. Montalto, M.B., J.D. Benson, and G.A. Martinez. Nutrient intakes of formula-fed infants and infants fed cow's milk. *Pediatrics* 75 (1985):343–50.

21. Committee on Nutrition, American Academy of Pediatrics. The use of whole cow's milk in infancy. *Pediatrics* 72 (1983):253–55.

22. Parraga, I.M., et al. Feeding patterns of urban black infants. *Journal of the American Dietetic Association* 88 (1988):796–800.

23. Lambert and Legacé, L. *Feeding your child.* New York: Beaufort Books, Inc., 1982.

24. Jelliffee, E. Infant feeding practices: Associated iatrogenic and commerciogenic disease. *Pediatric Clinics of North America* 24 (1977):49.

25. Kare, M., and G. Beauchamp. The role of taste in the infant diet. *American Journal of Clinical Nutrition* 41 (1985):418–22.

26. Lawless, H. Sensory development in children: Research in taste and olfaction. *Journal of the American Dietetic Association* 85 (1985):577–82.

27. Adair, L.S. The infant's ability to self-regulate caloric intake: A case study. *Journal of the American Dietetic Association* 84 (1984):543–46.

28. Filer, J. Modified food starch—An update. *Journal of the American Dietetic Association* 88 (1988):342–44.

29. Committee on Nutrition, American Academy of Pediatrics. *Review of safety and suitability of modified food starches in infant foods.* Evanston: American Academy of Pediatrics, 1978.

30. Endres, J., et al. Dietary sodium intake of infants fed commercially prepared baby food and table food. *Journal of the American Dietetic Association* 87 (1987):750–53.

31. Harris, C.S., et al. Childhood asphyxiation by food. A national analysis and overview. *Journal of the American Medical Association* 251 (1984):2231–35.

32. Committee on Nutrition, American Academy of Pediatrics. On the feeding of supplemental foods to infants. *Pediatrics* 65 (1980):1178–81.

33. Heterocyclic amines have wide-ranging effects on health. *Food Chemical News* 30, no. 19 (1988):36.

34. Komuvesh, M. *Infant nutrition. A guide for professionals.* Ontario: Ministry of Health, 1984.

35. Committee on Nutrition, American Academy of Pediatrics. Nutritional aspects of obesity in infancy and childhood. *Pediatrics* 68 (1981):880–82.

36. Woolman, P.G. Feeding practices in infancy and prevalence of obesity in preschool children. *Journal of the American Dietetic Association* 84 (1984):436–38.
37. Committee on Nutrition, American Academy of Pediatrics. Toward a prudent diet for children. *Pediatrics* 71 (1983):78–79, 883.
38. Taubman, B. Clinical trial of the treatment of colic by modification of parent-infant interaction. *Pediatrics* 74 (1984):998–1003.
39. Jakobsson, I., and T. Lindberg. Cow's milk proteins cause infantile colic in breast-fed infants: A double-blind crossover study. *Pediatrics* 71 (1983):268–71.
40. Davidson, M. Causes and management of colic in infancy. *Nutrition and the MD* 9, no. 11 (1983):1–3.
41. ———. Role of parenteral nutrition in the very-low-birth-weight infant. *Nutrition Reviews* 45 (1987):105–07.
42. Anderson, G.H., S.A. Atkinson, and M.H. Bryan. Energy and macronutrient content of human milk during early lactation from mothers giving birth prematurely and at term. *American Journal of Clinical Nutrition* 34 (1981):258–65.
43. Galeano, N.F., and C.C. Roy. Feeding the premature infant. In *Nutrition for special needs in infancy. Protein hydrolysates.* F. Lifshitz. New York: Marcel Dekker, Inc., 1985.
44. Satter, E.M. The feeding relationship. *Journal of the American Dietetic Association* 86 (1986):352–56.
45. Birch, L.L. The role of experience in children's food acceptance patterns. *Journal of the American Dietetic Association Supplement* 87 (1987):S36–S40.
46. Dietz, W.H. Childhood and adolescent obesity. In Frankle, R.T. and Yang, M. *Obesity and weight control. The health professionals guide to understanding and treatment,* edited by R.T. Frankle and M. Yang. Rockville: Aspen Publications Inc., 1988.
47. National Dairy Council. Adolescent nutrition: Issues and challenges. *Dairy Council Digest* 58, no. 4 (July–August 1987).
48. Story, M., and R.W. Blum. Adolescent nutrition: Self-perceived deficiencies and needs of practitioners working with youth. *Journal of the American Dietetic Association* 88 (1988):591–94.
49. Palla, B., and I.F. Litt. Medical complications of eating disorders in adolescents. *Pediatrics* 81 (1988):613–23.
50. Jaluvka, L. Teen-age shoppers. *IGA Grocergram* 62 (1988):19–21.

CHAPTER
5
NUTRITION FOR THE ADULT

Objectives

After studying this chapter, you will be able to
- explain how the preferences and needs of adults are influenced by physiological, psychosocial, and economic changes which occur during the aging process.
- identify specific changes that occur in nutritional needs for adults, highlighting nutrients for which a greater need exists.
- describe the challenges faced in nutritional assessment.
- list the major support services available for adults.
- identify nursing interventions related to the dietary management of the adult.

Overview

During the earlier stages of life, the body's major emphasis is growth and maturation. Energy from food is funneled to support the needs of growing tissues. Once individuals reach their third decade of life, the focus of the body changes. Maintenance of homeostasis becomes the body's primary concern (1). Because the caloric requirements of homeostasis are less than growth, eating and exercise patterns need to change. As indiviuals age, it becomes more difficult to maintain homeostasis under stress such as illness. Therefore, the elderly are more vulnerable to various infectious diseases and food-borne illness. In this chapter, the transition from growth to the maintenance period is presented. Particular attention is focused on the individual aged 55 and older.

THE EARLY YEARS OF ADULTHOOD

During the early years of adulthood, life-styles become well established, careers take hold, and new responsibilities are assumed, making this time of life very rewarding (2). From a nutritional aspect, most vitamin and mineral needs remain fairly stable. Only a few vitamins that are tied to energy requirements decline (see Appendix B). The major decline occurs in caloric needs, resulting from a decrease in basal-metabolic rate as well as a decline in physical activity. Unfortunately, many individuals do not alter food intake, gain weight gradually over a period of years, and enter middle age overweight and, consequently, at greater risk for developing cardiovascular disease and diabetes mellitus. Additionally, it is clear that not only the amount of food eaten, but also the composition of the diet can put adults at risk for major chronic diseases. Numerous intervention programs over the years have been targeted to the early years of adulthood in an effort to avert problems in later life.

The Dietary Guidelines for Americans (see Chapter 1) are excellent recommendations for the young adult. The maintenance of desirable weight cannot be stressed enough, and regular physical activity should be maintained as the individual enters older adulthood.

THE OLDER ADULT

The older adult population is the fastest-growing segment of our society. By the year 2000, approximately one-third of the U.S. population will be at least age 55. In the U.S., we have very little past experience for dealing with an aging society. The reason is simple. In 1900, the average life expectancy was 47 years. In 1985, it increased to 75 years. Thus, in the past, many people did not reach old age. They died from the results of diseases that are now treatable, and there was also a high infant mortality rate.

Today, older adults can be divided into three age segments: individuals 55–64 years, those aged 65–74 years, and those aged 75 years and older (3). Growth in the older-population segments is illus-

trated by current figures and future projections. In 1987, 27 million Americans were older than 65 years. This will increase to 35 million by the year 2000. Of the 35 million people aged 65 and older, 5 million individuals are expected to be 85 years and older (4).

How do maturing adults view themselves? According to the American Association of Retired Persons (AARP), most people, no matter how long they live, define old as about 10 years older than they are. The essence of this view has both positive and negative implications. On the bright side, the majority of individuals past the young adult stage of life are in good health, live independently, and look forward to the future. The darker side hints of the stereotypic view that illness, dependency, and frailty are often associated with "old age." Actually, the older population is subject to numerous misconceptions in our society, even though the myths of aging have been debunked through careful research of our elders.

MYTHS OF AGING

Common myths about aging pervade our society: Old age begins at 65; the elderly are in poor health; the elderly are poor; and the elderly are similar to one another (5).

The myth that old age begins at 65 can be traced to the common age at which most people are expected to retire. In fact, we are currently seeing a cyclic life plan in the U.S. rather than a linear life plan (6). As illustrated in Figure 5-1, according to the linear life plan, educational years are followed by working years. Leisure is a time of life reserved for the period following the working years. The current view, the cyclic life plan intersperses education, work, and leisure with fewer age demarcations. In the U.S. today, early retirement is on the increase; however, individuals may still be involved in activities such as consultation or may begin a second career (3). The age of 65 no longer signifies the end to one's usefulness.

AARP reports that the second myth about the health of older adults is easily debunked when the statistics are viewed. Only 3% of individuals 50–64

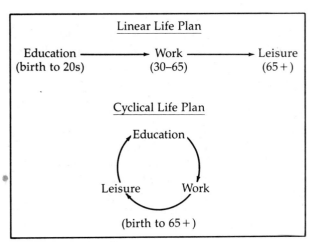

Figure 5-1. Life plans.

need assistance in performing personal care or home-management activities. The figure rises to 7% for those in the 65–74 range, and only at 85 and older does a large percentage (40%) require assistance.

What does the economic picture of the older adult look like? While there continues to be serious pockets of poverty among the elderly, not all older adults are poor. Approximately 12% of those 50 and older have incomes below the poverty line, and 13% are near poor (7). The remainder enjoy adequate incomes.

No group has as many differences as older adults. Differences among individuals increase with age, reflecting their life experiences. There is also a tremendous variation in the aging process, making it unfair to generalize about all older individuals.

A PROFILE OF TODAY'S OLDER ADULT

Today's older adults have a younger view of themselves than did people in the past. They do not appreciate being marketed to as "old." The majority of older individuals are women, because they usually survive their husbands. For every 100 women aged 55–64, there are 88 males, and in the 85-plus range, there are only 42 males for every 100 females. They are a heterogeneous group with vast variations in food intake. For example, older per-

sons who live with another person and are physically and socially active tend to eat a more-varied and better-quality diet (8, 9). Greater financial resources and higher academic achievement are related to a greater variety in food intake. At the other end of the spectrum are the older persons who are homebound, physically or mentally disabled, living alone, and poor. These individuals often have a substandard nutrient intake and lack access to dental and medical care (10).

Nutrition and Health Concerns

The vitamin and mineral concerns of older adults are reflected in their nutrient-supplementation patterns. A study involving low-income individuals, primarily Caucasian elders in Nevada aged 60–94, showed a high incidence (66%) of food supplement use (11). Vitamins C and E were the supplements of choice. In this study, women were twice as likely as men to use supplements. Also, supplement intake was not related to income. Other studies conducted in different parts of the country yielded similar findings of a high frequency of supplement use among elderly individuals (12, 13). Mostly self-prescribed, the vitamins in the studies included A, C, E, B_{12}, and B_6. A disturbing fact about vitamin supplementation in the elderly is that the supplements most often used include nutrients that are adequate in the diet (14). A more disturbing fact is the potentially toxic dosage a number of individuals consistently take.

When specifically questioned, the elderly give varied reasons for taking supplements, and some reasons have no bearing on the vitamin's function in the body. In other cases, the benefits of taking supplements are overestimated. It has been suggested that older adults are particularly vulnerable to vitamin misuse because they are very concerned about their health. They often mistake normal aging-associated changes with a decline in health, and believe that vitamins will alleviate the problem.

Many elderly are so concerned about their health that they often fall victim to health-care fraud. Health-care fraud includes the major categories of arthritis remedies, questionable cancer cures, and youth cures (promises of hair restoration, renewed energy, antiaging, increased sexual potency, etc.). Approximately 60% of the victims of health-care fraud in the United States are the elderly (15).

Health-related factors are influential in determining food purchases. Older adults read food labels and are particularly sensitive to kilocalorie, fat, sodium, and calcium content. They look for foods low in cholesterol and saturated fat, low in salt, and low in kilocalories, thus accommodating their changing nutrient needs, their desire to maintain good health, and their dietary changes necessitated by the presence of chronic diseases.

Older adults like foods that are a good value for the price, easy to chew, and simple to prepare. They report a higher incidence of food intolerances than younger individuals because of the changes in the body systems (16). The vegetable category is the most frequently cited food group that causes intolerance. Nutrient intake need not be affected, however, since fruit consumption increases with age. Compared with younger individuals who are 18–29 and who report eating approximately five servings of fruit per week, adults 60 and older report an intake of 8.5 servings weekly (17).

Shopping habits and needs of this group are being recognized by retailers. Older adults shop for food more frequently than younger age groups, like to shop in the morning hours, are very service-oriented, and look for smaller packages (18). Some supermarkets now have benches, motorized carts, and training programs for employees detailing how to better serve the older population. Major sources of nutrition information for this group are the media—print, television, and radio—rather than health professionals.

The preferences, needs, and nutritional status of older adults are directly influenced by changes that occur during the aging process. Physiological, psychosocial, and economic changes can have profound effects on dietary intake.

POSSIBLE NURSING DIAGNOSES

Knowledge deficit related to
- understanding of the relationship between adequate nutrition and the physiological changes associated with aging.
- interaction of drugs (prescribed or over-the-counter) and nutrients;
- community resources that may be available to supplement nutritional needs.

Noncompliance related to
- lack of understanding of the role of adequate nutrition and the prevention of common age-related changes, such as decreased intestinal motility (constipation), osteoporosis (increase in number of fractures).
- lack of resources (financial and transportational) to provide for adequate nutritional needs.
- established food habits and practices.

Potential alteration in bowel elimination (constipation) related to
- decreased intestinal motility.
- decreased bulk food in the intestine.

Potential activity intolerance related to inability to secure and prepare food.

Potential alteration in home management related to inability to secure, store, and prepare food for adequate nutrition.

Potential alteration in health maintenance related to lack of knowledge to provide optimum nutrition.

Potential inadequate coping (individual or family) related to stress resulting from physiological changes associated with the aging process.

CHANGES THAT OCCUR WITH AGE

Physiological Changes

In general, physiological changes occur at different rates. The changes that occur are not noticeable in the resting state but are quite evident when the body is stressed (See Table 5-1).

The outward sign of the skin's loss of elasticity and turgor is wrinkles, which have little effect on physiological needs but can impact adversely on the psychological state of the individual. A decreased muscle mass results in a lowered energy requirement through the combined effects of a decreased basal-metabolic rate and a decreased activity level. As one ages, lean body mass declines and is replaced by fat tissue. The lower metabolic requirements of fat tissue have an impact on total energy needs.

Throughout life, bones undergo a remodeling process that involves absorption and deposition of minerals. During the third or fourth decade of life, absorption is greater than deposition, resulting in bone loss. Bone loss occurs in all individuals as part of the aging process; however, it appears to be more rapid in females, especially postmenopausal Caucasian females. Severe bone loss, or osteoporosis, is a disease influenced by a number of

Table 5-1. BIOLOGICAL CHANGES WITH AGE

SYSTEM	CHANGES WITH AGE
Integumentary	Decreased elasticity of skin
Muscular	Atrophy (decrease in muscle mass)
Skeletal	Decrease in bone mass
Digestive	Dentition changes (loss of teeth, improperly fitting dentures)
	Decreased motility
	Decreased acid/enzyme secretion
Endocrine	Glandular changes (decreased estrogen, decreased testosterone)
Circulatory	Increased rigidity of arterial wall
	Decreased myocardial contractility
	Decreased cardiac output
	Increased peripheral resistance at rest
Respiratory	Decreased lung compliance
Urinary	Decreased kidney filtration
Reproductive	Female: Menopause
	Male: Male Menopause
Nervous	Decreased sense of taste and smell, decreased reaction time, and changes in vision and hearing

factors such as age, lack of physical activity, inadequate calcium intake, and changes in hormonal state. The specific hormonal changes involve the slight decrease in testosterone in males and the marked decline in estrogen in females. As a result of the osteoporosis, older persons are more prone to fractures.

Alterations in the process of digestion as a result of aging are illustrated in Figure 5-2. The digestive process begins in the mouth, and dietary intake can be adversely affected by changes in dentition. Loss of some or all teeth occurs in most older individuals. Not all toothless individuals wear dentures, and sometimes dentures are ill fitting. Problems with chewing can result in a decreased intake of foods that require more chewing, such as meat. Further, a decline in saliva and the salivary enzyme ptyalin can result in inadequate lubrication of food (19).

The next phase of digestion occurs in the stomach. Older individuals excrete less hydrochloric

acid and pepsin in the stomach, and approximately 50% of older adults are afflicted with atrophic gastritis. The acidity of the stomach has an impact on the absorption of some nutrients. Food leaves the stomach as chyme and enters the intestinal tract. Here, decreased enzyme secretion as well as a decline in the mucosal surface area with age can affect food digestion and nutrient absorption. Additionally, muscle layers in the tract thin with age, leading to the formation of intestinal diverticula and a decline in motility (see Chapter 7). In some individuals, constipation can be a problem caused by the altered gastrointestinal motility (movement) combined with a decreased fluid intake, low-fiber diets, inactivity, and medications.

Glucose tolerance declines with age due to a lower insulin release in response to a glucose load coupled with a decline in tissue sensitivity (20). (Type II diabetes mellitus is discussed in Chapter 13.) Alterations in the function of the thymus gland may play a role in the changed immunity (decreased levels of antibodies) observed in older individuals.

Changes in the cardiovascular system limit the body's ability to adapt to physical activity and emotional stress. Also, systolic blood and diastolic pressure increases after age 65 due to the increased rigidity of the arterial walls (19). Lung capacity decreases by approximately 40% throughout life. Normal activity is not hindered by the lower-lung capacity; however, performance during exercise declines due to the decrease in both lung capacity and muscle mass.

The structure and function of the kidney decline in adulthood. In most older individuals, renal blood flow and glomerular filtration rate decrease by 50% during the 30–80-year age span. Tubular function also decreases, and the entire kidney shrinks (21). The shrinking kidney is less able to concentrate the urine and conserve water during deprivation. As a result, older individuals are very susceptible to dehydration. Diminished thirst sensations combine with, often, a voluntary fluid restriction to avoid frequent trips to the bathroom. Recent studies cast doubt on the inevitable decline in kidney function, since the deterioration is not

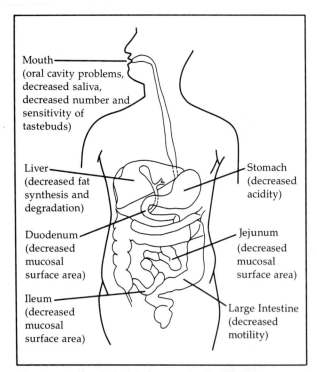

Mouth
(oral cavity problems, decreased saliva, decreased number and sensitivity of tastebuds)

Liver
(decreased fat synthesis and degradation)

Duodenum
(decreased mucosal surface area)

Ileum
(decreased mucosal surface area)

Stomach
(decreased acidity)

Jejunum
(decreased mucosal surface area)

Large Intestine
(decreased motility)

Figure 5-2. Age-related changes in the digestive tract.

universal. Environmental factors such as hypertension, atherosclerosis, diabetes mellitus, infections, and drugs are thought to play a role.

As mentioned previously, both males and females undergo climacteric changes. The female experiences decreases in estrogen levels while the male produces less testosterone. Finally, the nervous system undergoes quite a bit of change resulting in alterations in taste, smell, hearing and vision. As one ages, the number of taste buds declines. While some investigators maintain that the loss results in a decline in the perception of taste, others have shown that the taste sensation is compensated by remembered sensory experiences. Changes in the sensation of taste are more often due to dentures covering many of the taste buds. Olfactory sensitivity declines, which may adversely affect eating enjoyment.

A slow decrease in hearing acuity (presbycusis) occurs, characterized by the inability to hear tones of high frequency and distinguish speech patterns from background noise. Total loss of hearing occurs in about one-third of older adults, with an increased frequency in males.

The aging cornea yellows, resulting in difficulty distinguishing pastel colors. Also, less violet light registers in the aging eye, making it difficult to distinguish blues and greens. Every persons over age 65 suffers some loss in adaptation to the dark, ability to focus, and ability to resolve images. Severe visual impairment caused by senile macular degeneration, glaucoma, and cataracts affects 15% of the older population.

Psychosocial Changes

No drastic personality changes generally occur during the normal aging process. Older individuals frequently work through the acceptance of their own death but must also cope with the loss of relatives, friends, and the loss of a spouse. The loss of an offspring is the most difficult to handle followed by loss of a spouse.

Loss of mobility resulting from chronic illness, arthritis, as well as from changes in hearing, vision, and movement can cause feelings of dependence and social isolation. Retirement may have

quite different effects. Some individuals experience a loss of self-esteem if they identify themselves solely by their work. Decreased income may also be a factor in the psychological changes associated with aging. Others experience a renewed sense of vigor to pursue interests that have been on hold for years. The passage of the burden of child rearing may also have different effects on different people. Some couples feel depressed and lonely, while others are thrilled to have the freedom to spend more time on themselves.

Economic Changes

Even greater than the fear of death for this age group is the fear of economic deprivation (19). Some individuals must make adjustments to live on a fixed income in the face of rising costs. However, individuals 55 and older actually account for 77% of the financial assets in the United States (22). Three-fourths of the elderly own their own homes, and with the cessation of house payments and the financial obligation of child rearing, discretionary income actually increases in this age group. However, a catastrophic illness or chronic disease requiring extended care can quickly and seriously deplete savings accumulated over a lifetime.

Nutritional Needs

Individuals over the age of 51 are treated as one group with respect to nutritional recommendations. Efforts were expended to change the 1980 RDA age categories. It seemed more appropriate to divide the 51-and-older age group into two groups: those aged 50–69, and those aged 70 years and older. The age recommendations were part of the total revisions recommended for the 1980 RDAs. Unfortunately, the changes were not included in the 1989 RDAs because it was felt that data is insufficient to support separate RDAs for individuals 70 years and older. Still, researchers view the older segment as having varied nutrient needs.

Protein, Fat, Carbohydrate, and Fluid Needs. Nitrogen-balance studies in the elderly have yielded contradictory results. The protein RDA of 0.8 g per kilogram body weight appears to be sufficient for maintaining nitrogen balance for this age group. A recent study of healthy older adults showed an average protein intake of 1.02–1.06 g per kilogram body weight (23).

Fat in the diet has different effects at different ages. It appears that serum total cholesterol stabilizes in males after age 60 and in females after age 70 (24). While elevated cholesterol continues to be pathologic, it has less predictive value for coronary heart disease in older versus younger persons (25). Other factors, particularly high blood pressure, are more predictive of coronary heart disease in older adults. Because fat is a concentrated source of kilocalories, it is often modified in the diet to lower total caloric intake. In addition, gall bladder abnormalities appear to strike this age segment more frequently than other age groups. Gall bladder problems may require restriction of total fat intake (20).

The ability to metabolize carbohydrate declines with age. Impaired glucose tolerance not only occurs through the normal aging process, but also can be a result of medications such as steroids. Current recommendations are to encourage the intake of complex rather than simple carbohydrate, with an emphasis on high-fiber foods, if tolerated.

Because of changes that occur in the kidney, special attention should be given to fluid needs. An intake of 30 ml per kilogram of body weight is recommended. While older adults living in community settings have no problem achieving adequate fluid intake, those in nursing homes and hospitals need to be offered water at regular intervals to prevent dehydration.

Vitamin Needs. Surveys indicate that intake of vitamin A among older adults often depends on socioeconomic status and gender. Older adults with higher incomes consume more vitamin A, and males have a greater vitamin A intake than females. Surveys have also shown that up to 65% of the elderly have vitamin-A intakes that are less than two-thirds of the 1989 RDA (800 R.E.). Even so, the serum vitamin-A values are normal in the majority, indicating better absorption coupled with a possibly lower need (26).

Vitamin-D intake and utilization constitute a unique problem in the elderly. Intakes less than two-thirds of the RDA (5 mcg) have been reported

in 60%–74% of older adults (26). In addition, metabolic changes profoundly affect vitamin-D metabolism. The process of aging results in a substantial decline in the activation of vitamin D by the kidney. There is also often a lack of sun exposure, thereby decreasing vitamin-D synthesis in the skin. As a result, vitamin-D requirements may be increased in older adults. Vitamin D is essential for the absorption of calcium. This relationship is described later in this chapter.

Problems with vitamin K cannot be traced to inadequate diets but rather to medications such as local-acting antiinfective agents that reduce vitamin-K producing bacteria in the intestines (24). Data conflicts with respect to vitamin E. Because vitamin E is the least toxic of the fat-soluble vitamins, abusive doses are often taken based on promises that it can do everything from arresting clinical problems to retarding the aging process. Hale et al. (27) demonstrated little effect of vitamin E on clinical disorders or hematologic and biochemical parameters. Whether or not vitamin E retards the oxidation processes thought to be associated with aging is unclear.

A wide variation in the intake of the water-soluble vitamin C is evident in the older population. Low intake, not decreased absorption, results in low vitamin-C status in the older person (26). Low vitamin C intake is often found in individuals of lower socioeconomic status.

The 1989 RDA for folate is 200 mcg for males and 180 mcg for females 51 years and older. In the past, the RDA for folate was much higher. However, it is now recognized that adequate folate status can be maintained on lower dietary intakes. However, only 3%–7% had low serum folate levels. Folic-acid absorption decreases with atrophic gastritis, but it is believed that bacterial folate synthesis may compensate (26). A higher pH level, as a result of decreased acidity, allows bacterial overgrowth. The increased numbers of bacteria produce enough folate to compensate for faulty absorption. Folate status is more related to socioeconomic status and health status than to aging per se.

Thiamin and riboflavin intakes vary widely. Physiologically, thiamin needs are associated with kilocalorie intakes that decline with age. Aging changes in absorption of these vitamins are not evident. Niacin needs are based on caloric intake and are unchanged from young adulthood (6.6 niacin equivalents/1,000 kcal).

Vitamin-B_6 needs may be increased with age (26). Not only are intakes usually well below recommended levels, but aging also has an effect of lowering the levels of physiologically active forms of vitamin B_6. Changes in absorption and metabolism also occur. Still, the data is not clear enough to recommend an increased intake.

A decrease in serum vitamin B_{12} occurs with increasing age, but it appears to be a problem for only those individuals with atrophic gastritis. A decrease occurs in hydrochloric-acid release in the stomach, which causes three effects: a decrease in the release of food-bound vitmin B_{12}, lower bioavailability of vitamin B_{12} resulting from the binding and changes in bacteria in the upper gastrointestinal tract, and a decrease in IF release, an essential compound for vitamin-B_{12} absorption. Because a large portion of the elderly population is affected by the problem of atrophic gastritis, vitamin-B_{12} needs may be increased in this subset. Many of these persons will manifest anemia.

Mineral Needs. The National Institutes of Health Consensus Development Conference on Osteoporosis recommended an increase in calcium intake from the RDA of 800 mg to 1000–1500 mg per day to prevent osteoporosis in males and postmenopausal females (28). With advancing age, dietary calcium absorption decreases, which is believed to result from a decreased level of calcitriol, the active form of vitamin D. Also, survey findings consistently show less than adequate intakes of calcium. The observation is particularly serious because adaptation to low intakes of calcium decreases as age increases. These factors along with other factors such as decreased estrogen levels lead to the increased incidence in fractures in older persons. (A detailed description of osteoporosis is included in Chapter 14.)

Decreased stomach acidity results in a decreased absorption of nonheme iron; however, iron requirements are lower in old age than at any other time of life. Anemia is therefore not a result of aging, but its occurrence is associated with chronic disease processes and medications.

With respect to nutrient requirements, it is evident that some vitamin and mineral needs increase. At greatest risk for specific nutritional problems in the group of noninstitutionalized elderly are those individuals with lower incomes, those on medications that interfere with nutrient metabolism, and those with chronic diseases (24, 29).

SPECIAL PROBLEMS AFFECTING OLDER ADULTS

Chronic Disease

The 27 million Americans aged 65 and over incur 29% of health-care costs (30). Chronic-disease conditions account for many cases of lengthy and debilitating illnesses. The most common chronic disease is arteriosclerotic heart disease (19). Combined hypertension (systolic blood pressure 140 mm Hg or higher and diastolic pressure 90 mm Hg or higher) is estimated to afflict 64% of persons 65–74 years old (31). Isolated systolic hypertension and diastolic hypertension are associated with an increased morbidity and mortality rate in people over 85 years of age. Cancer and diabetes mellitus Type II are other diseases that afflict older individuals. A chronic condition causing a great restriction in activity is arthritis, the most frequently reported condition among persons 45 years of age and over. Arthritis affects one-fourth of persons 45–64 and almost half of those older than 65 (32).

Drug-Nutrient Interactions

A critical factor affecting the nutritional status of older adults is the use of medications, both prescribed and over-the-counter (Table 5-2). Older adults consume at least 50% of all drugs used in the U.S. (33). Those living independently may take three or more drugs. Individuals in long-term care may average more than 10 drugs that are prescribed to treat three or more medical problems.

The reasons for drug-nutrient interactions are varied, and include chronic and multiple drug use,

Table 5-2. DRUG-NUTRIENT INTERACTIONS

DRUG	NUTRIENTS ADVERSELY AFFECTED
Analgesics	Iron
Antacids	Phosphate, calcium, vitamin D, folate
Antiinflammatory agents	fat, vitamin B_{12}, folate
Antibiotics	Calcium, vitamin K
Anticoagulants	Vitamin K
Anticonvulsants	Folate, vitamin D
Antihypertensive agents	Vitamin B_6
Antituberculosis agents	Vitamin B_6, niacin, vitamin D
Antiulcer agents	Vitamin B_{12}
Chemotherapeutic agents	Folate
Diuretics	Potassium, calcium, zinc, magnesium
Hypocholesterolemic agents	Fats, vitamins A, K, and B_{12}
Laxatives	Potassium, fat, calcium
Tranquilizers	Riboflavin

Adapted from Table 4 in Roe, D.A.: Therapeutic effects of drug-nutrient interactions in the elderly. Copyright The American Dietetic Association. Reprinted by permission from *Journal of the American Dietetic Association*, Vol. 85:174, 1985.

age-related physiological changes, such as a slower hepatic metabolism, which slows the rate of drug metabolism, and drug misuse and abuse. The most commonly used drugs in the older age group are cardiovascular agents, analgesics, laxatives, antacids, sedatives, and tranquilizers (33).

It is necessary to consider not only the effect that drugs have on nutrient status, but also the effect that food has on drug metabolism. A number of antibiotics (erythromycin, penicillins, tetra-cycline) are less well absorbed if taken with food or close to meal time. The poor absorption is attributed to complexes formed between the medications and minerals in the food. Once complexed, the medication cannot be absorbed. On the other hand, some drugs are better absorbed when taken with food. When phenytoin (Dilantin) is administered with food, its time in the stomach is increased, allowing for better dissolution and a more appropriate rate of delivery to the small intestine. Some drugs must be taken with food to prevent gastric irritation (Dilantin). Protein content of the diet appears to be an important nutritional variable that influences the rate of drug metabolism (33). Higher protein content of the diet is associated with an increased rate of metabolism of some drugs and vice versa. Instruct persons taking drugs to ask the pharmacist whether drugs should be taken with or without food, or whether certain foods will adversely interact with prescribed drugs.

NUTRITION ASSESSMENT OF OLDER ADULTS

Biochemical Indices

Most biochemical standards used to judge the nutritional status of the elderly population are inferred from studies on a younger population. This causes some confusion and can draw inaccurate pictures of nutritional health. Low albumin levels are not necessarily an indication of problems with protein nutriture. Albumin declines with age due to a decline in synthesis. Some advocate that 3.2 mg/dl rather than 3.5 mg/dl be used as a cut-off point (34).

In one study, plasma-zinc levels in hospitalized elderly showed lower than normal levels. However, zinc deficiency was not supported by other zinc status parameters. Plasma zinc tends to decrease with age due to the decrease in serum albumin, because 60%–70% of circulating zinc is bound to albumin (35). The lower levels of zinc may be responsible for the decreased acuity in the sense of taste.

Accurate hemoglobin measurements are also a problem. Hemoglobin levels below standards for younger individuals are not necessarily indicative of iron deficiency anemia. There appears to be an anemia of aging that is not explained by a deficiency of iron, vitamin B_{12}, vitamin B_6, or folate (34).

Urinary creatinine measurements are usually associated with skeletal muscle mass. It is unknown what the relationship between creatinine excretion and body composition should be in the elderly because of the decline in renal function that occurs in individuals as they age.

Biochemical assessment and decisions for the elderly should be made on the basis of more than one type of biochemical data. In the case of iron, for example, hematocrit, mean corpuscular hemoglobin, serum-iron and serum-transferrin values can be measured in addition to hemoglobin measurements before a diagnosis of iron deficiency is made. Obviously, continued research on the elderly should lead to the development of age-specific standards.

Anthropometry

Weight decreases in later years. Cross-sectional data shows that in males, weight normally increases until age 40–50, and then it declines. In females, weight increases until age 50–60 before showing a decrease (19). Distinguishing between an age-related decrease and pathological changes requires a discussion of dietary intake and weight measurements on a regular basis. Another change that occurs with age is a decrease in height due to loss of bone.

Body composition is often quickly assessed with skinfold measurements. Problems can be encountered because of the changes in lean body mass, body fat, body-fat distribution, skin thickness, turgor, elasticity, and compressibility (36). Because of the age-related changes, nutritional status should not be measured with a single standard. Other body sites should be used for skinfold measurements in addition to the triceps. Other measures such as mid- to upper-arm circumference can be used in addition to the skinfold measures. Provisional tables have been released listing norms for triceps skinfold thickness and mid-arm muscle circumference in the elderly (37).

Dietary Intake

The 24-hour recall and one-day food records are methods used to assess dietary intake. Both methods have been found to be equally effective in assessing dietary intake in noninstitutionalized older adults (38). Research involving hospitalized elderly, however, has identified that recall ability is a problem (39). When requesting older adults to complete questionnaires or keep food records, consideration should be given to vision problems, education level, mobility impairments resulting from arthritis or stroke, and living arrangements.

In addition to the questions about foods that older adults eat, questions should be included concerning the use of vitamin and mineral supplements. The dietary assessment should also be concerned with medications, both prescribed and over-the-counter, that the individual is taking. As detailed previously, medications can alter nutritional status. In addition to specific nutrient concerns, side effects of drugs, such as alterations in taste, nausea, vomiting, heartburn, and anorexia can significantly impair nutritional status.

NUTRITION AND SUPPORT SERVICES FOR OLDER ADULTS

Title III-C of the Older Americans Act

In 1972, a nutrition program for older adults was developed under Title VII of the Older Americans Act. In 1978, it was reorganized under Title III-C and is known as the Nutrition Program for the Elderly. The program includes congregate and home-delivered meals to older persons. The Administration on Aging manages the delivery of meals through state and local agencies on aging. Meals are provided to individuals 60 and older and their spouses, regardless of age. No income requirements exist for participation. Participants receive a minimum of one meal per day, five days per week. According to the National Association of Area Agencies on Aging, home and community meals ranked high in services assessed to be essential to the health maintenance of noninstitutionalized older adults (40).

Recipients of home-delivered meals were studied in New York State with the finding that continuance on the program differed depending on the reason for enrollment (41). Persons who utilized the program for a short duration included elderly with acute and terminal illnesses who had a temporary need for the services during recuperation. Clients using the program for a moderate duration

suffered from coronary heart disease, respiratory disease, hip fractures, and mental illness, which improved with medical care. Long-duration clients had chronic debilitating illnesses that permanently impaired mobility, such as stroke and diabetes mellitus. Because of the increasing trend toward earlier discharge of patients from the hospital, it was believed that this service filled a nutritional gap to aid in recovery. This program also served as a substitute for institutionalization for long-duration clients.

Congregate (group) meals at churches and senior community centers supply a large percentage of dietary intake for some individuals. For other individuals, the meals satisfy more of a social than nutritional need (42).

Food Stamps

The Food Stamp Program is targeted to the low-income elderly. Unfortunately, recent work has been unable to demonstrate an effect of participation in the program on energy or iron status in the U.S. elderly poor (43, 44). Many older persons may not be aware of the availability of food stamps or are too proud to apply for them.

Home Health Care

Home health care is reserved for individuals who require medical care but do not require hospitalization. It generally involves regular home visits by a registered nurse, a licensed practical nurse, a nursing assistant, a home health aide, or a nutritionist. The individual is eligible for reimbursement of some costs by Medicare if prescribed by the physician. Major benefits of home health care include retaining independence and living in the home setting.

Home medical care is expected to triple in growth in the 1990s. The major consumers are expected to be older, frail persons who are at nutritional risk as a result of multiple medical problems and drug intake (45).

HOUSING OPTIONS FOR OLDER ADULTS

The housing options open to older adults are varied, and the choice depends on medical needs as well as personal preference. In *match-up home sharing*, the home owner with room to spare in his or her home is matched with a home seeker. *Shared-living residences* are homes in which a number of unrelated individuals live together. Each person has a private bedroom, but meals, chores, and the cost of managing the house are shared. No medical care is provided. *Accessory apartments* are separate apartments built onto a single-family house. The units are completely independent in that private living, sleeping, and kitchen and bathroom facilities are provided. When children desire to have their parents close to them yet understand the need for independence and privacy, this option is a possibility. *ECHO units* (elder cottage housing opportunities) may be another alternative. ECHO units are small, freestanding homes placed on the same property as the primary residence. The units are installed for a parent and removed when they are no longer needed. Zoning regulations have an impact on whether or not ECHO units are possible.

Home equity conversion is a financial procedure that helps older homeowners use the equity in their homes without moving. Some older adults are "brick rich and cash poor," meaning that they own their own homes but have problems with cash flow. Home equity conversion might be a beneficial option in such a case.

Retirement Communities are self-contained complexes that provide private living quarters as well as shared facilities, such as an auditorium, dining rooms, and activity rooms. A professional staff is present, including nurses, dietitians, and social workers. Retirement communities vary widely. Some include more than one level of care and have age restrictions, while others do not.

If extensive and extended health care is needed, a nursing home, or skilled-nursing facility, may be the best solution. A nursing home provides 24-hour medical care, and admission is by a physician's order. Medicare and Medicaid, as well as private insurance companies, reimburse some of the skilled-nursing facility expenses. It is clear that more options for living arrangements are open to older adults today than in the past.

NURSING INTERVENTIONS
RELATED TO DIETARY MANAGEMENT

- Work closely with the dietitian or nutritionist and the physician as may be required to assist the older adult in achieving optimum nutrition.
- Act as a resource person in providing information related to the physiologic demands associated with the aging process and the role of adequate nutrition; conducting dietary assessments; referring individuals and/or families to the appropriate community agencies for additional assistance (e.g., financial, medical, and nutritional); and working with counselors, dietitians, dietetic technicians, nursing assistants in providing nutritional information to older adults.
- Assess for potential nutritional problems associated with older adults in the varied settings in which the nurse works (e.g., hospital, school, clinic, office, and community).
- Instruct persons on cooking tips to encourage good nutrition (e.g., easy-to-prepare recipes, and use of herbs and spices to enhance flavors).
- Instruct persons on tips to conserve energy while cooking or preparing food (e.g., by sitting and using foot stools).

TOPIC OF INTEREST

What will the next generation of the elderly be like? It has been said that the "Baby Boomer" generation (individuals born between 1946 and 1964) will become serious about aging when their parents require care (6). This group likes youth so much that they want to take it into old age. "The Graying of America" will become "The Tinting of America" (6). Because tomorrow's older population will be better educated than their elders, they will not tolerate services that do not respect their background and knowledge. They will be healthier and wealthier than their elders because of medical advances, preventive approaches and more white-collar jobs that have better benefits. The size of this generation will give it a tremendous amount of power. Products and services for this segment will proliferate, making the U.S. an age-oriented rather than a youth-oriented society.

SPOTLIGHT ON LEARNING

You work for a home-health agency, and one of your visits is with Mr. Horgan, who is 82 years old and lives alone. He has arthritis, chronic constipation, and hypertension. He has been taking aspirin for the arthritis, and his blood pressure is under control through medication (a diuretic).

1. List the factors that have an impact on Mr. Horgan's dietary intake.
2. What suggestions can you make to Mr. Horgan to ensure adequate nutrient intake?

REVIEW QUESTIONS

1. Older Americans rely on which of the following as their major nutrition information source?
   a. nutritionists
   b. nurses
   c. families
   d. the media

2. As one ages, what is the body's primary concern?
   a. maturation
   b. homostasis
   c. energy use
   d. healing

3. What causes the lower energy requirement of older adults?
   a. decreased basal metabolism and physical activity
   b. decreased gastric motility
   c. decreased nutrient needs
   d. increased absorption and utilization of kilocalories

4. Which of the following is not a myth about aging?
  a. old age begins at age 65
  b. the elderly are in poor health
  c. the elderly are dissimilar to one another
  d. the elderly are poor

5. As a result of changes in the aging kidney, older individuals are more susceptible to which of the following?
  a. highly concentrated urine
  b. dehydration
  c. potassium retention
  d. decreased glucose tolerance

6. For which of the following nutrients is there an increased need as a result of
  aging?
  a. vitamin C
  b. vitamin K
  c. vitamin A
  d. vitamin D

7. Which of the following changes does not affect taking skinfold measurements
  in the older population?
  a. height
  b. skin thickness
  c. body fat
  d. lean body mass

8. Which drugs affect the absorption of fat-soluble nutrients?
  a. antacids
  b. penicillin
  c. colchicine
  d. mineral oil

9. Which of the following is irrelevant in a dietary assessment?
  a. prescribed and over-the-counter medications
  b. vitamin and mineral supplementation
  c. living arrangements
  d. income

10. Which program offers a minimum of one hot meal per day, five days per week,
  to participants?
  a. home health care
  b. food stamps
  c. congregate meals
  d. WIC

ACTIVITIES

1. Arrange a field trip to a congregate-meal site to learn about the types of foods served and the nutritional parameters that must be fulfilled.

2. Invite a representative from the American Association for Retired Persons to speak about the history of the group and the types of activities planned.

3. Develop a food that would perfectly fit the needs of older adults. Consider nutritional, packaging, storage, and preparation aspects.

4. Visit a nursing home and interview the staff about (a) the most common medical problems of the residents; (b) dietary challenges; and (c) foods most commonly liked and disliked by the residents. Also, observe clients in an Alzheimer's unit during mealtime.

5. Experience some of the changes that can occur with age.* Divide the class into three groups. Group 1 should separate into pairs. Each member of the pair should place cotton into his or her ears. Seated with backs facing each other, each should try to carry on a conversation. Group 2 students should drop a few unpopped popcorn kernels into their shoes and walk around the perimeter of the classroom. Each person in Group 3 should tie two fingers of the dominant hand together. Try to open tamper-evident packages with the fingers tied together.

Thought Question: How did you feel in each situation?

*Some of these ideas are from the seminar Marketing to Older Consumers, sponsored by the American Society on Aging.

REFERENCES

1. Sandstead, H.H. Some relations between nutrition and aging. *Journal of the American Dietetic Association* 85 (1985): 171–72.
2. Owen, A.Y., and R.T. Frankle. *Nutrition in the community. The art of delivering services.* 2d ed. St. Louis: Times Mirror/Mosby College Publishing, 1986.
3. Papa, A. A closer look at the mature market. *Nutrition Week* 17, no. 10 (1987): 4–5.
4. Hannigan, K.J. Meeting the needs of an aging market. *Food Engineering* February 1987: 78–84.
5. Dychtwald, K., and M. Zitter. The truth about elders. *Healthcare Forum* 30, no. 1 (1987).

6. Dychtwald, K. Marketing to older consumers. Seminar sponsored by the American Society on Aging, New York City, May 1988.

7. American Association of Retired Persons. *Truth about aging. Guidelines for accurate communications.* Washington, D.C.: The American Association of Retired Persons, 1986.

8. Fanelli, M.T., and K.J. Stevenhagen. Characterizing consumption patterns by food frequency methods: Core foods and variety of foods in the diets of older Americans. *Journal of the American Dietetic Association* 85 (1985):1570–76.

9. Grotkowski, M.L., and L.S. Sims. Nutritional knowledge, attitudes, and dietary practices of the elderly. *Journal of the American Dietetic Association* 72 (1978):499–505.

10. ———. Many frail elderly get inadequate food according to Cornell study. *Journal of the American Dietetic Association* 86 (1986):647.

11. Read, M.H., and A.S. Graney. Food supplement usage by the elderly. *Journal of the American Dietetic Association* 80 (1982):250–53.

12. Ranno, B.S., G.M. Wardlaw, and C.J. Geiger. What characterizes elderly women who overuse vitamin and mineral supplements? *Journal of the American Dietetic Association* 88 (1988):347–48.

13. Gray, G.E., et al. Vitamin supplement use in a southern California retirement community. *Journal of the American Dietetic Association* 86 (1986):800–802.

14. Belts, N.M., and V.M. Vivian. The dietary intake of the noninstitutionalized elderly. *Journal of Nutrition for the Elderly* 3 (1984):3–11.

15. Quackery. A $10 billion scandal. A Report by the Chairman of the Subcommittee on Health and Long-Term Care of the Select Committee on Aging, House of Representatives, 98th Congress, 2nd Session, May 31, 1984. Comm. Pub. No. 98-435. Washington, D.C.: GPO, 1984.

16. Zimmerman, S.A., and M.M. Krondl. Perceived intolerance of vegetables among the elderly. *Journal of the American Dietetic Association* 86 (1986):1047–51.

17. ———. Fruit consumption. *Journal of Nutrition for the Elderly* 6 (1986):73–74.

18. Donnegan, P. Older shoppers: A super market. *Progressive Grocer* August 1986: 91–98.

19. Ross Laboratories. *Aging and nutrition.* Columbus: Ross Laboratories, 1983.

20. Bidlack, W.R., et al. Nutrition and the elderly. *Food Technology* 40 (1986):81–88.

21. Rudman, D. Kidney senescence: A model for aging. *Nutrition Reviews* 46 (1988):209–214.

22. Poisson, A. The age wave. *Business Credit* 90, no. 1 (1988).

23. Munro, H.N., et al. Protein nutriture of a group of free-living elderly. *American Journal of Clinical Nutrition* 46 (1987):586–92.

24. Chernoff, R., and D.A. Lipschitz. Nutrition and aging. In *Modern nutrition in health and disease,* edited by M.E. Shils and V.R. Young. Philadelphia: Lea and Febiger, 1988.

25. Smith, D.A., W. Karmally, and V. Brown. Treating hyperlipidemia, part I: Whether and when in the elderly. *Geriatrics* 42 (1987):33–42.

26. Suter, P.M., and R.M. Russell. Vitamin requirements of the elderly. *American Journal of Clinical Nutrition* 45 (1987):501–12.

27. Hale, W.E., et al. Vitamin E. effect on symptoms and laboratory values in the elderly. *Journal of the American Dietetic Association* 86 (1986):625–29.

28. National Institutes of Health. Consensus development conference statement. Osteoporosis, 1984. *Journal of the American Medical Association* 252 (1984):799–802.

29. Foltz, M.B., and A.S. Ryan. Aging population presents marketing opportunities for dietitians. *Journal of the American Dietetic Association* 87 (1987):633–35.

30. Lecos, C. Diet and the elderly. *FDA Consumer*. HHS Pub. No. (FDA) 85-2201. December 1984–January 1985. Rockville: Department of Health and Human Services, Public Health Service, FDA.

31. ———. Statement on hypertension in the elderly: The working group on hypertension in the elderly. *Journal of the American Medical Association* 256 (1986):70.

32. ———. Prevalence of chronic diseases in U.S., '79–'81. *Nutrition Week* 18, no. 25 (1988):7.

33. Roe, D.A. Therapeutic effects of drug-nutrient interactions in the elderly. *Journal of the American Dietetic Association* 85 (1985):174–85.

34. Russell, R. *The problem of evaluating nutritional status of the elderly*. Chapel Hill: University of North Carolina, Institute of Nutrition, 1983.

35. Patterson, P.G., D.A. Christensen, and D. Robertson. Zinc levels of hospitalized elderly. *Journal of the American Dietetic Association* 85 (1985):186–91.

36. Falciglia, G., J. O'Connor, and E. Gedling. Upper-arm anthropometric norms in elderly white subjects. *Journal of the American Dietetic Association* 88 (1988):569–74.

37. Chumlea, W.C., et al. Prediction of body weight for the nonambulatory elderly from anthropometry. *Journal of the American Dietetic Association* 88 (1988):564–68.

38. Fanelli, M.T., and K.J. Stevenhagen. Consistency of energy and nutrient intakes of older adults: 24-hour recall vs. 1-day food record. *Journal of the American Dietetic Association* 86 (1986):665–67.

39. Evans, H.K., and D.J. Gines. Dietary recall method comparison for hospitalized elderly subjects. *Journal of the American Dietetic Association* 85 (1985):202–05.

40. ———. Nutrition services vital in elderly health care. *Nutrition Week* 17, no. 45 (1987):4–5.

41. Frongillo Jr., E.A., et al. Continuance of elderly on home-delivered meal programs. *American Journal of Public Health* 77 (1987):1176–79.

42. Holahan, K.B., and M.E. Kunkel. Contribution of the Title III meals program to nutrient intake of participants. *Journal of Nutrition for the Elderly* 6 (1986):45–54.

43. Lopez, L.M., and J-P. Habicht. Food stamps and the iron status of the U.S. elderly poor. *Journal of the American Dietetic Association* 87 (1987):598–603.

44. Lopez, L.M., and J-P. Habicht. Food stamps and the energy status of the U.S. elderly poor. *Journal of the American Dietetic Association* 87 (1987):1020–24.

45. Posner, B.E.M., C.G. Smigelski, and M.M. Krachenfels. Dietary characteristics and nutrient intake in an urban homebound population. *Journal of the American Dietetic Association* 87 (1987):452–56.

PART
TWO

CLINICAL ASPECTS
OF
NUTRITION

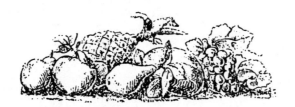

CHAPTER
6

NUTRITION AND THE PATIENT UNDER PHYSIOLOGICAL STRESS

Objectives

After studying this chapter, you will be able to
- describe the pathophysiological changes associated with excessive stress.
- differentiate between fasting in a healthy and stressed patient.
- describe the catabolic effects of fever and infection.
- list the problems associated with a persistent negative nitrogen balance (lasting for two to three weeks).
- discuss catabolism as a defense mechanism for the body.
- differentiate among the nutritional needs for patients in mild, moderate, and severe stress situations: surgery, infection, fever, burns, and fractures.
- identify nursing interventions for nutritional disorders associated with mild, moderate, and severe stress situations.

Overview

Physiological stress can occur when the body's natural defense system is mobilized in response to trauma, induced and controlled (surgery) or accidental (soft-tissue injury, fractures, or burns), infection, and fever. An altered metabolic state is created, and the severity of the condition determines the ability of the body to respond without causing a detrimental effect on the individual.

THE METABOLIC RESPONSE TO STRESS

Normally, the healthy person is able to withstand periods of increased stress, fasting, or starvation for short periods of time. Liver glycogen reserves are mobilized during the first 24 hours. Protein, mainly from skeletal muscles, is broken down, deaminated (in the liver), and used for energy. The excess nitrogen is excreted in the urine, and a negative nitrogen balance results (nitrogen output exceeds nitrogen intake). After several days, the body attempts to conserve protein and begins to break down the fat stores; fatty acids become the primary fuel source. As fatty acids are broken down, excess ketones are the by-product.

The metabolic response to stress is catabolic, with significant changes occurring as the result of hormonal stimulation. The system for the breakdown of carbohydrate, protein, and fats into the simple substances for energy use and the excretion of by-products are activated. In order to support this process, the body must accelerate the metabolic state, creating a hypermetabolic state. The pulse increases, body temperature may increase, and there is an increased need for oxygen in the tissues. If the catabolic process should continue without support, complications would result in shock and ultimately death. Table 6-1 illustrates the classification of catabolism indicating the differing energy requirements for selected patients.

The metabolic response pattern is directly proportional to the severity of the insult to the body. Elective surgery for the normal, healthy person will have minimal impact on the homeostatic mechanisms of the body, whereas a 35% BSA (body surface area) burn or a severe infection for an infant or a debilitated person may have catastrophic effects.

When the body begins to overcome the injury and tissues are regenerated and healing occurs, the process is referred to as the building or anabolic phase of metabolism. Support for the person must continue through this period in order to prevent relapse.

Kudsk et al. have identified several stages of response to injury or trauma (1). These phases of

Table 6-1. CLASSIFICATION OF CATABOLISM

CLINICAL SITUATION	DEGREE OF CATABOLISM	UREA (g/day)	INCREASE OF RESTING METABOLIC RATE OVER BMR (%)	TOTAL ENERGY REQUIREMENT (kcal)
Person in bed	1° (normal)	<5	none	1800
Uncomplicated surgery	2° (mild)	5–10	0–20	1800–2200
Multiple fractures or trauma	3° (mod)	10–15	20–50	2200–2700
Acute major infections or major burns	4° (severe)	>15	50–125	2700–4000 or more

(From M.V. Krause and L.K. Mahan, *Food and Nutrition in Diet Therapy: A Textbook of Nutritional Care* (Philadelphia: W.B. Saunders Company, 1984). Reprinted with permission.)

Table 6-2. STAGES OF RESPONSE FOLLOWING TRAUMA

STAGE	TIME DURATION
Acute	24 hours
Intermediate	24–96 hours
Adaptive	14–21 days
Chronic	months

Source: Adapted from K.A. Kudsk, J.M. Stone, and G.F. Sheldon, "Nutrition and Trauma in Burns," *Surgical Clinics of North America* 62(1982):183–92.

response and time parameters can help to predict the changes that result in the metabolic process following the initial injury and during healing (Table 6-2). Nutritional needs during these stages will also vary. In this section, the discussion will center on the body's response and the nutritional needs related to surgery, infection, fever, trauma, burns, and fractures.

Nutritional Assessment

The nutritional assessment can be of value in identifying the metabolic and energy needs prior to trauma and determining the effect of the trauma on the need for modifications to conserve protein, reverse the potential negative nitrogen balance, and provide the needed energy.

The assessment includes a variety of measurements, physical examination, diet history, and anthropometric (e.g., height, weight, skinfolds, discussed in Chapter 11), biochemical (laboratory tests), and immunologic studies.

Nutritional Implications Related to Surgery

Preoperative Period. For most patients, postoperative recovery with decreased risk of complications is directly related to the nutritional state in the preoperative period. Nutritional assessment is performed and nutritional therapy is instituted, in some instances, several weeks before hospitalization. Pre- and postoperative nutritional needs can

be identified and predicted through an analysis of the data gathered during the nutritional assessment. Obese patients may be encouraged to lose weight prior to surgery. Obesity predisposes patients to a variety of complications, including poor wound closure and infection.

The type of surgery performed determines the actual preoperative preparation. In general, most patients are NPO (nothing by mouth) for 8–12 hours prior to surgery. The diet, unless otherwise prescribed, should provide ample nutrients (glucose, amino acids, vitamins, and minerals) and liberal quantities of fluids.

Postoperative Period. The type of surgical procedure, anesthesia, and the patient response determine the point at which oral intake is resumed. Hydration along with minimal kilocalorie intake is provided through intravenous fluids. Some patients are permitted to eat the evening following a simple surgical procedure. Most patients undergoing major surgery may be permitted to resume oral intake when peristalsis is reestablished (24 hours or longer). The diet prescription and progression are determined by the physician (see Chapter 6 for a description of dietary progression).

If patients are unable to ingest oral feedings, enteral or parenteral feeding may be prescribed. Enteral feeding, considered to be an aggressive therapy, is also known as tube feeding. All enteral feedings use the digestive tract. Parenteral feedings, including total parenteral nutrition (TPN) provide nutrients directly into the bloodstream, bypassing the intestine. Parenteral feedings also bypass the liver, since they are not routed through the portal system. Despite these drawbacks, parenteral nutrition has been extremely valuable in reversing the catabolic processes in critically ill patients.

The trauma associated with surgical intervention creates a state of hypermetabolism. The catabolic state must be reversed with adequate nutrients, especially protein, to provide amino acids necessary for healing and carbohydrates to meet the increased energy needs. Vitamin and mineral replacement is also essential.

The majority of patients who undergo elective surgery have a quick recovery and are able to achieve a state of anabolism with good nutritional support. Negative nitrogen balance is usually reversed about the fifth postoperative day.

The patients who have a more complicated and prolonged recovery require more detailed and specialized nutritional support. The nutritional support may entail enteral and/or parenteral feeding initially or in conjunction with oral intake. Increased protein and kilocalorie intake is mandatory for the stressed patient in order to reverse the negative nitrogen balance.

POSSIBLE NURSING DIAGNOSES

Potential alteration in nutrition; less than body requirements related to
- decreased dietary intake (resulting from nausea, vomiting, pain, diet restrictions).
- increased need for nutrients to support the healing process.

Potential for wound infection related to
- break in skin barrier.
- altered immune response.

Alteration in comfort (pain).

Potential alteration in elimination; constipation related to
- decreased peristalsis.
- surgical procedure, anesthesia.
- analgesic medications.
- immobility.
- possible fluid deficit.

NURSING INTERVENTIONS FOR NUTRITIONAL DISORDERS

Potential alteration in nutrition, less than body requirements related to
- **decreased dietary intake (resulting from nausea, vomiting, pain, diet restrictions).**
- **increased need for nutrients to support the healing process.**

Preoperative Phase
- Encourage adequate intake of nutrients, protein, carbohydrates, vitamins and minerals.

Continued

NURSING INTERVENTIONS (continued)
- Urge liberal fluid intake, 8–10 glasses of fluid per day prior to NPO order.
- Record food and fluid intake.
- Note signs of fear and apprehension which may alter appetite.
- Maintain NPO status as prescribed in order to prevent regurgitation and potential aspiration of stomach contents.

Postoperative Phase
- Maintain hydration as prescribed, initially with intravenous fluids.
- Monitor intake and output, note signs of excessive loss or fluid overload.
- Recall that food intake may be delayed for several days depending upon the type of surgery. Follow the individual's progress to avoid malnutrition related to prolonged continuation of the NPO or liquid diet prescription.
- Keep oral mucous membranes moist by means of good oral hygiene.

Potential for wound infection related to
- **break in skin barrier.**
- **altered immune response.**

- Monitor laboratory reports; for example, note levels of nitrogen, electrolytes (sodium, potassium), red blood cells, and white blood cells.

- Note signs of impending complications, such as bleeding or sepsis.

Alteration in comfort related to incisional pain.

- Offer analgesic medications as prescribed. The patient who experiences minimal pain may be able to cooperate more readily with treatment protocols.
- Encourage ambulation as prescribed to increase intestinal motility and to prevent losses of calcium.

Potential alteration in elimination, constipation related to
- **decreased peristalsis.**
- **surgical procedure, anesthesia.**
- **analgesic medications.**
- **immobility.**
- **possible fluid deficit.**

- Listen for bowel sounds. Physician will resume orders for oral intake after bowel sounds have returned.
- Offer oral fluids and foods as prescribed; that is, clear liquid (see Chapter 7) to regular or specific diet determined by the type of surgical intervention.
- Encourage ambulation as prescribed to increase intestinal motility and to prevent losses of calcium.

Nutritional Implications Related to Infection

The response of the body to invasion by microorganisms is determined by the potency of the invasive organism and the ability of the body to mobilize a defense. (Figure 6-1 illustrates the interrelationship of malnutrition and infection.)

When microorganisms invade the body, the process of phagocytosis (increase in the number of white blood cells) occurs. The white blood cells migrate to the point of entry, and an inflammatory response begins. Metabolism is increased, and the body undergoes a number of hormonal and biochemical changes.

Hormonal changes enable the body to mobilize the stores of glycogen and promote the breakdown of proteins and fats for energy. A negative nitrogen balance may result. When the body is in sepsis (massive infection), the hormonal regulating mechanisms may malfunction. Despite increased amounts of insulin, hyperglycemia may exist and

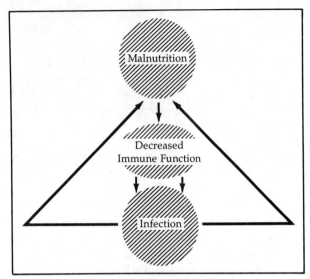

Figure 6-1. The interrelationship of malnutrition and infection.
(From J.F. Hansbrough, R.L. Zapata-Sirvent, and V.M. Peterson, "Immunodilution Following Burn Injury," *Surgical Clinics of North America* 67 (1987):69–92. Reprinted with permission.)

the body may not be able to utilize either glucose or fatty acids as fuel. Large quantities of lean tissue mass (protein) may be broken down for energy. This protein breakdown creates an even larger negative nitrogen balance.

Not only are large quantities of nitrogen lost, but also potassium, magnesium, and phosphorus may be lost as a result of cellular destruction. Sodium and fluids may be retained due to the influence of aldosterone (mineralocorticoid) and ADH (antidiuretic hormone). Zinc and iron, which are important factors in the immunologic response of the body, also seem to be of benefit to the growth of microorganisms. In order to make these substances unavailable to the infectious organisms, the minerals may be stored in the body until the infection is controlled.

The toxins given off by the microorganisms act as pyrogens and cause fever. The body thermostat located in the hypothalamus is reset to a higher level to create an environment that may be unsuita-ble to the invading microorganisms. Fever will be discussed in the next section.

The immediate goal of nutritional therapy for a person with an infection is weight maintenance. Generally, a diet that is high in protein and high in kilocalories is prescribed.

The catabolic process in a mild to moderate infection may increase energy needs 20%–30%. In severe infections, energy needs may increase to approximately 50% of the basal-metabolic needs (2). (See Figure 6-2.)

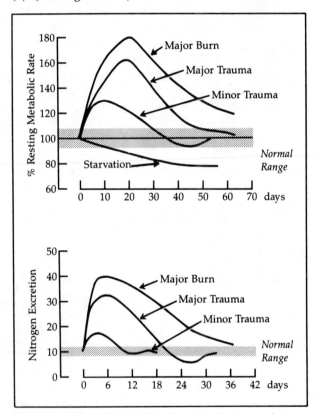

Figure 6-2. The relationship of metabolic rate and nitrogen excretion to the extent of injury.
(From W.W. Souba and D.W. Wilmore, "Diet and nutrition in the care of the patient with surgery, trauma, and sepsis," in *Modern Nutrition in Health and Disease*, edited by M.E. Shils and V.R. Young (Philadelphia: Lea and Febiger, 1988), D.W. Wilmore, "Percentage of resting metabolic rate and nitrogen excretion," *Metabolic Management of Critically Ill*, (New York: Plenum Publishing Corporation, 1977). Reprinted with permission.)

Ideally, nutrients are replaced in relation to the amount of nitrogen loss. Approximately 16% of the intake kilocalories should come from protein sources. This quantity is based on a ratio of 150:1 (kilocalories to nitrogen) (3). Protein of high biological value should be included.

The diet prescription will be determined by the physician. Patients with severe sepsis may receive parenteral or enteral feedings until it is possible to consume oral feedings. Enteral feeding as opposed to parenteral feeding is the optimal route for intake of nutrients if the gastrointestinal tract is functioning (4). If a person has not been able to tolerate oral or enteral feedings, it is important to offer small, dilute amounts of clear liquids in order to prevent dehydration.

POSSIBLE NURSING DIAGNOSES

Potential alteration in nutrition; less than body requirements related to
- increased metabolic rate.
- infection.
- anorexia.
- fever.

Potential fluid-volume alteration (excess or deficit) related to
- sodium retention (excess).
- fever (deficit).
- diaphoresis (deficit).

Potential alteration in body temperature related to infection.

Potential activity intolerance related to weakness and fatigue associated with catabolic process.

NURSING INTERVENTIONS
FOR NUTRITIONAL DISORDERS

Work closely with the dietitian, physician, and patient to determine the dietary needs to promote anabolism.

Potential alteration in nutrition; less than body requirements related to
- **increased metabolic rate.**
- **infection.**
- **anorexia.**
- **fever.**

- Offer small quantities of food at more frequent intervals (6–8 feedings per day) if regular meal intake and snacks are not tolerated.
- Weigh daily to determine the effectiveness of diet.
- Administer mineral and vitamin supplements as prescribed.

Continued

NURSING INTERVENTIONS *(continued)*

Potential fluid-volume alteration (excess or deficit) related to
- **sodium retention (excess).**
- **fever (deficit).**
- **diaphoresis (deficit).**

- Encourage increased fluid intake, 2000–3000 ml/day as prescribed.
- Observe for side effects of antiinfective drugs. Diarrhea, nausea, and vomiting may require alteration in oral intake.
- Weigh daily to determine the effectiveness of diet. Be alert for fluid retention as opposed to nutritional weight gain in the critically ill patient.

Potential alteration in body temperature related to infection.

- Monitor laboratory reports to note increased white blood count.
- Monitor vital signs to detect the presence of fever. Infection will increase fluid needs of the patient.

Potential activity intolerance related to weakness and fatigue associated with catabolic process.

- Instruct the patient to continue with prescribed diet through convalescence. Activity levels may increase as the infection is controlled.

Nutritional Implications Related to Fever

Body temperature is the balance between heat produced and heat lost during metabolic processes in the body. Normal body temperature varies in relation to a number of physiological factors, such as excitement, exercise, digestion, and increased environmental temperatures. Body temperature also normally fluctuates throughout the day. The lowest temperature generally occurs during sleep in the early morning hours, and the highest temperature occurs in the late afternoon.

Fever is an elevation of body temperature above the normal range (36°C–37.4°C or 96.8°F–99.3°F). Fever can result from a variety of causes: inflammatory processes within the body, infections, trauma, CNS (central nervous system) disorders, dehydration, or from a number of unknown causes.

Endogenous pyrogens are formed in response to a microbial toxin or other stimuli. Prostaglandins are among the substances produced in the body that stimulate the thermoreceptor site in the anterior hypothalamus. The thermostatic set point in the hypothalamus is reset above the normal 37°C (98.6°F). Drugs such as acetylsalicylic acid (aspirin) and acetaminophen (Tylenol) are effective in treating fever because they inhibit prostaglandin synthesis.

In some instances, a fever can be beneficial. Fever generally creates an environment that is not suitable to microbial growth. Depending on the type and concentration of the microorganism and the health status of the host, normal body defense systems, including fever, can be augmented to help overcome the attack on the body. Rest, fluid intake, and adequate nutrition may help a person overcome the infection. If the host is unable to mobilize the necessary defenses, illness may result.

Fever is a symptom, and accurate measurement of the increases in body temperature may provide important clues in fighting disease. Adequate management of the fever is essential in order to reverse the catabolic process. High fevers produce a marked catabolic effect on the body (Figure 6-3.)

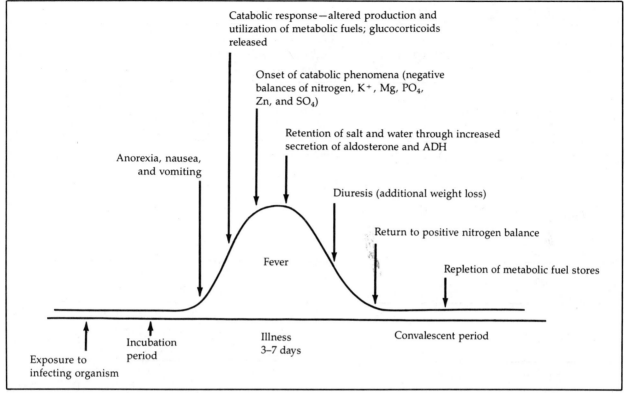

Catabolic response—altered production and utilization of metabolic fuels; glucocorticoids released

Onset of catabolic phenomena (negative balances of nitrogen, K^+, Mg, PO_4, Zn, and SO_4)

Retention of salt and water through increased secretion of aldosterone and ADH

Diuresis (additional weight loss)

Anorexia, nausea, and vomiting

Return to positive nitrogen balance

Fever

Repletion of metabolic fuel stores

Exposure to infecting organism

Incubation period

Illness 3–7 days

Convalescent period

Figure 6-3. The catabolic response to infection.
(From M.V. Krause and L.K. Mahan, *Food, Nutrition and Diet Therapy: A Textbook of Nutritional Care* (Philadelphia: W.B. Saunders Company, 1984) and W.R. Beisel, "The influence of infection or injury on nutritional requirements during adolescence," in *Nutrient Requirements in Adolescence,* edited by J.I. McKigney and H.N. Munro (Cambridge, MA: MIT Press, 1976.) Reprinted with permission.)

For every degree rise in body temperature, the metabolic rate increases. One degree Celsius causes a 10%–13% rise in metabolic rate; 1°F causes approximately a 7% rise in metabolic rate. A prolonged fever of 40°C (104°F) may increase metabolic rate by 40%. If the fever is accompanied by restlessness, the metabolic needs may even be greater.

Insulin requirements may be increased due to the increased need and availability of glucose for energy. Lack of, or inadequate insulin production in the diabetic patient intensifies the process of catabolism because glucose cannot be used for energy. The fat and muscle tissues are then catabolized as alternate energy sources. Exoge-

nous insulin may be prescribed for the diabetic patient during periods of increased stress (see Chapter 13).

Diet therapy during fever will be determined by the physician in relation to the cause and duration of the pathological process. Basically, the diet should be high in protein, high kilocalorie, with increased amounts of B-complex vitamins, as well as vitamins A and C (5).

Fluid replacement is essential because of the losses associated with hyperventilation and diaphoresis. A 30-year-old male weighing 70 kg with a fever of 103°F would need approximately 3000 ml of fluid intake per day (6). Infants and the elderly may respond more dramatically to fluid changes associ-

Table 6-3. BASELINE FLUID REQUIREMENTS IN TEMPERATE CLIMATE

ADULTS based on "ideal" weight for height and age, ± 20% of ideal weight)		
	AGE	AVERAGE WATER REQUIREMENTS (ml/kg/day)
Average	20–55	35
Young Active	16–30	40
Older	55–75 ±	30
Elderly	75	25
CHILDREN (over 5 kg body weight to age 18)		
		AVERAGE WATER REQUIREMENTS (ml/kg/day)
First 10 kg of body weight		100
Second 10 kg of body weight		50
Weight above 20 kg		25

From H.T. Randall, "Water, Electrolytes and Acid-Base Balance," In *Modern Nutrition in Health and Disease*, edited by M.E. Shils and V.R. Young. (Philadelphia: Lea and Febiger, 1988). Reprinted with permission.

ated with fever. Using the data in Table 6-3, the nurse can calculate approximate fluid needs for individual patients.

Sodium and potassium losses may also be increased during fever. Monitoring of the serum levels of the electrolytes will help determine the amount of deficit. Sodium replacement is possible through the use of salty broths, bouillon, pretzels, and liberal use of salt on foods. Fruit juices and milk are good sources of potassium.

Initially, a person with a fever may be anorectic.

A great deal of encouragement is needed to entice the person to consume even part of the needed nutrients and fluids. Bland diets that contain foods that are easily digested may be more readily tolerated. Frequent, small feedings should be offered until the person is able to eat three meals and a bedtime snack. Diet progression to a high protein, high kilocalorie diet should be as rapid as possible. Enteral and/or parenteral feedings may be necessary for those persons who cannot consume oral feedings.

POSSIBLE NURSING DIAGNOSES

Potential alteration in body temperature related to
- infection.
- trauma.
- dehydration.

Potential alteration in fluid volume; deficit related to
- infection.
- fever.
- diaphoresis.

Potential alteration in nutrition related to
- fever.
- infection.
- anorexia.

NURSING INTERVENTIONS FOR NUTRITIONAL DISORDERS

Work closely with the dietitian, physician, and patient to determine the dietary needs necessary to reverse the catabolic process of fever (high protein, high kilocalorie, with vitamin and mineral supplements).

Potential alteration in body temperature related to
- **infection.**
- **trauma.**
- **dehydration.**

- Encourage increased fluid intake as prescribed (3000–5000 ml per day) to meet basal needs and aid in the renal excretion of toxins.
- Monitor laboratory reports. Pay close attention to alterations in white blood count and electrolytes.

Potential alteration in fluid volume; deficit related to
- **infection.**
- **fever.**
- **diaphoresis.**

- Monitor intake and output to determine hydration needs of the patient.
- Be alert for side effects of antiinfective drugs. Diarrhea, nausea, and vomiting may require alteration in fluid intake.

Potential alteration in nutrition related to
- **fever.**
- **infection.**
- **anorexia.**

Continued

NURSING INTERVENTIONS *(continued)*

- Offer small amounts of easily digested foods at frequent intervals until three meals and a snack are tolerated.
- Weigh daily to determine fluid and nutrient needs.
- Instruct the patient to:
    take antipyretic drugs, such as aspirin, with food to prevent gastric irritation;

continue the prescribed diet through convalescence (activity levels may increase as fever or infection subsides);

take vitamin and mineral supplements as prescribed, if foods do not provide sufficient intake.

Nutritional Implications Related to Burns

Thermal injury to body tissues constitutes a major threat to the host by inducing severe stress. The hypermetabolic state is created by the destruction of body tissue, losses of large quantities of protein, fluids, and electrolytes. Immune responses within the host are diminished and the potential for infection is high. As with other forms of trauma, the extent and severity of the burn determine the amount of catabolic response by the body.

The age of the person and presence of any other associated illness may play a role in the severity of the situation. Smaller-surface-area burns may be fatal to the elderly, chronically ill, or infants. (Review the pathophysiology associated with severe stress or trauma included in this chapter.)

Burns constitute a grave stress situation for the patient. Fluid loss creates a major concern during the first 12–24 hours postburn. After the initial assessment, the primary emphases are cardiovascular resuscitation and restoration of circulating blood volume. Nutritional support is provided after the patient has been stabilized.

Fluid replacement is essential to prevent hypovolemia (decreased blood volume) because blood and serum leak from the capillaries in the area of the burn due to injury to the capillary as well as impaired cell-membrane function. Edema also occurs in other parts of the body due to changes in the permeability of the capillaries in general (7).

Crystalloid solutions such as lactated Ringer's are commonly used to replace fluid loss in the initial period postburn. Glucose solutions are not well tolerated because of the glucose intolerance associated with catabolism. The Parkland formula (3–5 ml/kg body weight × percent of BSA burned) is currently widely used in the United States to determine the amount of fluids to be replaced. Half the calculated fluid loss is replaced during the first eight hours postburn. The remaining fluid is administered evenly over the next 16 hours. A burn involving 40% of the total BSA for a male who weighs 70 kg may require 13 liters of fluid in the first 24 hours (8).

During the second 24-hour period postburn, capillary leaks begin to heal. When this healing occurs, fluids are generally replaced with colloid (plasma or albumin) solutions for approximately eight hours, followed by 5% dextrose in water as needed. Colloid solutions are used to draw edema from the tissues of the body into the vascular tree.

Urinary output is maintained at no less than 30–50 ml per hour for adults or one milliliter per kilogram of body weight per hour for children. Output that is less than these parameters indicates inadequate renal perfusion. Diuresis usually begins after the second day.

Researchers have found that infection with systemic sepsis is the major cause of death in severely burned patients (9). The burn patient is particularly prone to infection because massive areas of the first line of defense (the intact skin and mucous membrane in the gastrointestinal and respiratory tracts) may have been broken. The patient may also face repeated surgical procedures for debridement of the eschar (scab composed of nonliving tissue, which may constrict circulation in the area of the burn). Treatment may involve the use of antibiotic prophylaxis, debridement, and skin grafting. Supportive care, including adequate nutrition, is essential.

Severely burned patients may be treated with cimetidine (Tagamet) and antacids because of the tendency to form stress ulcers (see Chapter 7). Stress ulcers of the gastrointestinal tract are frequently referred to as Curlings' ulcers if the ulceration occurs in conjunction with burns.

After the systems of the body are functioning, nutritional emphasis begins. Patients with severe burns may be NPO for 48 hours or more. When there is evidence of intestinal peristalsis, oral feedings may be prescribed. The patient will frequently be given clear fluids with progression to a high kilocalorie, high protein diet with necessary mineral and vitamin supplements as indicated. Enteral or parenteral feedings may be necessary for some patients, depending on the extent of the injury and the involvement of the respiratory and/or alimentary tracts in the burned areas.

Due to the hypermetabolic process initiated by the burn, kilocalories must be sufficient to enable the body to rebuild the damaged tissues. It is estimated that a burn can increase the metabolic rate two to two-and-a-half times the resting metabolic rate (10).

A formula that is used to calculate the needed kilocalories is (3):

> Adults: 25 kcal × preburn weight (kg) + 40 kcal × percent burn.
> Children: 40–60 kcal × preburn weight (kg) + 40 kcal × percent burn.

Using the first formula, an adult who weighs 70 kg with 40% BSA burns would require approximately 3350 kcal (3).

The optimum ratio of kilocalories to nitrogen is still unknown. Patients with severe burns may lose more than 200 g of protein per day during the first few weeks after injury. Researchers are not clear as to the level of protein required to minimize the catabolic process (10).

The physician will prescribe a level of dietary protein based on the determination of renal and hepatic function. Individual calculations are needed for each patient.

POSSIBLE NURSING DIAGNOSES

Potential fluid-volume alteration (deficit in 12–48 hours or excess after 48 hours).

Potential alteration in nutrition; less than body requirements related to
- increased catabolic response.
- anorexia due to pain or infection.
- inability to ingest adequate nutrients.

Potential alteration in elimination; constipation related to
- fluid shifts.
- paralytic ileus.

- analgesic medications.
- inadequate intake of nutrients.

Knowledge deficit related to
- fluid requirements.
- nutritional requirements.

NURSING INTERVENTIONS FOR NUTRITIONAL DISORDERS

Work closely with the dietitian, physician, and patient to determine the dietary needs in order to reverse the catabolic process associated with burns.

Potential fluid-volume deficit (12–48 hours).
Potential fluid-volume excess (after 48 hours).

- Monitor urinary output every hour until stable.
- Monitor laboratory reports at frequent intervals.
- Record preburn weight because postburn weight may be inaccurate because of, for example, edema or dressings.
- Record all intake and output. Nutrients and fluids are essential to reverse the catabolic process and prevent complications.
- Monitor vital signs to note impending complications, such as shock or sepsis.
- Offer oral electrolyte solutions to the less severely burned person. Water may further upset the fluid and electrolyte imbalance.

Potential alteration in elimination; constipation related to
- **fluid shifts.**
- **paralytic ileus.**
- **analgesic medications.**
- **inadequate intake of nutrients.**

- Assess for bowel sounds.
- Offer foods rich in fiber to prevent constipation, if not contraindicated.

Potential alteration in nutrition; less than body requirements related to
- **increased catabolic response.**

- **anorexia due to pain or infection.**
- **inability to ingest adequate nutrients.**

- Observe for gastrointestinal upset. Bleeding, for example, may indicate the presence of stress-ulcer formation.
- Observe for signs of potassium deficit due to massive cellular injury (thirst, muscle weakness, dizziness, confusion, EKG changes).
- Administer electrolyte and vitamin supplements as prescribed.
- Schedule dressing changes at times other than prior to meals because of potential for anorexia.
- Offer small high kilocalorie, high protein feedings at frequent intervals (if tolerated). High kilocalorie, high protein commercial formulas, such as Ensure Plus HN and Traumacal, may be offered.

Knowledge deficit related to
- **fluid requirements.**
- **nutritional requirements**

- Instruct the patient to
    learn techniques for enteral administration of nutrients (tube feedings) if necessary.
    consume a high kilocalorie, high protein diet through the period of convalescence to ensure adequate repair and healing of tissues.
    use nutritious snacks (yogurt, half sandwich of meat with milk, custard) to supplement meals if necessary.
    take mineral and vitamin supplements as prescribed.
    continue to consume 8–10 glasses of fluid per day, if possible.

Nutritional Implications Related to Fractures

A fracture is a break in the continuity of a bone. Most fractures are the result of a traumatic injury associated with a home–related accident, recreational injury (stress fracture associated with repeated injury to the foot during jogging), motor vehicle accidents, or on-the-job injuries. Elderly persons may be more prone to fractures due to osteoporosis (loss of bone mass). (Refer to Chapter 14 for a discussion of osteoporosis.) Pathologic fractures, such as those associated with osteoporosis or other disease processes, such as cancer of the bone or metastasis from another site, result from normal activities or minimal injury that would usually not injure healthy bone.

Soft-tissue injury in the area of the fracture usually results because the strong muscles, ligaments, and tendons in the area of the fracture cause the bone fragments to separate following injury. The bleeding that is associated with the tissue trauma may actually be the first step in the healing process.

A hematoma forms and thrombocytes together with fibroblasts work to form a fibrin network to "wall off" the area so that the normal inflammatory response of the body can be effective. Immobilization of an extremity facilitates the healing process. Since bony tissue is involved, osteoblasts (bone-forming cells) migrate to the walled-off area and begin to form granulation tissue. The capillary network in the damaged area increases so that additional nutrients and mineral salts (calcium and phosphorus) can be brought to the site. The granulation phase leads to the development of callus, the bony material that aids in the healing of the fracture, and is ultimately replaced by true bone. Depending on the severity of the fracture, the healing process may take from three to six months or more.

Bone healing is an intricate process involving a number of local and systemic responses. The type of bone involved, the age of the patient (children generally heal faster), and the presence of other diseases, such as diabetes mellitus, may alter the healing process.

Treatment of fractures involves closed or open (surgical) reduction of the fracture; internal fixation with pins, screws, intermedullary nails, or wires; and immobilization with a cast, brace, or elastic bandage, depending on the severity.

Because of the complex mechanisms involved in the healing process, a negative nitrogen balance can occur if sufficient kilocalories or protein are not available to supply the body's needs. The loss of nitrogen (protein) is accompanied by losses of calcium (primarily due to immobility), phosphorus, potassium, and sulfur. If infection and fever are also present, as described earlier in this chapter, the catabolic process may be accelerated.

The diet should provide adequate kilocalories and increased protein intake to foster an anabolic state required for the healing process. Calcium supplements are usually withheld until the patient has some degree of mobility in order to prevent the excess calcium from precipitating out in the urine and forming calculi (stones).

Vitamin supplements may also be necessary. Vitamin C is important in the formation of collagen substances to foster healing and increased capillary building. Vitamin D allows the body to utilize the available calcium and phosphorus. Fluid volume should be adequate (2500–3000 ml per day unless contraindicated) so that waste products, especially those resulting from immobility and demineralization of bone, are excreted.

POSSIBLE NURSING DIAGNOSES

Potential alteration in nutrition; less than body requirements related to
- decreased dietary intake.
- pain.
- increased need to support healing process.

Alteration in comfort; pain related to tissue trauma.

Potential alteration in elimination; constipation, secondary to trauma or surgery related to
- immobility.
- possible fluid deficit.
- inadequate fiber intake.

Potential impaired home-maintenance management related to physical immobility.

NURSING INTERVENTIONS FOR NUTRITIONAL DISORDERS

Work closely with the patient and dietitian to plan a diet that provides sufficient kilocalories to allow the body to use protein intake for new bone synthesis.

Potential alteration in nutrition; less than body requirements related to
- **decreased dietary intake.**
- **pain.**
- **increased need to support healing process.**

- Encourage adequate intake of nutrients (especially protein and vitamins C and D).
- Provide between-meal supplements as necessary.
- Offer analgesic medications as prescribed so that the patient may cooperate with treatment protocols.
- Monitor laboratory reports; note levels of nitrogen, electrolytes (calcium, phosphorus, potassium), and white blood cells. Hypercalcemia may be present due to demineralization of bone associated with immobility.

Alteration in comfort; pain related to tissue trauma.

- Offer analgesic medications as prescribed.

Potential alteration in elimination; constipation, secondary to trauma or surgery related to
- **immobility.**
- **possible fluid deficit.**
- **inadequate fiber intake.**

- Encourage adequate intake of sufficient fiber in the diet to prevent constipation.
- Urge liberal fluid intake (8–10 glasses of fluid per day) to prevent urinary stasis and constipation.

Potential impaired home-maintenance management related to physical immobility.

- Assess degree of immobility and ability to provide self-care (food preparation).
- Arrange for Meals On Wheels, if necessary.

TOPIC OF INTEREST

Numerous commercial supplements have been formulated to meet the high nutritional requirements of patients under metabolic stress. See Table 6-4 for available products and the characteristics of each.

Table 6-4. SUPPLEMENTS USED FOR PATIENTS UNDER METABOLIC STRESS

PRODUCT	MANUFACTURER	KCALS/ 8 OZ.	PROTEIN	FAT	CHO
			—% of kcal—		
Traumacal	Mead Johnson	355	22 sodium and calcium caseinate	40 soy oil, MCT* oil	38 corn syrup, sugar
Ensure Plus	Ross Labs	355	14.7 sodium and calcium caseinate	32 corn oil	53.3 corn syrup, sucrose
Ensure Plus HN	Ross Labs	355	16.7 sodium and calcium caseinate	30 corn oil	53.3 hydro-lyzed corn-starch, sucrose
Precision Isotein HN	Sandoz Nutrition	350	23 delac-tosed lactal-bumin, sodium caseinate	25 soy oil, MCT*	52 malto-dextrin, fructose

*Medium-chain triglyceride

SPOTLIGHT ON LEARNING

Jack Jones, age 25, is recovering from a 20% body burn. His preburn weight was 80 kg. Jack has been dismissed from the hospital, and you are making a home visit to assess his knowledge of the dietary regimen that is required. Jack lives alone and admits that he rarely cooks. He says that he does not eat breakfast regularly and that his friends drop off foods from the local fast-food restaurants for lunch and dinner. He usually eats a sandwich (roast beef, hamburger) and french fries and drinks soda. Sometimes he eats pizza. He is getting bored with the food but does not know what to do.

1. What are some of the actions you can take to help Jack meet his dietary needs?
2. What suggestions do you have for Jack?

Hint. Formula for calculating necessary kilocalories is 25 kcal × preburn weight (kg) + 40 kcal × percent burn.

REVIEW QUESTIONS

1. Protein contains an element that differs from other energy nutrients. Identify that element.
  a. oxygen
  b. hydrogen
  c. nitrogen
  d. carbon

2. During the first day of fasting, the body depends primarily on which of the following to produce energy?
  a. amino acids
  b. glycogen
  c. fatty acids
  d. fat

3. Which of the following measurements is not included in nutritional assessment?
  a. height
  b. weight
  c. skinfolds
  d. bone thickness

4. Why are most patients NPO for 8–12 hours prior to surgery?
   a. to deplete the body of excess nitrogen
   b. to prevent potential aspiration of stomach contents
   c. to prevent the loss of lean body tissue for energy
   d. to prevent the loss of calcium stores in the body

5. What type of diet is necessary in order to maintain positive nitrogen balance in a major stress condition such as severe sepsis or burn?
   a. high fiber, low carbohydrate
   b. high protein, high kilocalorie
   c. low carbohydrate, low fat
   d. low protein, high carbohydrate

6. A person on a high-protein diet should choose which of the following foods to receive the best source of protein?
   a. eggs
   b. peanut butter
   c. spinach
   d. whole-wheat bread

7. Why is a high-carbohydrate, high-protein diet beneficial for anabolism?
   a. carbohydrates can be used for energy
   b. protein utilization is increased
   c. protein will stabilize fluid loss
   d. carbohydrate increases fluid loss

8. During physiological stress, the body conserves which of the following?
   a. fat
   b. protein
   c. carbohydrate
   d. water

9. Through which of the following does the gastrointestinal tract respond to stress?
   a. increasing the blood supply
   b. increasing gastric secretions
   c. slowing secretions and muscular activity
   d. not reacting to the stress hormone secretion

10. When should nutritional support for the patient with a moderately severe burn usually occur?
    a. during the first 12 hours
    b. 24 hours postburn
    c. approximately 72 hours postburn
    d. 2 weeks postburn

ACTIVITIES

1. Explain the fallacy in the old saying: "Feed a cold and starve a fever."

2. Visit the library. Using a food composition table, make a list of snacks that provide increased amounts of protein, and vitamins A, B-complex, and C.

3. Calculate the energy needs of a child who weighs 25 kg and has sustained burns over 25% of her body.

4. A young woman with severe infection must consume 3000 ml of fluid each day. Plan a regimen that should allow her to consume the necessary fluid during her waking hours.

5. Obtain a diet history from a classmate, incluidng a one– to three–day food record, and calculate average kilocalorie and protein intake (using a food composition table). Calculate the protein and kilocalorie needs if a mild to moderate infection were present. What changes in the diet would be required to meet the recommended protein and kilocalorie levels?

REFERENCES

1. Kudsk, K.A., J.M. Stone, and G.F. Sheldon. Nutrition and trauma in burns. *Surgical Clinics of North America* 62(1982):183–92.
2. Souba, W.W., and D.W. Wilmore. Diet and nutrition in the care of the patient with surgery, trauma, and sepsis. In *Modern nutrition in health and disease,* 7th ed., edited by M.E. Shils and V.R. Young. Philadelphia: Lea and Febiger, 1988.
3. Robinson, C.H., et al. *Normal and therapeutic nutrition.* New York: Macmillan Publishing Company, 1986.
4. Apelgren, K.N., and D.W. Wilmore. Nutritional care of the critically ill. *Surgical Clinics of North America* 63(1983):497–506.
5. Krause, M.V., and L.K. Mahan. *Food, nutrition and diet therapy: A textbook of nutritional care.* Philadelphia: W.B. Saunders Company, 1984.
6. Randall, H.T. Water, electrolytes and acid-base balance. In *Modern nutrition in health and disease,* 7th ed., edited by M.E. Shils and V.R. Young. Philadelphia: Lea and Febiger, 1988.
7. Demling, R.H. Fluid replacement in burned patients. *Surgical Clinics of North America* 67(1987):15–29.
8. Krupp, M.A., M.J. Chatton, and L.M. Tierney, Jr. *Current medical diagnoses and treatment: 1986.* Los Altos: Lange Medical Publications, 1986.
9. Dasko, C.C., A. Luterman, and P.W. Curreri. Systemic antibiotic treatment in burned patients. *Surgical Clinics of North America* 67(1987):57–68.
10. Pasulka, P.S., and T.L. Wachtel. Nutritional considerations for the burned patient. *Surgical Clinics of North America* 67(1987):109–31.

CHAPTER
7

NUTRITION AND THE PATIENT WITH GASTROINTESTINAL DISORDERS

Objectives

After studying this chapter, you will be able to

- describe the dietary management for common problems of the gastrointestinal tract (e.g., nausea, vomiting, diarrhea, constipation, heartburn, and flatus).
- identify nursing interventions related to the nutritional disorders associated with the common problems.
- describe dietary management for selected dysfunctions of the gastrointestinal tract and accessory organs.
- identify nursing interventions for nutritional disorders associated with selected dysfunctions of the gastrointestinal tract and accessory organs.

Overview

Nutritional status can be affected in numerous ways when there is an alteration in the gastrointestinal tract. Common problems such as nausea and vomiting may temporarily, or over a long period, disrupt nutrient intake. Multiple alterations and dysfunctions may interfere with the digestion and/or absorption of nutrients or elimination of waste products.

COMMON GASTROINTESTINAL PROBLEMS

Everyone either has or will experience one or more of the common problems that affect the gastrointestinal tract: nausea and vomiting, diarrhea, constipation, heartburn, and gas (flatus). These conditions may be associated with a disease process, but for the greater majority of persons, they are transient conditions that are self-limiting and may have been precipitated by a change in lifestyle, such as travel or lack of sleep, or by brief exposure to a toxic or irritating substance such as contaminated food.

Nausea, vomiting, and diarrhea are forms of acute syndromes that affect the gastrointestinal tract. Even though the majority of conditions will be short-term, the nurse must be aware of the tremendous potential for dehydration and depletion of electrolytes associated with the loss of gastric and intestinal fluids.

Nausea and Vomiting

A person with repeated episodes of vomiting or diarrhea must be assessed for fluid and electrolyte losses by monitoring output; noting the appearance of the skin (poor turgor), mucous membranes (dry mouth and tongue), and eyes (sunken, with dark circles); and noting the presence of impending complications, such as abdominal pain and/or fever.

Treatment of nausea may consist of allowing the gastrointestinal tract to rest for several hours. Oral fluid replacement may be resumed when the nausea subsides. Fluid replacement may be concurrent during episodes of diarrhea. Small quantities of non-irritating, clear fluids, such as broth, tea, or gelatin, may be offered when feasible. Advise against the use of red-colored fluids or gelatin products, if possible. If vomiting is excessive and/or prolonged, the color may disguise the presence of bleeding. Intravenous fluid and electrolyte replacement may be necessary for infants, young children, or elderly individuals, who are more sensitive to internal shifts and losses of fluids and electrolytes.

The types of fluids that might be offered to a person on a clear liquid diet are:

- carbonated beverages
- clear or strained fruit juices (apple, cranberry, grape)
- clear broths, bouillon, consomme (fat-free)
- coffee or tea (with sugar, if desired)
- electrolyte-replacement solutions (Gatorade, Pedialyte)
- fruit ices
- gelatins
- hard sugar candies
- popsicles
- water or ice chips

A clear-liquid diet is nutritionally inadequate but can be used for a short time. Clear liquids primarily allay thirst and provide minimal kilocalories (energy) in the form of carbohydrates.

Initially, the person should be instructed to take only small amounts of fluid so as to avoid stimulating subsequent vomiting. After water is tolerated, suggest the use of broth, juices, or electrolyte replacement fluids such as Gatorade or Pedialyte, alone or used to prepare gelatin. Intake of large quantities of water or ice chips can replace fluid loss but may actually intensify the electrolyte loss. If a nutritionally adequate clear-liquid diet is needed, an elemental diet such as Vital High Nitrogen, Vivonex HN, or Criticare HN may be ordered by the physician.

If the fluids are tolerated by the patient, the doctor may order the clear-liquid diet to be upgraded to full-liquid, then soft or light, and, finally, a regular diet. See Table 7-1 for fluids and foods that are contained in full-liquid and soft diets.

Table 7-1. EXAMPLES OF FOODS INCLUDED ON FULL-LIQUID AND SOFT DIETS

FULL LIQUID DIETS	
FOOD GROUP	FOODS INCLUDED
Milk	any type of milk (if no lactose intolerance), ice cream, cream soups, plain yogurt, sherbets, puddings, custard
Meats	strained meat or poultry, eggs, cooked in custards; raw eggs should not be used in, for example, milk shakes or eggnog because of the potential for bacterial contamination[1]
Fruits/vegetables	fruit and vegetable juices, strained fruits and vegetables
Grains	cereal gruel
Fats	butter, margarine, cream if not fat-free diet
Other	any component or combination of clear liquids, sugars (honey, syrup, jelly, hard candy), salt or flavorings as tolerated, spices as tolerated
SOFT DIETS	
Milk	all milk and dairy products
Meat	all meat, poultry and fish, prepared by broiling, baking or roasting (not frying), eggs (except fried)
Fruits/vegetables	canned or cooked
Grains	all breads, pastas, noodles, rice, and cereals
Other	butter, margarine, spices, and desserts as tolerated

[1]Source: M.E. St. Louis, et al., "The Emergence of Grade A Eggs as a Major Source of Salmonella Enteritides Infections. New Implications for the Control of Salmonellosis." *Journal of the American Medical Association* 259, no. 14 (1988):2103–7.

POSSIBLE NURSING DIAGNOSES

Potential alteration in nutrition; less than body requirements, manifested by lack of desire to ingest foods related to nausea and vomiting.

Potential fluid deficit related to inadequate intake of fluids and vomiting.

NURSING INTERVENTIONS FOR NUTRITIONAL DISORDERS

Potential alteration in nutrition, less than body requirements manifested by lack of desire to ingest foods related to nausea and vomiting.

- Provide diet as prescribed, initially NPO (nothing by mouth) to prevent increased intestinal peristalsis.
- Determine food and fluid preferences when appropriate.
- Advise against the use of red-colored fluids or gelatin products since they may mask bleeding.
- Provide or assist with frequent oral hygiene to reduce unpleasant taste in the mouth, especially after vomiting.

Potential fluid deficit related to inadequate intake of fluids and vomiting.

- Monitor intake and output.
- Record weight.
- Monitor electrolytes and report abnormal values.
- Monitor for poor skin turgor, dry mouth, sunken eyes, and/or impending complications, such as abdominal pain and/or fever.

Diarrhea

Diarrhea, which is defined as an increase in the water content (in excess of 200 grams per day) and the number of stools, can be both acute and chronic (1). Acute diarrhea may be caused by irritation of the mucosal lining of the intestine. The inflammatory process that results causes a decrease in the transit time of the intestinal contents with decreased absorption and leads to the potential for loss of fluids and electrolytes. Chronic diarrhea, which may be associated with conditions like Crohn's disease, ulcerative colitis, malabsorption syndromes (lactose intolerance), or infectious process may also lead to fluid and electrolyte and acid-base imbalances (1). Pus and/or mucus may be present in stools of patients with chronic diarrhea.

Assessment of the patient includes determining the number and consistency of the stools and the presence of cramps or abdominal pain. It is important to listen for hyperactive, gurgling bowel sounds. Carefully note signs of dehydration similar to those listed above in the discussion of nausea and vomiting.

Goals for the care of the patient at home or in the hospital include reducing the number of stools per day. This may involve a combination of pharmacologic and diet therapy. Prevention of dehydration and skin breakdown (perianal) is essential. Diarrhea that persists for more than 48–72 hours should be reported to the physician. Infants, young children, elderly or debilitated persons need to be carefully monitored.

Mild, acute diarrhea may be managed initially with rest for the intestines in order to prevent increased peristalsis associated with food intake. When the person is able to tolerate fluids by mouth, clear liquids and then full liquids may be offered (see Table 7–1). Patients with severe diarrhea may require intravenous replacement.

Patients who suffer from chronic diarrhea may manifest a number of nutritional deficiencies. The physician will prescribe the diet best suited to the needs of the individual patient. It is important for the nurse and the dietitian to work closely with the patient to help meet the nutritional needs. Dietary modifications for persons with Crohn's disease, ulcerative colitis, and malabsorption syndromes are discussed later in this chapter.

POSSIBLE NURSING DIAGNOSES

Alteration in bowel elimination; diarrhea related to
- nutritional disorders.

- metabolic or endocrine disorders.
- dumping syndrome.
- infection.

NURSING INTERVENTIONS FOR NUTRITIONAL DISORDERS

Alteration in bowel elimination; diarrhea related to nutritional disorders, metabolic or endocrine disorders, dumping syndrome, infection.

- Monitor frequency and characteristics of stool.
- Listen for and record bowel sounds.

- Monitor intake and output and weight.
- Monitor electrolytes and record abnormal values.
- Instruct the patient in measures to prevent and control diarrhea and provide for necessary fluid intake.

Constipation

Constipation is difficult to define because of the subjective nature of the condition. Generally, constipation refers to infrequent or difficult passage of feces. Normal bowel movements may vary in number from 3–12 stools per week (2).

Inactivity or lack of physical exercise, diet that contains low fiber or highly refined foods, advancing age, drug therapy (e.g., iron salts, calcium, antacids containing aluminum, and antihypertensive agents), and laxative and enema abuse are among the many factors that may lead to the development of constipation.

Treatment of constipation depends on the cause. The majority of individuals benefit from establishing a routine of regular exercise, adequate fluid intake (8–10 glasses per day), increasing the fiber content of the diet, relaxation, and establishing a regular time for bowel movements. Many persons need to be instructed that it is not necessary to have a bowel movement every day.

Much research is currently being conducted as to the constituents of dietary fiber. Fibrous foods contain complex polysaccharides, both soluble (pectin and gums) and insoluble (cellulose, hemicellulose, and lignin) substances. The properties of the fiber content of plants vary with regard to the maturity of the plant fiber and the conditions under which it was grown (see Table 7–2).

Soluble fibers such as pectins are contained in citrus fruits and apples; gums are found in legumes, barley, and oats. Insoluble fibers include both noncarbohydrates, such as lignin, and carbohydrates, such as cellulose and hemicellulose. The insoluble carbohydrate fibers may be found in bran, whole-grain cereals and breads, and root vegetables, such as carrots and turnips. Lignin is found in wheat, fruits with edible seeds, and mature vegetables; as the plant cells age, more lignin is formed (3).

Fiber can be added to the diet by eating whole grains and raw fruits and vegetables. (See Table 7–3.) Cooked fruits and vegetables will also add fiber. Insoluble fiber has the ability to absorb fluid and, therefore, adds bulk and helps to soften the fecal matter in the intestinal lumen. Individuals who are not accustomed to eating fibrous foods should be cautioned to gradually increase the quantity of fiber consumed in order to prevent cramping and abdominal discomfort.

POSSIBLE NURSING DIAGNOSES

Alteration in bowel elimination; constipation related to
- inadequate food intake.
- inadequate fluid intake.
- irregular pattern for defecation.
- lack of exercise.

Knowledge deficit related to lack of understanding of proper food and fluid intake.

NURSING INTERVENTIONS FOR NUTRITIONAL DISORDERS

Alteration in bowel elimination; constipation related to inadequate food intake, inadequate fluid intake, irregular pattern for defecation, lack of exercise.

- Instruct the patient in possible ways to prevent constipation, such as:
  eat foods that contain fiber, such as fresh fruits, vegetables, and whole-grain cereals and breads;

  drink adequate fluids, at least 2000 ml per day;

  develop a regular program of exercise;

  develop a regular time for defecation.

Knowledge deficit related to lack of understanding of proper food and fluid intake.

- Instruct the patient in possible ways to prevent constipation.
- Inform the patient about normal bowel habits.
- Refer the patient to dietitian for dietary counseling, if necessary.

Table 7-2. CLASSIFICATION OF PLANT FIBER

FIBER	PRIMARY FRACTION	FOOD SOURCES
Polysaccharides		
Cellulose	insoluble	bran, whole-wheat breads, cereals, fruits, vegetables
Noncellulose		
Hemicellulose	insoluble	bran, whole-wheat breads, cereals
Pectins	soluble	apples, strawberries, citrus fruits
Gums, mucilages	soluble	oatmeal, legumes (dried beans, peas, lentils)
Nonpolysaccharides		
Lignin	insoluble	fruits with edible seeds (raspberries, strawberries, blackberries), mature vegetables, wheat

Sources:

J.L. Slavin, "Dietary Fiber: Classification, Chemical Analyses, and Food Sources," *Journal of the American Dietetic Association* 87, no. 9 (1987):1164–71.

J.W. Anderson and S.R. Bridges, "Dietary Fiber of Selected Foods." *American Journal of Clinical Nutrition* 47, no. 3 (1988):440–47.

Table 7-3. SOURCES OF FIBER

RICH SOURCES OF FOOD FIBER 4 g or more per serving (foods marked with an * have 6 g or more fiber per serving)		
	SERVING	CALORIES (rounded to the nearest 5)
Breads and cereals *All Bran *Bran Buds Bran Chex	⅓ cup–1 oz ⅓ cup–1 oz ⅔ cup–1 oz	70 75 90

Continued

Table 7-3. SOURCES OF FIBER (continued)

RICH SOURCES OF FOOD FIBER 4 g or more per serving (foods marked with an * have 6 g or more fiber per serving)		
	SERVING	CALORIES (rounded to the nearest 5)
Corn Bran	⅔ cup–1 oz	100
Cracklin' Bran	⅓ cup–1 oz	110
*100% Bran	½ cup–1 oz	75
Raisin Bran	¾ cup–1 oz	85
*Bran, unsweetened	¼ cup	35
Wheat germ, toasted, plain	¼ cup–1 oz	110
Legumes (cooked portions)		
Kidney beans	½ cup	110
Lima beans	½ cup	130
Navy beans	½ cup	110
Pinto beans	½ cup	110
White beans	½ cup	110
Fruits		
Blackberries	½ cup	35
Dried prunes	3	60
MODERATELY RICH SOURCES OF FOOD FIBER 1 to 3 g of fiber per serving		
	SERVING	CALORIES (rounded to the nearest 5)
Fruits		
Apple	1 medium	80
Apricot, fresh	3 medium	50
Apricot, dried	5 halves	40
Banana	1 medium	105
Blueberries	½ cup	40
Cantaloupe	¼ melon	50
Cherries	10	50
Dates, dried	3	70
Figs, dried	1 medium	50
Grapefruit	½	40

Continued

Table 7-3. SOURCES OF FIBER *(continued)*

MODERATELY RICH SOURCES OF FOOD FIBER 1 to 3 g of fiber per serving		
	SERVING	CALORIES (rounded to the nearest 5)
Orange	1 medium	60
Peach	1 medium	35
Pear	1 medium	100
Pineapple	½ cup	40
Raisins	¼ cup	110
Strawberries	1 cup	45
Breads and cereals		
Bran muffins	1 medium	105
Popcorn (air-popped)	1 cup	25
Whole-wheat bread	1 slice	60
Whole-wheat spaghetti	1 cup	120
40% bran flakes	⅔ cup–1 oz	90
Grapenuts	¼ cup–1 oz	100
Granola-type cereals	¼ cup–1 oz	125
Cheerio-type cereals	1¼ cup–1 oz	110
Most	⅓ cup–1 oz	95
Oatmeal, cooked	¾ cup	110
Shredded wheat	⅔ cup–1 oz	100
Total	1 cup–1 oz	100
Wheat Chex	⅔ cup–1 oz	105
Wheaties	1 cup–1 oz	100
Legumes (cooked) and nuts		
Chick peas (garbanzo beans)	½ cup	135
Lentils	½ cup	105
Almonds	10 nuts	80
Peanuts	10 nuts	105
Vegetables		
Artichoke	1 small	45
Asparagus	½ cup	30
Beans, green	½ cup	15
Brussels sprouts	½ cup	30
Cabbage, red and white	½ cup	15
Carrots	½ cup	25

Continued

Table 7-3. SOURCES OF FIBER (continued)

LOW SOURCES OF FOOD FIBER Less than 1 g of fiber per serving		
	SERVING	CALORIES (rounded to the nearest 5)
Cauliflower	½ cup	15
Corn	½ cup	70
Green peas	½ cup	55
Kale	½ cup	20
Parsnip	½ cup	50
Potato	1 medium	95
Spinach, cooked	½ cup	20
Spinach, raw	½ cup	5
Summer squash	½ cup	15
Sweet potato	½ medium	80
Turnip	½ cup	15
Bean sprouts (soy)	½ cup	15
Celery	½ cup	10
Tomato	1 medium	20

LOW SOURCES OF FOOD FIBER Less than 1 g of fiber per serving		
	SERVING	CALORIES (rounded to the nearest 5)
Breads and cereals		
White bread	1 slice	70
Spaghetti, cooked	1 cup	155
Brown rice, cooked	½ cup	90
White rice, cooked	½ cup	80
Corn flake-type cereals	1¼ cup–1 oz	110
Vegetables		
Lettuce, shredded	1 cup	10
Mushrooms, sliced	½ cup	10
Onions, sliced	½ cup	20
Pepper, green, sliced	½ cup	10
Fruits		
Grapes	20	30
Watermelon	1 cup	50

Table 7-3. SOURCES OF FIBER *(continued)*

	LOW SOURCES OF FOOD FIBER Less than 1 g of fiber per serving	
	SERVING	CALORIES (rounded to the nearest 5)
Fruit juices		
Apple	½ cup–4 oz	60
Grapefruit	½ cup–4 oz	50
Grape	½ cup–4 oz	80
Orange	½ cup–4 oz	55
Papaya	½ cup–4 oz	70

Source: U.S. Department of Health and Human Services, HHS, PHS, *Diet, Nutrition and Cancer Prevention. A Guide to Food Choices*, NIH Pub. No. 85-2711, 1984.

Heartburn

Heartburn (reflux esophagitis) or indigestion is caused by the reflux of the acid, gastric contents into the distal portion of the esophagus. Normally, the lower esophageal or cardiac sphincter (LES) prevents the regurgitation of the stomach contents. Certain substances such as alcohol, coffee, nicotine, high fat foods, carbonated beverages, chocolate and spices, such as peppermint, cause the LES to relax and regurgitation of stomach contents into the lower portion of the esophagus is possible.

Heartburn may be more prevalent during pregnancy and in patients who are obese because of increased intra-abdominal pressure. It may also be precipitated by changes in position, especially when bending over and/or lifting heavy objects.

Irritating foodstuffs like coffee, juices (orange or tomato), or spices may irritate the inflamed portion of the esophagus and cause the burning sensation.

Nutritional care may involve weight loss for the obese patient (see Chapter 15 for a discussion of eating disorders). Encourage the patient who is subject to episodes of heartburn to avoid the foods and other agents that may precipitate an attack. A person might be encouraged to eat smaller, more frequent meals. A diet that is high in protein and low in fat may also help to prevent heartburn by increasing LES pressure.

The use of baking soda as an antacid should be discouraged because it is systemic in nature and can predispose to alkalemia. Occasional use of nonsystemic over-the-counter (OTC) antacids (e.g., Mylanta, Maalox) may not be harmful to relieve discomfort. Common OTC antacids contain aluminum or magnesium as the active buffer. Using too much of an aluminum-based product may produce constipation; use of magnesium-based products may cause diarrhea.

POSSIBLE NURSING DIAGNOSES

Potential alteration in comfort; pain related to regurgitation of gastric-acid secretions.

Knowledge deficit related to lack of understanding of proper food intake.

NURSING INTERVENTIONS FOR NUTRITIONAL DISORDERS

Potential alteration in comfort; pain related to regurgitation of gastric acid secretions.

- Avoid the use of irritating substances such as coffee, juices (orange or tomato), or spices that may irritate the inflamed esophagus.
- Instruct the patient that occasional use of OTC antacids may be helpful in relieving discomfort (if not contraindicated).

Knowledge deficit related to lack of understanding of proper food intake.

- Instruct the patient to:
  eat slowly and chew all foods well;
  maintain an upright position and avoid strenuous exercise for at least 30 minutes to one hour after meals;
  avoid foods that cause the LES to relax, such as alcohol, coffee, high-fat foods, carbonated beverages, chocolate, and spices.

Flatus

Intestinal gas (flatus) and the problems related to it are highly individual and primarily subjective in nature. Gases in the intestine are the result of swallowing air (eating or drinking rapidly or with the mouth open), bacterial breakdown of food, and increased intestinal motility (less time for absorption of the gases into the bloodstream).

Certain foods, such as those in the legume family (peas and beans), onions, cabbage, apples, and melons, may cause problems for some people. Other potential gas-forming foods are beer, broccoli, cauliflower, cheese, milk products, and peanuts.

Suggestions for a person who suffers from too much gas might include:
- Avoiding foods that may produce gas;
- Limiting or avoiding the use of carbonated beverages;
- Avoiding drinking through straws;
- Limiting the amount of fat in the diet;
- Eating slowly.

If the person continues to complain of gaseousness after trying the above, it is important to consult a physician. The physician may want to determine if the flatus is related to a lactase deficiency. Lactose intolerance will be discussed under malabsorption syndromes later in this chapter.

POSSIBLE NURSING DIAGNOSES

Knowledge deficit related to
- dietary management.
- techniques to reduce air ingestion.

NURSING INTERVENTIONS FOR NUTRITIONAL DISORDERS

Knowledge deficit related to dietary management; techniques to reduce air ingestion.

- Instruct the patient to:
   avoid foods that may produce gas;

limit or avoid the use of carbonated beverages;

avoid drinking through straws;

limit the amount of fat in the diet;

eat slowly.

DYSFUNCTIONS OF THE GASTROINTESTINAL TRACT

Obstruction

Obstruction, either partial or complete, can occur anywhere within the gastrointestinal tract. This discussion focuses on the lower esophagus (achalasia or cardiospasm) and on the large intestine.

Achalasia. The cause for achalasia is unknown. Due to lack of peristalsis within the esophagus and stricture of the LES, the lower portion of the esophagus distends. Food becomes trapped in the dilated portion of the esophagus and is eventually regurgitated. The person manifests increasing difficulty in swallowing (dysphagia).

Mechanical dilation of the LES is attempted to relax the sphincter; however, occasionally, surgical intervention is necessary. Following dilation, the diet usually progresses from clear liquids to bland or regular as tolerated by the patient.

POSSIBLE NURSING DIAGNOSES

Potential alteration in nutrition; less than body requirements, related to dysphagia.

Alteration in comfort; heartburn related to regurgitation.

Knowledge deficit related to
- disease process.
- positioning after ingestion of food.
- dietary management.

NURSING INTERVENTIONS FOR NUTRITIONAL DISORDERS

Potential alteration in nutrition; less than body requirements related to dysphagia.

- Encourage the patient to eat slowly and chew all foods well.
- Limit foods that cause discomfort (those that increase lower esophageal sphincter pressure) and include foods that help to decrease lower esophageal pressure (e.g., fats, chocolate, and coffee).

Alteration in comfort; heartburn related to regurgitation.

- Maintain an upright position for at least 30 minutes to one hour after eating.
- Drink fluids with meals to reduce the viscosity of solid food. Fluids taken alone may accumulate at the lower esophageal sphincter.

Knowledge deficit related to
- **disease process.**
- **positioning after ingestion of food.**
- **dietary management.**

- Instruct the patient to:
  eat slowly and chew all foods well;

  maintain an upright position for at least 30 minutes to one hour after eating;

  drink fluids with meals to reduce the viscosity of solid foods (liquids taken alone do not require peristaltic action and may accumulate at the lower esophageal sphincter);

  avoid foods that increase lower esophageal sphincter pressure;

  ingest foods that help to decrease lower esophageal sphincter pressure (fats, chocolate, coffee) (whole milk should be served because of the higher fat content; alcoholic beverages may be beneficial for some patients; seek medical advice because of the "empty" kilocalories);

  utilize stress reduction techniques, especially before mealtime.

Intestinal Obstruction. Pathology within or outside the lumen of the bowel may impede the flow of fecal contents. The cause of the obstruction will determine the type of treatment.

Bowel obstructions may be mechanical, vascular, or neurogenic in origin. Mechanical obstruction may be due to conditions such as adhesions (scar tissue from previous abdominal surgery or infectious processes); strangulated hernia; volvulus (twisting of the intestine on itself); intussusception (telescoping of the bowel on itself); and tumors, intestinal or involving adjacent organs or structures. Vascular obstructions are due to an interference with the blood supply to a section of the intestine, such as a mesenteric thrombosis. Paralytic ileus is an example of neurogenic obstruction. The nerve supply to a portion of the intestine may be altered due to manipulation and edema associated with surgery; following severe infections such as peritonitis; or following shock, severe pain, or in association with spinal cord injury.

The level of obstruction within the intestinal tract will determine the degree of problem associated with the passage of feces. If the obstruction occurs in an area of the small intestine or involves the ascending colon, the obstruction may be far advanced before diagnosis is established because the fecal matter is in a liquid to semiliquid state and can easily flow past the obstruction. Vomiting, however, may be a sign of obstruction.

An impediment to the flow of feces in the descending or sigmoid portions of the colon will cause earlier symptoms of abdominal pain and/or rigidity and changes in the bowel patterns and the character of the stool. The function of the distal portion of the colon is to extract the remaining fluid from the stool and return the fluid to the general circulation. The longer the fecal material remains in contact with the mucosal surface, the more fluid will be absorbed. This same principle occurs in persons who suffer from constipation.

If a person shows signs of impending intestinal obstruction, it is important to instruct the person to refrain from oral intake and seek immediate medical attention. Treatment of intestinal obstruction frequently involves surgery. Dietary management following surgery is usually progressive, beginning with clear liquids after the gastric suction has been discontinued and peristalsis is established. Fecal diversion (colostomy or ileostomy) may be necessary to rest the bowel or create a new opening for the passage of stool. Ostomies and the nursing considerations related to diet will be discussed later in this chapter.

Paralytic ileus is treated conservatively. The bowel is allowed to rest, a nasogastric tube is inserted, and the patient is maintained on nothing by mouth status until peristalsis is reestablished. It is important for the nurse to listen for bowel sounds. When there is evidence that intestinal peristalsis is present, the physician will frequently order dietary progression, beginning with clear liquids.

POSSIBLE NURSING DIAGNOSES

Potential alteration in nutrition; less than body requirements related to decreased intake secondary to pain, nausea, vomiting, and diet restriction.

Anxiety related to possible surgical experience.

Knowledge deficit related to diet and fluid restrictions.

NURSING INTERVENTIONS FOR NUTRITIONAL DISORDERS

Potential alteration in nutrition; less than body requirements related to decreased intake secondary to pain, nausea, vomiting, and diet restriction.

- Assess the patient for signs of impending intestinal obstruction (pain, hyperactive or absence of bowel sounds, abdominal distention).

Anxiety related to possible surgical experience.

- Provide nursing care as dictated by the type of treatment for the obstruction (See Chapter 6 for "Nursing Interventions for Nutritional Disorders" following surgery).

Continued

NURSING INTERVENTIONS *(continued)*
Knowledge deficit related to diet and fluid restrictions.

- Instruct the patient to refrain from oral intake until diagnosis is confirmed by the physician.

Inflammation

Inflammation can occur anywhere within the gastrointestinal tract. This discussion focuses on inflammation within the stomach (gastritis) and inflammatory bowel disease (Crohn's disease—regional enteritis and ulcerative colitis). Ostomies (colostomy and ileostomy) are also discussed.

Gastritis. Gastritis is an inflammation of the stomach characterized by a number of subjective symptoms, including anorexia and epigastric distress and nausea, with or without vomiting.

Causes of gastritis may be varied. The irritation may be due to stress, food, spices, infectious organisms or their toxins, alcohol, drugs such as aspirin, and may be associated with aging. The inflammation of the mucosa may lead to erosion and potential bleeding.

Treatment is related to prevention or elimination of the causative agent, if possible. Dietary management usually focuses on allowing the stomach to rest for 24–48 hours. Parenteral fluid replacement may be necessary for some patients. When fluids can be tolerated orally, the diet progresses from clear liquids to a bland diet. Once the symptoms have been relieved, the physician will generally allow a regular diet.

POSSIBLE NURSING DIAGNOSES

Alteration in nutrition; less than body requirements related to nausea.

Alteration in comfort related to epigastric distress.

Potential fluid-volume deficit related to nausea and vomiting.

NURSING INTERVENTIONS FOR NUTRITIONAL DISORDERS

Alteration in nutrition; less than body requirements related to nausea.

- Instruct the patient to:
    eat four to six smaller meals per day;

    drink ample fluids as prescribed;

    avoid the use of substances that are known to cause irritation (e.g., alcohol, nicotine, caffeine, broth, aspirin);

    understand the relationship of milk and milk products to increased gastrin formation (discussed later in this chapter in the section on peptic ulcer disease);

    create a relaxing atmosphere, especially at mealtime.

Continued

NURSING INTERVENTIONS *(continued)*

Potential fluid-volume deficit related to nausea and vomiting.

- Monitor fluid intake and output.
- Advise the patient to drink fluids as prescribed.

Alteration in comfort related to epigastric distress.

- Advise the patient to avoid food substances that cause gastric distress and resume a bland diet as prescribed.
- Caution the patient to seek medical advice before self-medicating with OTC antacids.

Inflammatory Bowel Disease. Crohn's disease (regional enteritis) and ulcerative colitis are frequently referred to as inflammatory bowel disease (IBD). The two conditions are similar in that they may cause widespread inflammation within the intestinal tract and ultimately can lead to severe malnutrition. They are, however, different pathological processes that frequently involve different portions of the intestine. Both diseases can affect persons of all ages but are common in young adults.

Ulcerative colitis is characterized by widespread inflammation and bleeding. It frequently begins in the rectum and lower intestine and progresses upward; it involves the mucosal lining.

Crohn's disease can occur anywhere in the gastrointestinal tract, but primarily involves the terminal ileum and the cecum (proximal colon). It is characterized by a "cobblestone" appearance inside the intestine, since the inflammation and subsequent ulceration involve all layers of the mucosa and submucosa. Not all inflammatory processes within the intestine are necessarily contiguous (adjacent to each other); the inflammatory processes may occur in patches separated by normal intestinal segments.

Nutritional support for the patient with IBD may be complex. Medical management combined with bowel rest is the usual treatment approach during the acute phase. Elemental diets and TPN permit the maintenance of nutritional status while allowing the bowel to rest. Risks associated with other treatment, primarily surgical intervention, are greatly reduced. Recently, the therapeutic value of bowel rest has been questioned, because the colon atrophies during this period. Research is currently being conducted on the addition of soluble fibers to the dietary regime, since these may prevent colonic atrophy without producing fecal bulk (4).

Anemia may be present in the patient who suffers blood loss; therefore, supplements of iron, folic acid, and parenteral vitamin B_{12} may be needed. Sulfasalazine, which is a drug of choice in the treatment of IBD, can interfere with the absorption of folic acid. This drug should be given between meals to avoid problems associated with the absorption of folates.

Due to the chronic nature of Crohn's disease, the dietary management is slightly different. TPN or elemental diets are used during the acute phase to promote bowel rest. Elemental diets consist of small peptides or purified amino acids as the protein source, simple sugars as the carbohydrate source, and a limited amount of oils, medium-chain triglycerides, and/or fatty acids as the fat source. Frequently, patients with IBD malabsorb protein and fat and are lactose intolerant (5).

In order to prevent further catabolism and negative nitrogen balance, the diet should contain 1.0–1.5 g protein and 40–50 kcals per kilogram ideal body weight (6). Multivitamin and mineral supplements may also be needed. The water soluble B vitamins are not stored, and there is an increased need for vitamin C to aid in healing. If diarrhea is severe, potassium supplements will be ordered. Iron and calcium will also be replaced.

If the person with IBD is being treated with steroid drugs, it is important to provide a calcium supplement along with vitamin D. The vitamin D will aid in the utilization of calcium and both will counteract the demineralizing effects of steroid drugs.

POSSIBLE NURSING DIAGNOSES

Alteration in nutrition; less than body requirements related to:
- diarrhea.
- pain after eating.

Fluid-volume deficit related to
- diarrhea.
- inadequate fluid intake.

Alteration in comfort related to the inflamed intestine.

Potential for impairment of skin integrity, perianal, related to diarrhea.

Knowledge deficit related to dietary restriction.

NURSING INTERVENTIONS FOR NUTRITIONAL DISORDERS

Work closely with the physician and dietitian to help the patient to achieve the nutritional goals.

Alteration in nutrition; less than body requirements related to:
- **diarrhea.**
- **pain after eating.**

- Advise the patient to eat frequent, small meals to avoid discomfort.
- Caution the patient to avoid those foods that are known irritants.
- Suggest that the patient eat foods rich in potassium, such as potatoes and bananas.

Fluid-volume deficit related to:
- **diarrhea.**
- **inadequate fluid intake.**

- Monitor fluid intake and output.
- Encourage adequate fluid intake, 8–10 glasses per day, especially if on sulfasalazine therapy.
- Advise the patient to be alert for fluid retention if taking steroid drugs.

Alteration in comfort related to the inflamed intestine.

- Caution the patient to avoid foods that are known irritants.

Potential for impairment of skin integrity, perianal; related to diarrhea.

- Advise that the patient eat foods that are high in protein value to facilitate skin repair.

Continued

NURSING INTERVENTIONS *(continued)*

Knowledge deficit related to dietary restriction.

- Instruct the patient to:
  chill elemental diets or combine with fruit juices to increase palatability;

  eat frequent, small meals to avoid possible discomfort;

avoid foods that are known irritants;

increase intake of potassium when diarrhea persists;

understand the relationship between food intake and increased peristalsis and the possible need to defecate during mealtime (ulcerative colitis, particularly); resume meal when able, and take multivitamin and mineral supplements as prescribed.

Ostomies. When it is necessary for the surgeon to remove large sections of the small and/or large intestine in an attempt to treat Crohn's disease, ulcerative colitis, cancer or other obstruction, or severe trauma, it may be necessary to divert the flow of fecal contents. The opening that is created on the abdominal wall is referred to as an ostomy.

If the ileum is anastomosed (surgically attached) to the abdominal wall, an ileostomy is created. If a portion of the colon (ascending, transverse, descending, or sigmoid) is anastomosed, the surgical procedure creates a colostomy. The higher up the intestinal tract, i.e., ileostomy versus colostomy, the more liquid and consequently more irritating is the effluent (intestinal contents) that drains from the stoma (opening on the abdominal wall) (Figure 7-1).

Dietary management is similar for both the colostomy and the ileostomy patient. Ideally, the person will be able to tolerate a regular diet that has been modified to the specific needs of that person. The person must understand the nutritional requirements of the type of ostomy and the effects of specific foods on establishing and maintaining bowel control.

If the person had not been chronically ill prior to surgery or if TPN was used in the preoperative period, the person may be in state of adequate nutrition. The malnourished person must be watched closely during the postoperative period, and inadequate nutrients must be replaced in order for healing to occur.

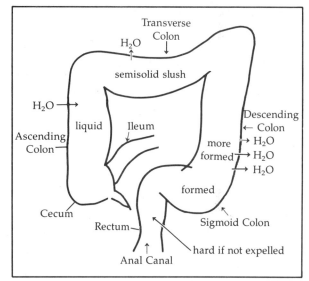

Figure 7-1. Consistency of fecal material in the colon and rectum.

Most patients who have an ostomy are primarily concerned with diet. In the early postoperative period, the diet will progress from the period of intravenous fluids and bowel rest, nothing by mouth, to clear liquids and ultimately to a modified, regular high-protein, high-carbohydrate diet.

Foods should be added one at a time to determine the effect of specific foodstuffs on production of gas, diarrhea, or constipation. As a general rule, the person who has had an ostomy must limit the intake of high-fiber foods and those that are laxative in nature (e.g., prunes and squash). (See Table 7-4.) The person must experiment with the diet to determine the ideal.

Because of the tendency for intestinal blockage, the person with an ileostomy must be extremely careful to avoid high-fiber foods, especially those with kernels and nuts. An increase in the formation of gas and subsequent odor is also a problem. Liberal fluid intake is advised for all ostomy patients, especially those with an ileostomy. Multivitamin and mineral supplements may be required by the person with an ileostomy.

Table 7-4. POTENTIAL PROBLEM FOODS FOR THE PERSON WITH AN ILEOSTOMY

OBSTRUCTION	CONSTIPATION	DIARRHEALIKE	ODOR PRODUCING	FLATUS PRODUCING
Apple peels	apples (also	baked beans	alcohol	dried beans
Asparagus	sauce)	beer	asparagus	beer
Celery (raw)	bananas	broccoli	baked beans	broccoli
Coleslaw	milk products	fried, greasy	cabbage	carbonated
Corn	peanut butter	foods	cheese	beverages
Greens (salad)	rice	fruits	eggs	cabbage
Lettuce	tapioca	(excessive)	fish	cheese
Nuts		grape juice	garlic	milk products
Peas		milk products	onions	peanuts
Popcorn		red wine	shellfish	onions
Raw vegetables		rich sauces		
Spinach		spicy foods		
Seeds				

(From L. Burrell, *Adult Nursing in Hospital and Community Settings* (East Norwalk: Appleton and Lange, 1990). Reprinted with permission.)

POSSIBLE NURSING DIAGNOSES

Potential alteration in nutrition; less than body requirements related to altered metabolic processes that necessitated the ostomy.

Knowledge deficit related to
• nutritional adaptation.
• odor control.

Potential for social isolation related to
• fear of loss of control.
• odor.
• disturbances in body image.

NURSING INTERVENTIONS FOR NUTRITIONAL DISORDERS

Work closely with the physician, dietitian, and other members of the health team to help the patient meet the nutritional needs.

Potential alteration in nutrition; less than body requirements related to altered metabolic processes that necessitated the ostomy.

- Carefully assess the patient's nutritional needs.

Knowledge deficit related to
- **nutritional adaptation.**
- **odor control.**

- Instruct the patient to:
    ingest liberal quantities of fluids, six to eight glasses per day;

    eat slowly to prevent swallowing of air;

    experiment with one new food at a time to determine the effect on the gastrointestinal tract;

    chew all foods well to prevent obstruction;

    avoid or limit foods that are known to cause intestinal gas;

avoid high-fiber foods, those that contain kernels and nuts (ileostomy);

ingest buttermilk or yogurt to help control fecal odors;

check with the physician to prescribe drugs that may control odor (chlorophyll or bismuth subgallate);

eat bananas or applesauce if stools are too loose; seek medical advice if diarrhea persists.

Potential for social isolation related to
- **fear of loss of control.**
- **odor.**
- **disturbances in body image.**

- Give the patient and family support throughout the process of developing an ideal diet.
- Suggest that the patient control odor by:
    avoiding or limiting foods known to cause intestinal gas;

    ingesting buttermilk or yogurt;

    check with the physician to prescribe drugs that may control odor (chlorophyll or bismuth subgallate).

Ulceration

Peptic-Ulcer Disease. Peptic-ulcer disease is an acute or chronic condition that produces ulcerations in the areas of the gastrointestinal tract where gastric secretions are present. The location of the ulceration, i.e., gastric or duodenal, denotes the anatomical location of the lesion. Stress ulcers are multiple, small lesions that form on the gastric mucosa. These are likely to occur when a person suffers severe trauma such as burns, undergoes prolonged surgery, or has severe blood loss. Changes in the microcirculation (inadequate blood supply to the gastric mucosa), and hence decreased mucosal resistance, may be the cause of this problem.

The cause of ulceration of the mucosa may be due to several factors, including an increase in gastric acid and pepsin formation and the decreased resistance of the gastric mucosa to the irritating effects of those secretions. Peptic ulcers may also occur when persons are being treated for other conditions such as arthritis, which may involve taking large doses of salicylates, steroids, or nonsteroidal antiinflammatory agents. Emotional stress may also play a role in the hypersecretion of gastric acids for some persons.

The classic symptom is pain or epigastric distress that occurs approximately one hour after meals and during the night. The pain is relieved by food or antacids. Confirmation of the diagnosis is made by radiologic and/or endoscopic visualization of the defect.

Treatment protocols have changed in recent years. Antacids (acid neutralizers) have traditionally and continue to be used to relieve discomfort. H-2 receptor antagonist drugs, ranitidine and cimetidine, which help to decrease gastric acid secretions, have been valuable adjuncts in treatment. Sucralfate is a local acting, mucosal protective agent that prevents further irritation by gastrin, pepsin, and bile.

The primary goals of nutritional therapy are to reduce and neutralize the gastric acidity, maintain the resistance of gastric mucosal tissue, and restore nutritional status (7). Dietary treatment protocols for peptic ulcers have changed markedly. A special diet is not needed for most patients.

The traditional ulcer diet that consisted, initially, of large quantities of milk and cream, followed by the addition of low-fiber foods and ultimately six feedings of bland nonirritating (chemical, mechanical, or thermal) foods, was used for many years. The liberal dietary approach began about 1971, and was based on research that indicated there was little difference in the amount of acid secreted when a person ate three meals versus six meals per day.

The liberal dietary emphasis focuses on the needs and responses of the individual person rather than on the diet. The person should be taught to eat balanced meals of moderate quantity. Foods that are known to be irritating or gas forming should be avoided (e.g., substances containing alcohol and caffeine). All foods should be chewed well to avoid mechanical irritation to the stomach lining. Most condiments have been found to be tolerated; however, spices such as black pepper and chili powder may be irritating to some people. It largely depends on the person, working with the dietitian and the nurse, to determine which foods cause problems.

Substances that are known to cause irritation and damage to the gastric lining, such as alcohol, salicylates, and nonsteroidal antiinflammatory agents should be used only under the direction of the physician.

Nicotine has been found to increase gastric-acid secretions and motility. Cigarette smoking should be avoided by persons known to have ulcers.

Many times, the nurse must help to dispel the myth that large quantities of milk help to cure an ulcer. It has been found that the ingestion of milk and milk products (protein and calcium) stimulate gastric-acid secretion. Milk may be included in the diet but might be taken with meals to prevent gastric irritation.

POSSIBLE NURSING DIAGNOSES

Alteration in comfort; pain related to ulceration secondary to increased gastric secretion.

Potential alteration in bowel elimination; constipation related to diet and side effects of medications.

Knowledge deficit related to dietary modifications.

NURSING INTERVENTIONS FOR NUTRITIONAL DISORDERS

Work closely with the patient and dietitian to help determine a diet plan best suited to the needs of the individual patient.

Alteration in comfort; pain related to ulceration secondary to increased gastric secretion.

- Advise the patient to eat regular meals of moderate size to prevent overdistention of the stomach and increase in gastric acid secretion.
- Help the patient understand the role of stress in relation to increased gastric-acid production.
- Caution the patient to seek medical advice if symptoms persist or if complications such as bleeding or severe abdominal pain occur.
- Advise the patient to take drugs such as cimetidine (Tagamet) with meals to ensure a more consistent therapeutic action.

Potential alteration in bowel elimination; constipation related to diet and side effects of medications.

- Advise the patient to drink liberal quantities of fluid to help prevent constipation.

Knowledge deficit related to dietary modifications.

- Instruct the patient to:
  eat slowly and chew all food well;

  eat regular meals of moderate size in order to prevent overdistention of the stomach and an increase in gastric acid secretion;

  drink milk with meals to decrease potential for gastric irritation because milk tends to increase gastric secretions;

  avoid the use of alcohol, caffeine, and nicotine;

  use stress-relieving techniques, if indicated; and

  seek medical advice if symptoms persist or if complications such as bleeding or severe abdominal pain should occur.

Surgical Treatment for Peptic Ulcer. If symptoms persist despite conservative medical treatment or if complications of hemorrhage or gastric-outlet obstruction occur, surgical intervention may be necessary. Subtotal gastric resection, with or without vagotomy is usually performed (see Figure 7–2). The Billroth I and II are examples of subtotal gastric resections. The vagotomy (severing of the vagus nerve) is performed to decrease stimulation of the parietal (acid-producing) cells of the stomach.

Dumping Syndrome. Following subtotal gastric resection, the food that enters the intestine from the stomach is no longer regulated by the pyloric sphincter. Food is able to rapidly empty into the small intestine. This concentrated food, which is literally "dumped" into the intestine, precipitates a number of symptoms; this is referred to as dumping syndrome.

The concentrated food is hypertonic, thus it draws fluid from the vascular system. Symptoms of dizziness, palpitations, abdominal fullness and cramping, and profuse perspiration usually occur approximately 30 minutes following a meal. After two to three hours, especially following a high carbohydrate meal, late-dumping syndrome can occur.

Late-dumping syndrome is caused by rapid entry of carbohydrates into the small intestine. The carbohydrate is absorbed, causing a rapid rise in the blood sugar and the subsequent release of a large quantity of insulin. The symptoms of dizziness, palpitations, and diaphoresis are a result of a hypoglycemic reaction.

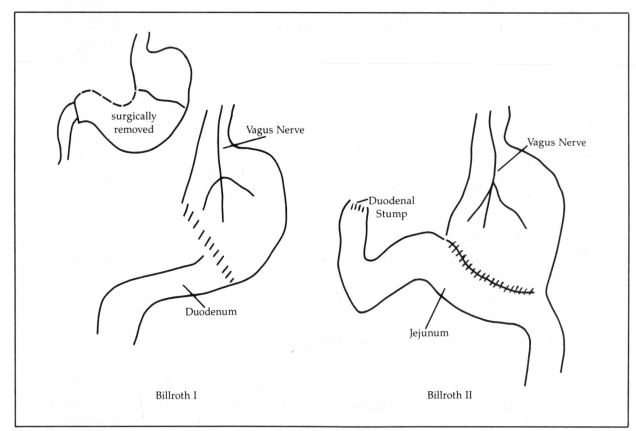

Figure 7-2. Types of gastric resections.

POSSIBLE NURSING DIAGNOSES

Potential alteration in nutrition; less than body requirements related to rapid gastric emptying.

Potential alteration in comfort related to hypoglycemic reaction.

NURSING INTERVENTIONS FOR NUTRITIONAL DISORDERS

Work closely with the patient and dietitian to determine the diet best suited to the needs of the patient.

Potential alteration in nutrition; less than body requirements related to rapid gastric emptying.

- Instruct the patient to:
  eat slowly and chew all foods well;

  eat meals of moderate size, at regular intervals;

  avoid concentrated carbohydrates (sugars, candy, pastries);

  drink fluids between meals;

  lie down for 30 minutes to one hour after meals to prevent rapid emptying of the stomach.

Potential alteration in comfort related to hypoglycemic reaction.

- Interventions listed in previous sections also apply here.

Weakness in Musculature

Both hiatal hernia and diverticulosis are examples of weakness and subsequent defect in a muscle wall. (See Figure 7–3). A defect in the diaphragm (congenital or acquired) can allow a portion of the stomach to enter the chest and is called hiatal hernia. Diverticulosis can occur when the intestinal mucosa protrudes through a defect in the muscular wall surrounding the intestine and creates a pouch in which fecal material can become trapped.

Hiatal Hernia. Because of the muscular defect, hiatal hernia can produce symptoms similar to heartburn (discussed previously in this chapter). The cause of the muscle weakness is frequently unknown; however, factors that cause an increase

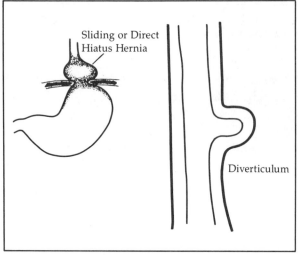

Figure 7-3. Weakness in musculature. (Hiatus hernia from M.J. Miller, *Pathophysiology: Principles of Disease* (Philadelphia: W.B. Saunders Company, 1983). Reprinted with permission.)

in intra-abdominal pressure (obesity, pregnancy, tight clothing, chronic cough, and straining to have a bowel movement) may predispose to the condition where a weakness is already present.

Treatment of hiatal hernia may consist of conservative measures such as decreasing intra-abdominal pressure, controlling pain and discomfort associated with heartburn, and maintaining an upright position following eating. A more aggressive approach is surgical repair of the diaphragm.

Dietary management includes eating small, bland meals more frequently; four to six meals per day will help to prevent gastric distention. Fluids should be taken between meals to help prevent regurgitation and overdistention of the stomach. Foods that tend to decrease the patency of the LES should be avoided (coffee, peppermint, alcohol, and fats). Foods and/or fluids that may irritate the inflamed portion of the esophagus and cardiac end of the stomach should not be ingested.

POSSIBLE NURSING DIAGNOSES

Potential alteration in comfort; pain related to gastric-acid reflux.

Potential alteration in nutrition; less than body requirements related to
- gastric acid reflux.
- anorexia.
- dysphagia.

Knowledge deficit related to
- muscular defect.
- diet management.
- position following meals.
- increased intra-abdominal pressure caused by excess weight or pregnancy.

NURSING INTERVENTIONS
FOR NUTRITIONAL DISORDERS

Work closely with the patient and dietitian to determine the diet best suited to the needs of the patient.

Potential alteration in comfort: pain related to gastric acid reflux.

- Advise the patient to:
  eat small amounts of food more frequently (four to six meals per day) to prevent overdistention of the stomach;

Continued

NURSING INTERVENTIONS *(continued)*

drink fluids between meals or take only a few sips with meals;

maintain an upright position for one to two hours following meals;

refrain from eating within two hours of bedtime;

sleep with the head of the bed elevated (elevate head of the bed using four- to six-inch cement blocks);

prevent constipation by eating adequate fiber and drinking sufficient fluids;

avoid foods that decrease the LES pressure (coffee, alcohol, fats);

take medications (antacids, H-2 receptor antagonists) as prescribed by the physician;

prevent increases in intra-abdominal pressure.

Potential alteration in nutrition; less than body requirements related to
- **gastric acid reflux.**
- **anorexia.**
- **dysphagia.**

- Interventions listed in the previous section also apply here.

Knowledge deficit related to
- **muscular defect.**
- **diet management.**
- **position following meals.**
- **increased intra-abdominal pressure due to excess weight or pregnancy.**

- Instruct the patient to follow the interventions listed in the previous section.

Diverticular Disease. A diverticulum is a herniation or saclike outpouching of the intestinal mucosa. These weaknesses of the lumen can occur where the blood vessels penetrate the muscular and mucosal layers of the intestine.

Diverticular disease can involve several phases. Diverticulosis refers to the nonsymptomatic presence of diverticula on the colon. Diverticulitis is an acute inflammatory process in which a microperforation occurs at the tip of the diverticulum. The contents of the colon can then seep out causing inflammation of the adjacent tissues. Diverticular disease is predominantly a disease of older age. Fifty percent of all persons in their 90s may have diverticula (8).

Treatment of diverticular disease is aimed at preventing or postponing complications. If diverticulitis is present, conservative measures are used initially in an attempt to rest the bowel and control the inflammation and infection. Surgical intervention (bowel resection or temporary colostomy) may be needed to treat obstruction, abscess, or fistula formation.

In order to decrease the pressure within the colon and prevent the formation of additional diverticula or complications involving existing diverticula, the person is encouraged to increase the amount of fiber in the diet. This can be accomplished by eating foods that are high in fiber (see Table 7–3) and by using psyllium hydrophilic muciloid laxatives (e.g., Metamucil, Konsyl). Fluid intake should also be increased to 8–10 glasses per day. Patients may recall that in the past, diverticular disease was treated with low fiber diets.

During periods of acute inflammation, the physician will prescribe bowel rest, nothing by mouth, with gradual progression to regular diet when sufficient healing has occurred (see the discussion of nutritional care for inflammatory bowel disease in this chapter).

POSSIBLE NURSING DIAGNOSES

Potential alteration in bowel elimination; constipation related to low-dietary-fiber intake.

Knowledge deficit related to
- anatomical defect.
- dietary management.
- signs and symptoms of complications.

Alteration in comfort related to intestinal inflammatory process (diverticulitis).

NURSING INTERVENTIONS FOR NUTRITIONAL DISORDERS

Work closely with the patient and dietitian to develop a diet best suited to the needs of the individual.

Potential alteration in bowel elimination; constipation related to low-dietary-fiber intake.

- Help the patient understand the rationale for the change in dietary management from low-fiber to high-fiber foods.

Knowledge deficit related to
- **anatomical defect.**
- **dietary management.**
- **signs and symptoms of complications.**

- Instruct the patient to:
      eat a diet that is rich in fiber; dietary fiber intake should be increased gradually to prevent abdominal cramping;

   drink 8–10 glasses of water per day to enhance the action of fiber;

   avoid constipation and the use of strong laxatives;

   avoid activities and restrictive clothing (e.g., improper lifting techniques and tight belts) that can increase intra-abdominal pressure.

Alteration in comfort related to intestinal inflammatory process (diverticulitis).

(Refer to "Nursing Interventions for Nutritional Disorders" pertaining to inflammatory bowel disease in this chapter.)

Weakness in Blood Vessels

Hemorrhoids. Hemorrhoids are masses of dilated and/or ruptured blood vessels that lie beneath the lining of the skin in the anal area. The hemorrhoids may be located internal or external to the anal sphincter and can cause varying amounts of pain and discomfort.

Treatment can be conservative, especially in the early stages. Symptomatic relief of discomfort through the use of a variety of OTC preparations and dietary management are possible. Surgical intervention may be necessary for those persons who have large, prolapsed internal hemorrhoids or for those persons whose symptoms have become progressively worse.

Dietary management should focus on prevention of discomfort. A diet that is rich in fiber should be encouraged, along with increased fluid intake to enhance the action of the fiber in preventing constipation (refer to the section on constipation in this chapter). Regular eating habits and mealtimes, as well as regular times for defecation, should be encouraged.

POSSIBLE NURSING DIAGNOSES

Potential alteration in comfort; pain related to defecation.

Potential alteration in bowel elimination; constipation related to fear of pain on defecation.

Knowledge deficit related to
- relationship of diet and pathophysiology.
- bowel elimination.

NURSING INTERVENTIONS FOR NUTRITIONAL DISORDERS

Work closely with patient and dietitian to develop a dietary plan suitable to the patient's needs.

Potential alteration in comfort; pain related to defecation.

- Encourage the patient to drink adequate fluids (8–10 glasses per day) to help keep stools soft.

Potential alteration in bowel elimination; constipation related to fear of pain on defecation.

- Advise the patient to eat foods that are high in fiber content to enhance bowel elimination.

Knowledge deficit related to
- **relationship of diet and pathophysiology.**
- **bowel elimination.**
- Instruct the patient to:
  eat a diet rich in fiber;
  drink liberal quantities of fluids (8–10 glasses per day);
  develop a regular exercise pattern;
  develop a regular pattern for bowel elimination.

Malabsorption

Malabsorption syndromes are characterized by the inability of the gastrointestinal tract to digest and absorb certain nutrients. Symptoms of malabsorption syndromes are varied. The person may manifest mild nutritional deficiency with minimal symptoms or weight loss, multiple nutrient deficiencies, and foul-smelling, diarrhealike stools. Symptoms vary with the type of nutrient deficiency. This discussion focuses on lactose or milk intolerance (disaccharide deficiency) and celiac sprue (gluten-related intolerance).

Celiac Sprue. Celiac sprue is a disease of the small intestine characterized by the malabsorption of all nutrients, especially fats. The disease is frequently discovered in infancy when cereals (gluten-containing grains) are introduced into the diet, but it can occur in adults.

Malabsorption occurs because the villi on the mucosal surface of the small intestine become atrophied, and transport of nutrients to the bloodstream is diminished. Celiac spru occurs in sensitive individuals after intestinal exposure to gluten. The severity of the disease correlates with the extent of the intestinal involvement.

Treatment involves the strict elimination of gluten-containing substances from the diet. Multivitamin and mineral supplements are usually ordered. Corticosteroids may be ordered for some patients to decrease the inflammatory process and aid in the absorption of nutrients.

A gluten-free diet omits glutamine-bound protein fractions (glutenin and gliadin) from the diet. Grains such as wheat, rye, barley, and oats are not permitted. It is important to read product labels to determine whether any of the offending substances are present. Corn, rice, soy, and potatoes are permitted in a gluten-free diet and can be incorporated into a diet plan. Recipes using permitted ingredients are available from a variety of sources.

Even though there is extensive damage to the intestinal villi and the villi continue to be destroyed if gluten is consumed, children seem to respond to the gluten-free diet better than adults and return to normal absorption. Adults generally manifest more villi damage and may later develop gastrointestinal carcinomas and lymphomas (7).

Lactose Intolerance. Lactase (enzyme that converts lactose into glucose and galactose) deficiency, congenital or acquired, produces a syndrome referred to as lactose or milk intolerance. Symptoms of lactose intolerance vary from minor abdominal bloating to abdominal cramps and pain and severe diarrhea. The unabsorbed lactose (milk sugar) in the intestine creates an osmotic effect and pulls fluid from the bloodstream to cause diarrhea. Lactose intolerance is frequently associated with other mucosal diseases of the intestine (regional enteritis) or following duodenal surgery.

Treatment is based on decreasing or omitting the amount of lactose in the diet. Dietary management is determined by the age of the patient. The availability of soybean and lactose-free formulas for infants and lactose-hydrolyzed milk and milk products has been an asset for the person on a lactose-restricted diet. Mineral and multivitamin supplements may be necessary, especially vitamin D and calcium.

Some individuals are able to tolerate only small amounts of lactose; for those persons, milk may be tolerated if it is offered with a meal rather than alone (7). It is important to read labels on all products to determine whether milk products are present among the ingredients. Breads, cakes, some candies (e.g., caramels, toffee, and milk chocolate), margarines, some salad dressings, and a variety of processed foods contain milk solids.

Yogurt, a fermented milk product that contains lactose, is tolerated by some individuals with lactose intolerance. The reason for this has been attributed to the autodigestion of lactose (via lactase activity) by the bacterial cultures used in yogurt production. The lactase activity of yogurt cultures may vary among brands (9).

POSSIBLE NURSING DIAGNOSES

Potential alteration in nutrition; less than body requirements related to
- inability to absorb nutrients.
- avoidance of food (gluten or milk products).

Potential alteration in bowel elimination; diarrhea related to excessive excretion of fats.

Potential fluid-volume deficit related to
- diarrhea.
- vomiting.

Potential alteration in comfort related to
- abdominal cramps.
- diarrhea.
- bloating.

Knowledge deficit related to
- pathophysiology of condition.
- dietary restrictions.

NURSING INTERVENTIONS
FOR NUTRITIONAL DISORDERS

Work closely with the patient, family, and dietitian to develop a dietary plan suitable to the patient's needs.

Potential alteration in nutrition; less than body requirements related to
- **inability to absorb nutrients.**
- **avoidance of food (gluten or milk products).**

- Advise the patient to follow the diet outlined by the dietitian to maintain optimum nutrition.

Potential alteration in bowel elimination; diarrhea related to excessive excretion of fats.

- Advise the patient to follow the dietary plan.

Potential fluid-volume deficit related to
- **diarrhea.**
- **vomiting.**

- Caution the patient to avoid offending foods.
- Encourage adequate fluid intake (8–10 glasses per day) when nausea is not present.

Potential alteration in comfort related to
- **abdominal cramps.**
- **diarrhea.**
- **bloating.**

- Caution the patient to avoid offending foods.

Continued

DYSFUNCTIONS OF ACCESSORY ORGANS

Liver

The liver is a complex and vitally important organ. With the exception of the long-chain fatty acids, all substances that have been digested are transported and transformed, and some are stored, by the liver for systemic use or excreted (see Figure 7–4).

Dysfunction of the liver can lead to major metabolic impairment. The major dysfunctions associated with the liver described in this section are inflammation of cells leading to hepatitis; death of cells, cirrhosis; and complications of liver disease, hepatic encephalopathy.

Hepatitis. Hepatitis is characterized by inflammation of the liver. The inflammatory process can be caused by a virus that is transmitted by the fecal-oral route and is known as Type A hepatitis. Type B hepatitis is usually transmitted by viral infected blood or blood products. The antigen for hepatitis B, however, is found in most body secretions. High-risk populations for hepatitis B are homosexuals, intravenous drug users, and medical

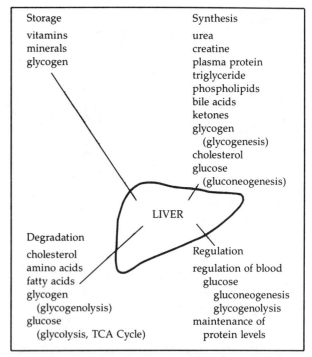

Figure 7-4. A sampling of liver functions.
Source: R.L. Pike and M.L. Brown, *Nutrition: An Integrated Approach,* 3d ed. (New York: John Wiley and Sons, Inc., 1984).

professionals. Technicians in laboratories or blood banks as well as physicians and nurses in hemodialysis centers are among the risk populations. Non-A/non-B hepatitis is frequently associated with posttransfusion disease.

The inflammatory process within the liver ultimately causes degeneration and death of liver cells. Under normal circumstances, the liver has the unique ability to regenerate cells, and liver function can be restored.

Symptoms of hepatitis may include anorexia, nausea and vomiting, epigastric discomfort, diarrhea or constipation, and fever. Jaundice may be present with the initial symptoms or appear after 5–10 days. Treatment protocols are aimed at regeneration of the diseased liver. Bedrest and diet modifications are primary protocols. (See Table 7–5).

In the initial stages, if the patient is suffering from nausea and vomiting, intravenous solutions of 10% glucose may be used (2). When the patient is able to tolerate oral feedings, the diet is high in

kilocalories, carbohydrate, and protein. If jaundice is present, the fat intake may be low.

Increased kilocalories and carbohydrates help to provide energy to meet the need for increased nutrients because of the inflammation and fever. Increased protein will aid the body in regenerating the disease cells and in reversing the negative nitrogen balance associated with tissue destruction. There is disagreement as to whether fats should be restricted. It is now felt that fats do not need to be restricted below the level of 25%–30% of total energy, unless the person shows signs of an intolerance (7). Usual fat intake in the United States is approximately 40% of total kilocalories. Fats generally help to make the food more palatable, increase the energy content of the food, produce satiety, and may help to prevent constipation. The physician will prescribe the type of diet best suited to the patient's needs.

The patient needs to understand the role of the diet in the healing process. Because the person

Table 7-5. DIETARY GUIDELINES FOR SELECTED LIVER DISEASES

DISEASES	NUTRIENTS/DAY				
	KILOCALORIES	CHO (g)	Protein (g/kg)	Fat (g)	Vitamins/ Minerals
Hepatitis	3000–4000	300–400	1.5–2.0	150	Supplement
Cirrhosis	2000–3000	300–350	1.0–2.0	Moderate	Supplement
Encephalopathy (hepatic coma)	1800+	225+	Low*	60**	Supplement

Sources:

M.V. Krause and L.K. Mahan, *Food, Nutrition and Diet Therapy. A Textbook of Nutritional Care* (Philadelphia: W.B. Saunders Company, 1984).

The American Dietetic Association, *Manual of Clinical Dietetics* (Chicago: The American Dietetic Association, 1988).

C.H. Robinson, et al., *Normal and Therapeutic Nutrition* (New York: Macmillan Publishing Company, 1986).

*Level should increase as patient improves
**Level may be lower depending on severity

may be anorectic, it is important for the nurse to encourage adequate food intake. Smaller, more frequent meals may be beneficial. Assess whether the person becomes more tired and has a reduced appetite at the end of the day. Encourage the majority of the kilocalories to be consumed early in the day. Dry milk powder can be added to foods and beverages to enhance the kilocalorie and protein content.

Increased fluid intake is also advised. Encourage the person to drink at least 8–10 glasses of fluid per day. Vitamin supplements, including B vitamins, vitamin B-12, and vitamin K should be replaced. Vitamins are stored in the liver, and damaged cells cannot store adequate quantities.

Alcohol should be eliminated from the diet because it is difficult for the diseased liver to detoxify the substance. Following recovery from hepatitis, the person should refrain from alcohol intake for four to six months unless otherwise specified by the physician.

POSSIBLE NURSING DIAGNOSES

Potential alteration in nutrition; less than body requirements related to
- nausea and vomiting.
- anorexia.
- food intolerance.

Potential fluid-volume deficit related to
- nausea and vomiting.
- lack of desire to drink.

Alteration in comfort related to epigastric pain.

Activity intolerance related to decrease in energy metabolism.

Knowledge deficit related to
- pathophysiology of condition.
- nutritional requirements.
- alcohol consumption.

NURSING INTERVENTIONS FOR NUTRITIONAL DISORDERS

Work closely with the patient and dietitian to plan a diet that meets the nutritional needs of the diseased liver.

Potential alteration in nutrition; less than body requirements related to
- **nausea and vomiting.**
- **anorexia.**
- **food intolerance.**

- Encourage the patient to eat small meals at frequent intervals (four to six per day).
- Administer anitemetic drugs prior to meals, if prescribed.

Continued

NURSING INTERVENTIONS *(continued)*

Potential fluid-volume deficit related to
- **nausea and vomiting.**
- **lack of desire to drink.**

- Offer the patient fluids at frequent intervals, i.e., every time someone enters the room.

Alteration in comfort related to epigastric pain.

- Caution the patient to avoid eating large quantities of food at one time and restrict those foods that cause bloating.

Activity intolerance related to decrease in energy metabolism.

- Advise the patient to consume all the kilocalories as prescribed to meet the energy needs of the body.

Knowledge deficit related to
- **pathophysiology of condition.**
- **nutritional requirements.**
- **alcohol consumption.**

- Instruct the patient to:
  eat small, frequent meals (four to six per day);

  use dry milk powders in foods and beverages to increase protein and kilocalories;

  drink liberal quantities of fluids, 8–10 glasses per day;

  take multivitamin supplements as prescribed; and

  take frequent rest periods to conserve energy needed for cellular regeneration.

Cirrhosis. Cirrhosis of the liver is a serious and irreversible disease characterized by hepatocellular destruction that leads to the development of fibrotic or nonfunctional scar tissue. Any agent (toxin) or condition (disease process) that causes irreversible damage to the liver cells can cause cirrhosis. Many alcoholics develop cirrhosis because alcohol is a toxic agent that can damage cells despite adequate nutritional intake (10).

Symptoms of cirrhosis include weakness, weight loss and nausea in the earlier stages. In the later stages, epigastric distress, that may result from enlargement of the liver and/or ascites (serous fluid collection in the peritoneal cavity), and steatorrhea due to faulty digestion of fats may occur. Hematemesis may occur due to increased portal hypertension and subsequent pressure of the blood vessels of the esophagus.

Treatment, especially in the early stages, includes rest; correction of the nutritional deficiencies with adequate kilocalories, nutrients, and vitamins; and abstinence from alcohol. Dietary management includes meeting increased energy requirements by providing a high kilocalorie, high carbohydrate, normal protein, and low-to-moderate fat intake. Protein intake will vary depending on the amount of liver damage. Increased amounts of protein may precipitate encephalopathy (see discussion later in this chapter). Vitamin supplementation is essential. Water-soluble and fat-soluble vitamins must be replaced (see Table 7-5 for dietary guidance in cirrhosis).

If the person has ascites and peripheral edema, the diet will also be sodium and fluid restricted. Since many patients suffer from steatorrhea, medium-chain triglycerides may be substituted for the long-chain triglycerides in the diet.

Because of the epigastric distress and anorexia associated with cirrhosis, it is important to encourage adequate nutrient intake. Daily intake may need to be divided into six to eight small feedings. Frequently, the majority of kilocalories can be consumed early in the day before the person becomes too tired.

POSSIBLE NURSING DIAGNOSES

Potential alteration in nutrition; less than body requirements related to
- anorexia.
- impaired nutrient metabolism.
- impaired nutrient utilization.
- impaired storage of vitamins.
- epigastric pressure.

Potential alteration in bowel elimination; steatorrhea related to excess secretion of fats secondary to liver dysfunction.

Potential fluid-volume excess; peripheral edema and ascites related to
- portal hypertension.
- sodium retention.
- lower plasma colloid osmotic pressure.

Knowledge deficit related to
- nutritional needs.
- risks of alcohol intake.

NURSING INTERVENTIONS FOR NUTRITIONAL DISORDERS

Work closely with the patient and dietitian to plan a diet that meets the needs of the diseased liver.

Potential alteration in nutrition; less than body requirements related to
- **anorexia.**
- **impaired nutrient metabolism.**
- **impaired nutrient utilization.**
- **impaired storage of vitamins.**
- **epigastric pressure.**
- Instruct the patient to eat frequent, small meals (six to eight per day).
- Encourage the patient to take rest periods before meals.

Potential alteration in bowel elimination; steatorrhea related to excess secretion of fats secondary to liver dysfunction.
- Advise the patient to follow the dietary plan to avoid unnecessary discomfort.

Potential fluid-volume excess; peripheral edema and ascites related to
- **portal hypertension.**
- **sodium retention.**
- **lower plasma colloid osmotic pressure.**
- Consult the dietitian to adjust diet in relation to changing needs (i.e., if ascites and/or esophageal varices are present).
- Monitor fluid intake and output, and weigh patient daily.

Knowledge deficit related to
- **nutritional needs.**
- **risks of alcohol intake.**
- Instruct the patient to:
  eat frequent, small meals (six to eight per day);
  ingest maximum kilocalorie intake early in the day;
  record daily intake and weight;
  take frequent rest periods to conserve energy;
  avoid coarse or mechanically irritating foods if esophageal varices are present;
  take multivitamin supplements as prescribed.

Hepatic Encephalopathy. Hepatic encephalopathy (ammonia intoxication) is a complication that results from systemic circulation of blood that cannot be detoxified because of the amount of degeneration of liver tissue. Ammonia, a nitrogenous waste, accumulates in the bloodstream. Bacteria and enzymes that are present in the intestinal tract normally metabolize amino acids, and ammonia is a by-product of the deamination process. The damaged liver cells cannot convert the ammonia circulating in the bloodstream into urea (nontoxic waste). The ammonia buildup creates a toxic environment for the central nervous system.

Symptoms of the toxic effects of ammonia range from lethargy to severe coma. Other symptoms might include depression, memory loss, slurred speech, Kussmaul-type (slow, deep) respirations, hiccups and other neurological manifestations such as confusion, decreased level of consciousness, and asterixis (liver flap).

Treatment is primarily aimed at reducing the protein concentration in the intestine, thus lowering the ammonia levels in the bloodstream. A combination of therapies is used. Adequate or increased kilocalories are provided with high carbohydrate concentrations in the diet.

Drugs such as locally acting antibiotics (Neomycin) are helpful in preventing bacterial overgrowth in the intestine. Lactulose, an osmotic agent, inhibits the diffusion of ammonia from the intestine into the bloodstream and has a potent laxative action. Laxative agents help to cleanse the bowel of fecal matter that contains protein.

A low-protein diet will be ordered. It is particularly important to limit foods such as buttermilk, some cheeses, chicken, gelatin, ground beef, ham, peanut butter, potatoes, onions, and salami, which contain high quantities of ammonia (11).

POSSIBLE NURSING DIAGNOSES

Alteration in nutrition; less than body requirements related to impaired
- utilization of nutrients.
- storage of nutrients.
- storage of vitamins.
- neurological state.

Alteration in bowel elimination; diarrhea related to lactulose and antibiotic therapy.

Potential fluid-volume deficit related to diarrhea.

NURSING INTERVENTIONS
FOR NUTRITIONAL DISORDERS

Work closely with the patient and dietitian to develop a dietary plan that meets the needs of the diseased liver.

Alteration in nutrition; less than body requirements related to impaired
- **utilization of nutrients.**

Continued

NURSING INTERVENTIONS *(continued)*

- **storage of nutrients.**
- **storage of vitamins.**
- **neurological state.**

- Instruct the patient to:
  eat frequent, small meals (if appropriate) that are high in carbohydrate to meet energy needs;

  limit or avoid protein ingestion as prescribed;

  avoid use of the sweetener aspartame, an aromatic amino acid (12).

- Assess the ability of the patient to ingest foods by mouth and determine whether it is necessary to obtain an order to insert a feeding tube.

- Monitor mental status to note ammonia intoxication and impending coma.
- Position the patient to prevent aspiration of feedings, if tube feedings are used.

Alteration in bowel elimination; diarrhea related to lactulose and antibiotic therapy.

- Monitor intake and output.
- Offer oral fluids at frequent intervals.

Potential fluid-volume deficit related to diarrhea.

- Monitor intake and output.
- Monitor laboratory values of electrolytes to determine potential complications.

Gallbladder

The gallbladder functions to concentrate the bile that is formed in the liver. When fatty substances enter the intestine, cholecystokinin (hormone) sends feedback to the gallbladder to release the stored bile through the common bile duct, the ampulla of vater, and into the duodenum (see Figure 7-5). Bile aids in the digestion and absorption of fats.

Cholecystitis and Cholelithiasis. Cholecystitis is an inflammation of the gallbladder that may occur simultaneously with cholelithiasis (stones in the gallbladder). Escherichia coli is the most frequent offending organism (13). The bacteria can be blood or lymph borne. In addition to cholelithiasis, post-surgical adhesions, obstruction by tumors, or intensive fasting may predispose to the disease process.

Why certain persons form stones in the gallbladder is unknown. Approximately 20 million Americans suffer from gallbladder disease and approx-

imately 500,000 cholecystectomies (surgical removal of the gallbladder) are performed each year (14).

Gallstones are formed from excess cholesterol or excess bilirubin pigments. They may rest silent in the gallbladder or become lodged in a duct leading to the intestine and ultimately cause a blockage to the flow of bile.

Persons most likely to suffer from gallbladder disease are women, usually older than 40, who have borne several children. Obesity may also be associated with the development of the disease.

Symptoms of these dysfunctions of the gallbladder are similar so they are discussed together. Initially, the person may be asymptomatic or may suffer from severe, sharp, colicky-type pains in the upper right quadrant of the abdomen after eating. Pain may also be experienced in the shoulder area. Nausea and vomiting may be present. Belching and bloating may also be a source of distress. If

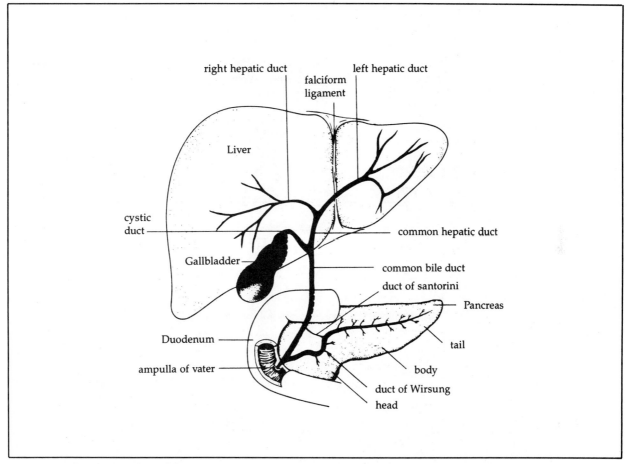

Figure 7-5. The relationship of the accessory organs.
(From M.J. Miller, *Pathophysiology: Principles of Disease* (Philadelphia: W.B. Saunders Company, 1983). Reprinted with permission.)

infection is present, the person will usually manifest a fever.

Treatment is based on the cause. Conservative management involves restricted fat intake in the diet. A low fat diet is generally ordered. A kilocalorie-restricted diet may also be ordered for the person who is obese. Small, frequent meals may be more readily tolerated by some persons because there is less stress on the gallbladder to supply bile needed for digestion.

In acute cases, surgery may be necessary. If the gallbladder is removed, bile is still formed by the liver, but the bile cannot be concentrated. The dietary regimen following surgery is usually progressive, NPO (nothing by mouth) to a low-fat diet. The fat restriction is usually ordered for approximately four to six weeks postoperatively. After that period of time, the person is instructed to gradually increase the amount of fat in the diet. The individual must determine which foods can be eaten without discomfort and which foods are to be avoided. As a general rule, concentrated fats are not well tolerated.

POSSIBLE NURSING DIAGNOSES

Potential alteration in nutrition; less than body requirements related to nausea and fat intolerance.

Potential fluid-volume deficit related to nausea and vomiting.

Alteration in comfort related to pain associated with biliary colic (spasms).

Potential for infection related to irritation due to obstruction of the flow of bile.

Knowledge deficit related to
- relationship of fat intake to pain and discomfort.
- hazards of obesity.

NURSING INTERVENTIONS FOR NUTRITIONAL DISORDERS

Work closely with the patient and dietitian to develop a dietary regimen that creates no discomfort.

Potential alteration in nutrition; less than body requirements related to nausea and fat intolerance.

- Instruct the patient to eat frequent, small meals and avoid those foods that contain concentrated fats.

Potential fluid-volume deficit related to nausea and vomiting.

- Offer antiemetic drugs as prescribed prior to meals.
- Encourage adequate fluid intake when the patient is not nauseated.

Alteration in comfort related to pain associated with biliary colic (spasms).

- Caution the patient to avoid those foods that precipitate discomfort, such as concentrated fats and spices.

Potential for infection related to irritation due to obstruction of the flow of bile.

- Note the color of the stool (pale) and urine (dark) to detect possible obstruction to flow of bile.

Knowledge deficit related to
- **relationship of fat intake to pain and discomfort.**
- **hazards of obesity.**

- Instruct the patient to:
    eat frequent, small meals;

    avoid foods that contain concentrated fats (fried foods);

    maintain a kilocalorie controlled diet, if indicated;

    take water-soluble forms of fat-soluble vitamins, if prescribed;

    use judgment in choosing foods that may be gas forming;

    eliminate foods from the diet that cause problems such as belching and bloating;

    avoid abuse of alcohol intake, which may precipitate pancreatitis.

Pancreas

The pancreas is intimately involved with the digestion of carbohydrate, protein, and fat. It has both exocrine (enzymes secreted into the intestine) and endocrine (internal hormonal secretion into the bloodstream) secretions. This section deals with pancreatitis. A discussion of the endocrine function of the pancreas is included in Chapter 13.

Pancreatitis. Pancreatitis (inflammation of the pancreas) is caused by obstruction of pancreatic secretions and leakage of secretions into pancreatic tissue with ultimate digestion of the pancreatic cells (see Figure 7-5). Autodigestion of the pancreas results because proteolytic enzymes are present in the exocrine secretions of the pancreas. Ultimately, a person can also develop insulin-dependent diabetes mellitus, as increasing numbers of cells in the islets of Langerhans are destroyed. Malabsorption syndromes and steatorrhea may also result.

Pancreatitis can be acute or chronic; chronic pancreatitis frequently follows recurrent episodes of acute pancreatitis. The primary symptom associated with pancreatitis is persistent epigastric pain that may radiate to the back. Other symptoms are nausea, vomiting, steatorrhea, and weight loss resulting from malabsorption of nutrients. Peritonitis may develop if the proteolytic enzymes leak into the peritoneal cavity.

Treatment is basically supportive; rest the pancreas and provide analgesics to control the pain. Oral foods and fluids are withheld, and nasogastric suction is used to prevent gastric secretions from entering and stimulating the small intestine. Hydration is maintained through the use of intravenous fluids. Electrolyte replacement must also be carefully monitored. Total parenteral nutrition may be used for those patients who are nutritionally deficient.

Frequent, small feedings of high-carbohydrate clear liquids may be offered when oral feeding is reestablished. Elemental feedings may be prescribed for some patients, since these feedings do not stimulate pancreatic secretions because they are hydrolyzed (predigested). Medium-chain triglycerides may be used to relieve steatorrhea and to help the person gain weight.

The diet will generally progress to a bland, low-fat, and ultimately, to a high-carbohydrate, high-protein, low-fat diet. Some individuals, especially those with chronic pancreatitis, require the use of oral pancreatic enzyme supplements. These supplements are given with food to aid in the digestive process. It may be necessary to encourage the patient to eat, since anorexia and nausea will continue to be problems. Offering favorite foods, if possible, may help.

POSSIBLE NURSING DIAGNOSES

Potential alteration in nutrition; less than body requirements related to
- nausea and vomiting.
- steatorrhea.
- diet restrictions.

Potential fluid-volume deficit related to
- nausea and vomiting.
- diarrhea.

Potential alteration in bowel elimination; steatorrhea related to excessive secretion of fats in the stool, secondary to deficient pancreatic enzymes.

Alteration in comfort; pain related to pancreatic discomfort and/or peritonitis.

Knowledge deficit related to
- pathophysiology and relationship to food intake.
- dietary management.
- alcohol consumption.

NURSING INTERVENTIONS
FOR NUTRITIONAL DISORDERS

Work closely with the patient and dietitian to develop a dietary plan to meet the nutritional needs through the various phases of the disease process.

Potential alteration in nutrition; less than body requirements related to
- **nausea and vomiting.**
- **steatorrhea.**
- **diet restrictions.**

- Encourage the patient to eat frequent, small meals and avoid intake of those foods that cause discomfort.
- Assess for signs of diabetes mellitus as a result of damage to the pancreatic tissue.
- Monitor for signs of hypocalcemia, which may accompany pancreatitis.

Potential fluid-volume deficit related to
- **nausea and vomiting.**
- **diarrhea.**

- Monitor fluid intake and output.
- Offer fluids at frequent intervals.

Potential alteration in bowel elimination; steatorrhea related to excessive secretion of fats in the stool, secondary to deficient pancreatic enzymes.

- Instruct the patient to take enzyme replacements with food and not to swallow capsules with hot liquids because heat destroys the enteric coating.

Alteration in comfort; pain related to pancreatic discomfort and/or peritonitis.

- Offer analgesic medications as prescribed.

Knowledge deficit related to
- **pathophysiology and relationship to food intake.**
- **dietary management.**
- **alcohol consumption.**

- Instruct the patient to:
  eat frequent, small meals when oral foods are tolerated;

  avoid the use of caffeine products and spices (gastric irritants);

  avoid the use of alcohol due to its damaging effect on pancreatic tissue;

  avoid nicotine, which stimulates pancreatic enzymes;

  maintain diet compliance in order to prevent subsequent attacks of pancreatitis.

TOPIC OF INTEREST

Interest in dietary fiber has grown in the last decade due to the positive health associations noted in epidemiological studies. In addition, the Surgeon General, the Federation of American Societies for Experimental Biology, and the National Academy of Sciences have all recommended that individuals increase their intake of fiber (15, 16, 17). The scientific groups have encouraged increased fiber intake through the inclusion of high-fiber foods rather than through the addition of isolated fibers to foods or fiber supplements. The effects of isolated fibers differ from the effects of fiber in native foods. Purified fibers caused an increase in chemically induced colon neoplasms in animal experiments (16). Additionally, no conclusive evidence exists that the fiber itself, rather than other components of foods in which fiber occurs naturally, exerts a protective effect with respect to chronic diseases (17). Increased intake of whole-grain cereals and breads, legumes, fruits, and vegetables remains the safest route for increasing fiber in the diet.

SPOTLIGHT ON LEARNING

Mrs. Oliver is a 72-year-old widow who lives alone. She must manage on a limited income and a small pension check. The doctor has told Mrs. Oliver that increasing the amount of fiber and fluid in her diet may help to prevent recurrent bouts of constipation. During one of her frequent visits to the Senior Citizens Center, Ms. Oliver asks you to help her think of ways to increase the fiber and fluid content in her diet. She complains that if she drinks fluids all day, she is "up all night."

Hint: Lunches may be available through the federally funded Congregate Meals Program at the Center.

1. What foods should be included in Ms. Oliver's diet on a daily basis?
2. How can fiber be added to the diet?
3. When should Ms. Oliver drink fluids in order to sleep without interruption?

REVIEW QUESTIONS

1. Jimmy is recovering from an acute episode of nausea and vomiting. The doctor has just ordered clear liquids. Jimmy's diet should not include which of the following?
   a. tea
   b. milk
   c. strained orange juice
   d. gelatin

2. During the acute phase of severe diarrhea, a person would receive which of the following diets?
   a. clear liquid
   b. full liquid
   c. bland
   d. soft, high fiber

3. What is the function of mucus in the stomach?
   a. activate gastrin
   b. neutralize stomach acid
   c. entrap bacteria
   d. protect stomach cells from gastric acid

4. What does negative nitrogen balance indicate?
   a. nitrogen is in equilibrium
   b. nitrogen is in excess of body needs
   c. nitrogen is low in relation to body needs
   d. has no physiological basis

5. Dietary fiber can be increased by adding which of the following to the diet?
   a. raw fruits and vegetables
   b. refined breads
   c. meats
   d. milk

6. Ms. Appleton returns to the clinic for her six-week postpartum checkup. She reports that she has been constipated. The nurse may suggest which of the following to minimize the problem?
   a. request an order for a laxative
   b. instruct the patient to take two teaspoons of mineral oil each day
   c. encourage the patient to drink two to three quarts of liquids daily
   d. instruct the patient to stop taking her iron supplements

7. Which of the following is not related to malabsorption syndromes?
   a. milk
   b. rice
   c. fat
   d. protein

8. Which diet is likely to be recommended in the late stages of cirrhosis?
   a. low protein, low kilocalorie
   b. high protein, high kilocalorie
   c. low protein, low sodium
   d. high protein, low potassium

9. Which is not a fat-soluble vitamin?
   a. A
   b. B complex
   c. D
   d. K

10. A 75-year-old woman is admitted to the nursing home. She has a history of diverticulosis. Which diet will most likely be recommended?
   a. pureed food
   b. low fiber
   c. high fiber
   d. high protein

ACTIVITIES

1. Plan a clear-liquid diet for a teenager who has been home recovering from stomach flu.

2. Identify five dos and five don'ts to prevent constipation in the elderly population in the nursing home.

3. Plan a dietary regimen to meet the needs of a woman who was recently diagnosed as having a duodenal ulcer. She needs six meals per day. She will be going back to work on the production line in the factory next week.

4. Go to the grocery store. Read the labels on several of the following products to determine the presence of milk or milk products and gluten: breads, cookies, candies, salad dressings, casserole mixes, soy sauce.

5. Prepare a diet assessment on a patient with cirrhosis of the liver. What dietary adjustments need to be made?

REFERENCES

1. Galambos, J.T., and T. Hersch. *Digestive diseases.* Boston: Butterworths, 1983.
2. Krupp, M.A., M.J. Chatton, and L.M. Tierney. *Current medical diagnoses and treatment: 1986.* Los Altos: Lange Medical Publishers, 1986.
3. Anderson, J.W. Physiological and metabolic effects of dietary fiber. *Federation Proceedings* 44 (1985):2902.
4. Rolandelli, R.H., et al. Comparison of parenteral nutrition and enteral feeding with pectin in experimental colitis in the rat. *American Journal of Clinical Nutrition* 47 (1988):715–21.

5. Hoppe, M.C., J. Descalso, and S.B. Kapp. Gastrointestinal disease: Nutritional implications. *Nursing Clinics of North America* 10 (1983):47–56.

6. Robinson, C.H., et al. *Normal and therapeutic nutrition.* New York: Macmillan Publishing Company, 1986.

7. Krause, M.V., and L.K. Mahan. *Food, nutrition and diet therapy. A textbook of nutritional care.* Philadelphia: W.B. Saunders Company, 1984.

8. Sleisenger, M.H., and J.S. Fordtran. *Gastrointestinal disease: Pathophysiology, diagnoses, management.* Philadelphia: W.B. Saunders Company, 1983.

9. Wytock, D.H., and J.A. DiPalma. All yogurts are not created equal. *American Journal of Clinical Nutrition* 47 (1988):454–57.

10. Achord, J.L. Malnutrition and the role of nutritional support in alcoholic liver disease. *American Journal of Gastroenterology* 82, no. 1 (1987):1–7.

11. Rudman, D., R.B. Smith, and A.A. Salam. Ammonia content of food. *American Journal of Clinical Nutrition* 26 (1973):487.

12. Uribe, M., M.A. Marquest, and G.G. Ramos. Treatment of chronic portal-systemic encephalopathy with vegetable and animal protein diets: A controlled crossover. *Digestive Disease Science* 27 (1982):12.

13. Lewis, S.M., and I.C. Collier. *Medical-surgical nursing: Assessment and management of clinical problems.* New York: McGraw-Hill Book Company, 1987.

14. Pancotto, F., D. Merrell, and A. Kelvin. Adult gastroenterology. In *Medicine and pediatrics in one book,* edited by J.D. Crapo, M.A. Hamilton, and S. Edgman. St. Louis: Hanley and Belfus, Inc., The C.V. Mosby Company, 1988.

15. The Surgeon General's report on nutrition and health. Summary and recommendations. Washington, D.C.: U.S. Department of Health and Human Services, Public Health Service, 1988.

16. Federation of American Societies for Experimental Biology. Physiological effects and health consequences of dietary fiber. Bethesda: Life Sciences Research Office, FASEB, 1987.

17. Committee on Diet and Health, Food and Nutrition Board, Commission on Life Sciences, National Research Council. *Diet and health. Implications for reducing chronic disease risk.* Washington, D.C.: National Academy Press, 1989.

CHAPTER
8

NUTRITION AND THE PATIENT WITH RENAL DISEASE

Objectives

After studying this chapter, you will be able to

- describe the metabolic consequences of glomerulonephritis, nephrosis, and renal calculi.
- explain the dietary management for patients with glomerulonephritis, nephrosis, and renal calculi.
- describe the metabolic consequences of renal failure (acute and chronic).
- list the components that are restricted in diets of individuals with acute or chronic renal failure who are not on dialysis and explain the rationale for the restrictions.
- explain the dietary rationale for a patient with acute or chronic renal failure not receiving dialysis.
- differentiate among the dietary approaches for individuals with renal failure who are using only diet to control uremia; undergoing hemodialysis; undergoing chronic intermittent or continuous ambulatory peritoneal dialysis; and recovering from renal transplantation.
- identify the reasons persons fail to adhere to the diet regimen in order to delay dialysis or while undergoing dialysis therapy.
- identify nursing interventions related to nutritional disorders associated with selected renal dysfunctions.

Overview

The kidney plays many crucial roles in the body. Disturbances in kidney function create havoc in many systems. In this chapter, normal kidney function is reviewed, and nutritional implications of kidney diseases are covered.

NORMAL KIDNEY FUNCTION

The kidney is an excretory, regulatory, and endocrine organ (1). As an excretory organ, the kidney rids the body of the end products of protein metabolism. Unlike carbohydrate and fat, which can be oxidized to carbon dioxide and water, protein catabolism results in the production of urea, uric acid, sulfate, creatinine, and organic acids. These by-products are of no use to the body and must be excreted.

The kidney's regulatory functions include adjustments to maintain the electrolyte, acid-base, fluid, and nutrient balances of the body. Electrolyte balance is maintained through active reabsorption and excretion of sodium, potassium, calcium, phosphorus, and chloride. The kidney regulates acid-base balance through its conservation of base groups and excretion of hydrogen ions. Fluid homeostasis is regulated by urine output, and nutrient balance is maintained through filtration and reabsorption of glucose and amino acids.

As an endocrine gland, the kidney secretes and/or is the site of action for a number of hormones, including renin, erythropoietin, and calcitriol. Renin acts on angiotensinogen, an important component in blood pressure regulation, as illustrated in Figure 8-1. Erythropoietin stimulates red-blood-cell production in the bone marrow, and calcitriol is the active form of vitamin D. The kidney is essential for converting vitamin D from an inactive to an active compound. (See Figure 8-2, page 190.)

The basic functional unit of the kidney is the nephron, and each kidney contains 1 million to 1.25 million of these units. It is in the various structures of the nephron that all blood is filtered, and electrolytes and nutrients are monitored, secreted, or reabsorbed, depending on the internal environment of the body. The pathway of blood through the kidney and the formation of urine is shown in Figure 8-3, page 191.

Blood enters the kidney through the renal artery. On the average, 1300 ml of whole blood or 700 ml of plasma flow through the kidney each minute (2). After the artery enters the kidney, extensive branching occurs, eventually giving rise to the afferent arterioles. The afferent arterioles supply blood to the glomeruli, tufts of capillaries located in structures called Bowman's capsules (see Figure 8-3). After being filtered by the glomeruli, blood leaves the structures via the efferent arterioles. The volume of plasma that filters through the glomeruli each minute is 125 ml, which adds up to approximately 180 l of plasma daily. This filtrate contains salt, sodium bicarbonate, glucose, free amino acids, vitamins C, K, and other valuable nutrients, as well as waste products such as urea and uric acid. The filtrate leaves Bowman's capsule, enters the proximal tubule, passes through the loop of Henle, continues through the distal tubule, and leaves the nephron via the collecting duct. Hormonal action, passive diffusion, active reabsorption, and selective secretion occur throughout the filtrate's passage through the nephron's structures. The final filtrate (urine) is quite different from the original filtrate in volume and composition. Only 1000–1500 ml of urine from the original 180 l of filtrate are excreted daily. The urine contains urea, sodium chloride, and other excretory products.

DISTURBANCES IN KIDNEY FUNCTION

Glomerulonephritis

Glomerulonephritis refers to an inflammatory process resulting from an infection that occurred

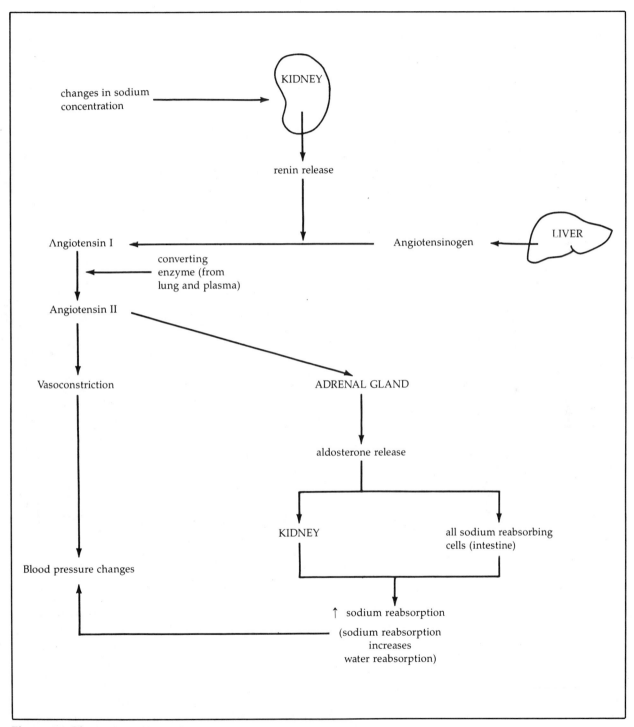

Figure 8-1. The renin-angiotensin system.

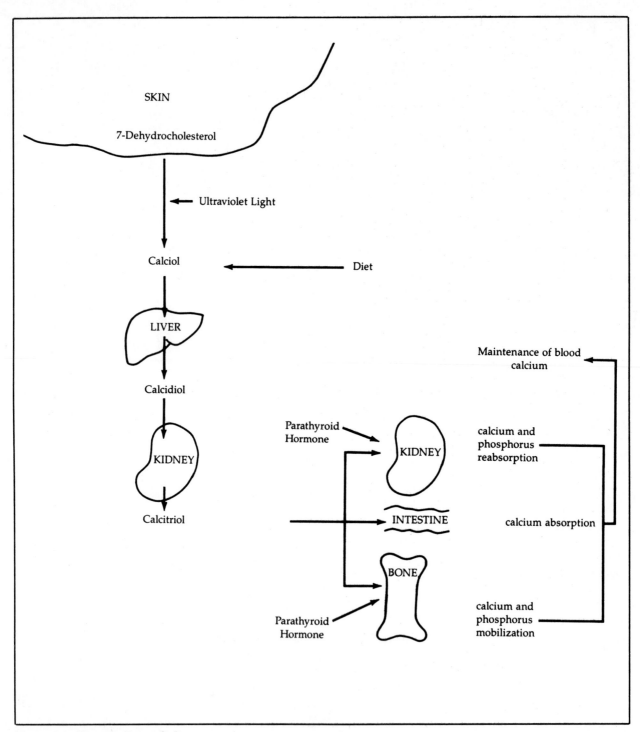

Figure 8-2. Vitamin-D metabolism.

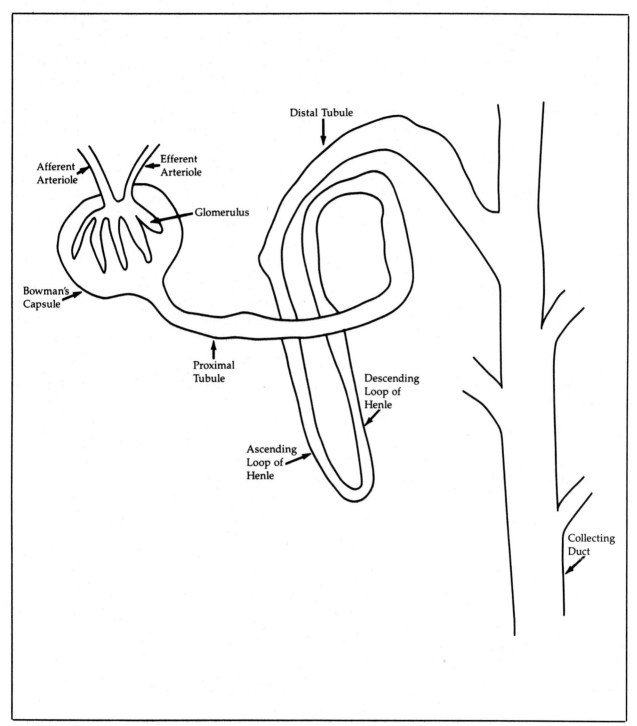

Figure 8-3. The nephron.

elsewhere in the body that disrupts the normal function of the glomerulus. Historically, glomerulonephritis has been classified as acute and chronic. With the newer methods of examining tissue and animal research, additional insights have been provided into the changes that occur in kidney tissue associated with glomerulonephritis. Many classifications are appearing, and changes will be noted in the future. Currently, one division is based on the etiology of the disease process, primary or secondary.

Primary glomerulonephritis is associated with changes and damage within the kidney itself. If another organ of the body is involved in precipitating the disease process, it is referred to as a secondary disorder. Secondary glomerulonephritis may occur following infectious diseases, such as streptococcal infections or hepatitis, or may be associated with other diseases, such as diabetes mellitus or lupus erythematosus.

Children frequently develop glomerulonephritis following a streptococcal infection, pharyngitis, or impetigo. In the case of poststreptococcal glomerulonephritis, immune complexes form as a result of an antigen-antibody reaction. Some of the complexes attach themselves to the basement membrane of the glomerulus. An inflammatory response is initiated, followed by scarring. The filtration surface of the membrane is altered, and the clinical signs become apparent.

Glomerulonephritis is characterized by hematuria, proteinuria, urinary sediment (including red-blood-cell casts), and low urinary sodium levels. The patient is usually hypertensive and edematous, and may have a decreased urinary output. Flank pain may be present, and the patient may complain of anorexia.

Treatment for this type of glomerulonephritis is supportive. The patient should have bed rest. If an infectious disease has been the cause, appropriate antibiotic therapy is used. Hypertension and edema are controlled by diuretics and/or antihypertensive drugs. Dialysis may be needed for some patients, especially if the glomerulonephritis exists for a prolonged period of time.

Dietary management usually involves adequate caloric intake to prevent tissue catabolism (2500–3500 kcal per day). Sodium and potassium intake are dependent on the serum levels of the electrolytes and the amount of edema. Protein levels of the diet may also be modified depending on the urinary protein loss and the amount of urinary output. If urine output is reduced, protein intake will be restricted. Once normal urine output has resumed, protein is added to the diet. Fluids are restricted when edema and oliguria are present. Fluid intake is usually limited to 500–600 ml (to account for water lost through the skin and lungs) plus the total urine and/or other fluid loss for the previous 24 hours. To ensure appropriate fluids are taken, the patient should also be weighed.

POSSIBLE NURSING DIAGNOSES

Alteration in nutrition; less than body requirements related to
- anorexia associated with disease process.
- decreased protein intake.

Potential fluid-volume excess related to edema and oliguria.

Self-care deficit, weakness related to disease process.

NURSING INTERVENTIONS FOR NUTRITIONAL DISORDERS

Work closely with the patient, physician, and dietitian to develop a dietary plan that will prevent further tissue breakdown.

Alteration in nutrition; less than body requirements related to
- **anorexia associated with disease process.**
- **decreased protein intake.**

- Instruct the patient to eat protein foods that have high biological value, such as meat, eggs, or milk, as prescribed.

Potential fluid-volume excess related to edema and oliguria.

- Keep accurate intake and output and daily weight measurements to help determine fluid intake.

- Monitor the results of laboratory tests which will provide indices for potential changes in the diet.
- Offer frequent mouth care, encourage the patient to chew gum and/or suck on hard candies to help alleviate thirst, if oral fluids are restricted.
- Encourage the patient to balance the prescribed fluid intake throughout the 24-hour day; some fluids should be taken during the night.

Self-care deficit; weakness related to disease process.

- Feed the patient, if necessary because of weakness.

Nephrosis

Nephrosis is a syndrome that affects both adults and children and results from increased glomerular permeability. It is likely to occur following diseases such as glomerulonephritis or systemic diseases, such as diabetes mellitus, or allergic or drug reactions.

Nephrosis is associated with a group of symptoms such as increased urinary protein, hypoalbuminemia, generalized edema, and hyperlipidemia (increased cholesterol). Large quantities of protein are lost through the glomerular membrane. Since the liver cannot replace the albumin at the rate it is being lost, hypoalbuminemia occurs. A decrease in the colloid oncotic pressure (the pressure created by the presence of protein) within the

blood vessels leads to a loss of volume in the vascular compartment and an increase in the third-space fluids (peritoneal cavity) and edema. As fluid volume is lost from the vascular tree, regulatory mechanisms (increased secretion of antidiuretic hormone and aldosterone) are enhanced. This contributes to the problem of fluid retention. Stimulation of the liver to produce additional proteins causes an increased production of lipoproteins manifested by hyperlipidemia.

Treatment protocols attempt to prevent further glomerular destruction. Plasma expanders, such as intravenous albumin, may be used to increase oncotic pressure within the blood vessels and thereby reduce edema formation. Diuretic drugs may be ordered to reduce edema and corticosteroids may be used to help stabilize the glomerular membrane and prevent further protein losses.

Dietary management is extremely important. Protein intake is largely dependent on glomerular filtration rate. Protein supplements such as Meritene or Citrotein may be ordered if the glomerular filtration rate is normal. If the glomerular filtration rate is decreased, protein intake may be limited. Unless there is hyperlipidemia, fat intake is not generally restricted. Adequate kilocalories should be provided to help reverse the catabolic state. Sodium restriction may be necessary to help reduce edema, concurrent with diuretic therapy.

POSSIBLE NURSING DIAGNOSES

Alteration in nutrition; less than body requirements related to anorexia associated with pressure from ascites.

Fluid-volume excess, edema, and ascites, related to decreased urine output.

NURSING INTERVENTIONS FOR NUTRITIONAL DISORDERS

Work closely with the patient, physician, and dietitian to develop a dietary plan that will enhance glomerular repair.

Alteration in nutrition; less than body requirements related to anorexia associated with pressure from ascites.

- Make the patient comfortable for meals; generally an upright position prevents pressure of ascites on the stomach.
- Entice the patient to eat prescribed kilocalories and protein.
- Encourage the family to bring favorite foods to the hospital.
- Offer fluids between meals and during the night to prevent over-distention of the stomach.

- Discuss the importance of dietary management, and reinforce written information that outlines methods for increasing kilocalories and restricting protein and sodium, if necessary.

Fluid-volume excess, edema, and ascites related to decreased urine output.

- Record intake and output and daily weight.
- Monitor vital signs to detect signs of hypovolemic shock associated with protein and fluid losses.
- Monitor results of laboratory tests that will provide clues to the prescribed dietary changes (sodium, potassium, urinary protein loss).

Renal Calculi

Calculi or stones can form anywhere within the urinary tract and may be fine and granular (sand-like) or large (filling the kidney pelvis). Calculi may be composed of calcium salts (including oxalates), uric acid, cystine, and struvite (magnesium ammonium phosphate). Calcium and uric-acid stones are the most common. If the stone is located in the kidney, it is referred to as a renal calculus. It is also possible for the patient to have ureteral and/or bladder stones. This discussion focuses on renal calculi; however, dietary-management principles are the same for all types of stones.

The pH of the urine, as well as the concentration and temperature of urine are all important in stone formation. A calculus can develop following an infection or stasis (causing concentration of urine). Organic matter or excess chemical substances can form the nucleus of a stone. Persons who live in certain areas of the United States are more prone to developing certain types of stones. For example, persons in the southeastern region are generally

Table 8-1. FOODS HIGH IN CALCIUM, OXALATES, AND PURINES

CALCIUM	OXALATES	PURINES

Milk and milk products
 	
Soybean curd
 	
Seafood
  sardines, canned salmon
  (with bone)
 	
Green leafy vegetables (low
  in oxalic acid)
  broccoli, kale
	Fruits
	  blackberries, concord
	  grapes, lemon and lime
	  peel, black raspberries,
	  rhubarb
	
	Vegetables
	  beets, celery, eggplant,
	  greens (swiss chard,
	  collard, dandelion,
	  escarole, pokeweed,
	  spinach), grits (white
	  corn), okra, green peppers,
	  sweet potatoes, rutabaga,
	  summer squash
	
	Other
	  beer, chocolate and cocoa,
	  peanuts, pecans, tea
		High Purine
		
		Bouillon
		  broth, consomme, gravies
		
		Meat extracts
		
		Organ meats
		  brain, heart, kidney, liver,
		  sweetbreads
		
		Seafood
		  mackerel, shrimp
		
		Vegetables
		  dried legumes, lentils
		
		Yeast
		  bakers, brewers
		
		Moderate Purine
		
		Meats, poultry, fish,
		  including shellfish (These
		  foods are limited to one to
		  two servings per week.)

Sources: M.V. Krause, and L.K. Mahan, *Food, Nutrition, and Diet Therapy* (Philadelphia: W.B. Saunders Company, 1984); C.H. Robinson, et al., *Normal and Therapeutic Nutrition* (New York: Macmillan Publishing Company, 1986); M.E. Shils, and V.R. Young (eds.) *Modern Nutrition in Health and Disease*, 7th ed. (Philadelphia: Lea & Febiger, 1988); and The American Dietetic Association, *Manual of Clinical Dietetics* (Chicago: The American Dietetic Association, 1988).

more prone to calcium oxalate stones because of the increase in the quantity of oxalates consumed in the diet (e.g., grits, greens, peanuts, and pecans). (See Table 8-1, page 195, for types of foods that may be implicated in the formation of calcium, oxalate, and uric-acid stones.) Persons who live in areas of the country where limestone is prevalent in the soil and water supply are more prone to developing calcium-base stones. Calcium stones may also develop in those patients with parathyroid disturbances and those with osteoporosis. Uric-acid stones may occur in those persons with gout or renal failure and in persons who use thiazide diuretics.

Stones may be "silent" or cause excruciating pain. Symptoms may include hematuria (microscopic or gross). If pain is present, it frequently radiates to the groin area. Patients may manifest a fever.

Urine is analyzed to determine excretion levels of calcium, oxalate, or uric acid; pH level; or infection. All urine is strained to note the presence of any small granular (sandlike) stones.

POSSIBLE NURSING DIAGNOSES

Alteration in nutrition; greater than body requirements related to increased levels of
- calcium.
- oxalate.
- uric acid.

Potential fluid-volume deficit related to need for forcing fluids.

Knowledge deficit related to dietary restrictions needed to prevent recurrence of calculi.

Potential noncompliance with dietary program to prevent recurrence of calculi.

NURSING INTERVENTIONS FOR NUTRITIONAL DISORDERS

Work closely with the patient, physician, and dietitian to develop a dietary plan that is modified to prevent additional calculi formation once the etiology of stone formation is identified.

Alteration in nutrition; greater than body requirements related to increased levels of
- calcium.
- oxalate.
- uric acid.

- Provide lists of foods to be included or excluded from the diet, depending on chemical composition of the stone (calcium, oxalate, or uric acid).
- Encourage the patient to follow the diet prescription.

Potential fluid-volume deficit related to need for forcing fluids.

- Encourage the patient to appreciably increase fluid intake to three to four liters per day to prevent stasis of urine.

Continued

NURSING INTERVENTIONS *(continued)*

Knowledge deficit related to dietary restrictions needed to prevent recurrence of calculi.

- Instruct the patient to:
    follow the diet regimen as outlined;

    balance fluid intake throughout a 24-hour period;

avoid dehydration; be alert for situations that might precipitate excess fluid losses (perspiration, vomiting, or diarrhea).

Potential noncompliance with dietary program to prevent recurrence of calculi.

- Encourage the patient to follow the diet prescription.

Renal Failure

Renal failure occurs when the metabolic demands of the body for excretion of waste products by the kidney cannot be met. Failure may occur suddenly (for example, following extensive body burns, exposure to or ingestion of toxic substances, including drugs or urinary-tract obstruction) and is referred to as acute renal failure. Acute renal failure is reversible if detected early, provided extensive kidney damage has not already occurred. Chronic renal failure occurs slowly and sometimes silently. It may be associated with diseases such as diabetes mellitus and hypertension. The resulting damage is irreversible.

Nurses are in a unique position to instruct persons in the ways to prevent potential damage to the kidney. Proper storage, use, and disposal of cleaning agents, chemical solvents, and insecticides in the home, industrial, and agricultural settings is one example. Instruction to parents of young children of the importance of medical follow-up for streptococcal infections is another example.

The assessment function of the nurse also plays a critical role in the early detection of renal failure following surgery or associated with severe trauma or burns. Monitoring renal function for patients with diabetes mellitus and hypertension is also essential.

Acute Renal Failure. Acute renal failure is the sudden cessation of urinary output resulting from a variety of possible causes. Currently, the causes are classified as prerenal, renal, or intrarenal, and postrenal. Prerenal causes of acute renal failure (ARF) include dehydration, hemorrhage, severe trauma or burns, and shock (surgical, traumatic or hypovolemic). Severe infections, toxic substances (including drugs and sudden occlusion of the blood supply to the kidney) may be classified as renal causes of ARF. Postrenal causes may include acute urinary-tract obstruction, such as urinary calculi or prostatic obstruction.

Failure of the kidney to excrete more than 400 ml of urine per 24-hour period may be caused by leakage of tubular fluid due to damage to the renal tubule, obstruction of the renal tubule with casts or other debris, alteration in the blood supply to the kidney, and disorders affecting the glomerulus.

Since two phases occur in the course of renal failure, it is essential to be alert to the changes that take place. The oliguric phase, during which urinary output may be diminished to as little as 20–30 ml per day or as much as 500 ml per day, may last for approximately two days to as long as six weeks. This phase is followed by the diuretic phase. The urine output may increase gradually to what may seem like a more adequate output. The urine that is excreted, however, may be largely extracellular fluid (minus the waste products), because the nephron unit may not be completely healed and the nitrogenous wastes and electrolytes may still be retained in the vascular tree.

Treatment is aimed at determining the cause of acute renal failure and reversing the process. Prompt treatment is essential to prevent further damage. Fluid volume and electrolyte, acid-base, and mineral balance must be maintained.

The goals of dietary management are to correct fluid and electrolyte imbalances and prevent further breakdown of body tissues, which causes an increase in nitrogenous wastes of endogenous origin. Fluid intake is limited to the 400–600 ml insensible fluid loss plus the total output from the previous 24-hour period. This applies to intravenous as well as oral fluid replacement. When diuresis begins to occur, fluid intake will be prescribed in proportion to the output and the patient's daily weight.

Energy demands are high and are provided through concentrated carbohydrates and lipids. In order to prevent negative nitrogen balance, approximately 2000–5000 kcal per day may be needed to prevent catabolism. (Refer to Chapter 6 for a discussion of physiologic stress.)

Unless the patient is undergoing dialysis, protein intake will be severely limited. Parenteral hyperalimentation, containing essential amino acids (partially synthesized by the kidney) and caloric support with concentrated glucose and lipids may be given.

Sodium is restricted until adequate kidney function returns. Non-dialyzed patients are restricted to 500–1000 mg sodium during the oliguric phase. If the patient is on dialysis, the restriction may be more liberal, 1500–2000 mg per day (3).

The patient's potassium levels must be carefully monitored. Replacement will be prescribed if a deficiency exists.

POSSIBLE NURSING DIAGNOSES

Potential alteration in fluid volume (excess or deficit) related to anuria/oliguria, diuresis, vomiting, diarrhea or fever.

Alteration in nutrition; less than body requirements related to anorexia and fatigue.

NURSING INTERVENTIONS FOR NUTRITIONAL DISORDERS

Work closely with the patient, physician, and dietitian to develop a dietary plan that will meet the nutritional needs without causing further damage to the kidney.

Potential alteration in fluid volume (excess or deficit) related to anuria/oliguria, diuresis, vomiting, diarrhea, or fever.

- Record intake and output and daily weight.
- Monitor vital signs; a rise in blood pressure may indicate fluid retention.

- Plan a regimen that will allow prescribed fluid intake to be consumed over a 24-hour day.

Alteration in nutrition; less than body requirements related to anorexia and fatigue.

- Encourage the patient to consume the prescribed kilocalories (2000–5000 kcal per day).

Chronic Renal Failure (End Stage). Renal diseases affect two nephron structures, the glomerulus or the renal tubules (4). No matter which structure is initially affected, the excretory and regulatory capabilities of the nephron eventually become involved, and the kidney fails to function adequately. Kidney diseases that may lead to chronic renal failure include chronic pyelonephritis, chronic glomerulonephritis, vascular kidney diseases, systemic diseases with renal manifestations, congenital abnormalities, and drug toxicities.

The large reserve capacity of the kidney is illustrated by the maintenance of homeostatic mechanisms even when 60% of the total nephrons are destroyed. Minimal excretory capacity continues until only approximately 10% of functioning nephrons remain (5). When this point is reached, the excretory and regulatory capabilities of the kidney are seriously compromised, and accumulation of waste products and metabolic aberrations occur. With the accumulation of toxic waste products in the tissues and blood (uremia), the final, common pathway of chronic, progressive kidney disease develops. Conservative treatment (diet) is used until the disease progresses to the point that dialysis or transplantation are the only choices to avoid death.

POSSIBLE NURSING DIAGNOSES

Alteration in nutrition; less than body requirements related to
- anorexia.
- nausea/vomiting.
- altered taste and/or smell.
- unpalatable food.

Potential or actual fluid-volume excess due to fluid and electrolyte imbalance related to renal dysfunction.

Knowledge deficit related to
- fluid restrictions.
- severe dietary restrictions.

Self-care deficit related to fatigue (inability to self-feed).

Renal function is often described in terms of glomerular filtration rate (GFR), or the volume of plasma filtered through the glomeruli in one minute. One method of measuring GFR is to measure creatinine clearance. Creatinine is a by-product of muscle metabolism and a normal constituent of urine. It is freely filtered by the glomerulus. A decrease in creatinine clearance is indicative of a decreased GFR.

Symptoms of uremia commonly appear at creatinine clearance rates of less than 25 ml per minute (normal GFR rate is 125 ml per minute). At this point, nitrogen retention in the form of increased urea, uric acid, and creatinine occurs. Serum or blood urea nitrogen (BUN), normally 10–20 mg/dl, climbs to 90–100 mg/dl or higher (3, 5).

Other biochemical abnormalities that appear in chronic renal failure are glucose intolerance, lipid disorders, aminoaciduria, altered hormone concentrations, anemia, hypocalcemia, electrolyte disturbances, altered protein concentrations, and acidosis. The primary defect leading to glucose intolerance in uremia is peripheral tissue resistance to insulin action, which leads to hyperglycemia as well as basal hyperinsulinemia (7).

Uremic individuals who are not on dialysis as well as those patients on dialysis exhibit a high incidence of atherosclerosis and cardiovascular disease (8). The exact mechanisms by which uremia leads to atherosclerosis are still unclear.

Numerous hormones are altered in uremia. Renin levels, which may affect blood pressure, may be normal, increased, or decreased (8). As stated previously, serum insulin is elevated. Also elevated are glucagon, growth hormone, gastrin, and parathyroid hormone due to impaired renal catabolism of the hormones as well as enhanced secretion in the abnormal homeostatic state observed in chronic renal failure (6). Some hormones originating in the kidney, such as erythropoietin and calcitriol, are decreased. Impaired production of erythropoietin in concert with toxic suppression of red-blood-cell production in the bone marrow and a shortening of the life of the red blood cell culminate in anemia, observed early in uremia (5). The depressed levels of calcitriol cause an inhibition of calcium absorption from the intestine resulting in low serum calcium (hypocalcemia).

Electrolyte balance is profoundly affected in chronic renal failure. Because the major route of phosphorus excretion is the kidney, serum phosphorus retention occurs with a loss of renal function. Hyperphosphatemia (elevated blood phosphorus) exacerbates the low serum calcium. Potassium is also excreted primarily through the kidney. In early renal failure, when urine production may be 1000 ml per day, hypokalemia (low blood potassium) may occur because tubular secretion of potassium increases, resulting in high losses through the urine. In addition, gastrointestinal secretion of potassium increases, allowing excretion of potassium via the feces. As urine production progressively declines, the danger of hyperkalemia (high serum potassium) increases. Sodium balance also changes as renal failure progresses. In the initial stages of kidney disease, the percentage of sodium reabsorbed in the renal tubule declines, and much sodium is lost in the urine. When end stage renal disease inevitably occurs (that is, when GFR is less than 4–10 ml per minute), patients can no longer excrete the sodium ingested, and they retain sodium along with fluid (8).

A decline in total protein, albumin, transferrin, and some components of complement (C_3) are observed in uremic patients, especially those who are wasted and malnourished. Altered plasma and muscle amino acids are also common. Acidosis, often seen in uremia, is due to the impaired ability of the kidney to excrete acidic metabolites as well as renal losses of bicarbonate.

The clinical manifestations of uremia include yellow discoloration and itching of the skin, anorexia, nausea, vomiting, diarrhea, sensory disturbances, and bone pain (5). Malnutrition and wasting are also common features associated with chronic renal failure.

Yellow discoloration and itching of the skin, as well as the gastrointestinal and sensory disturbances, are directly related to the accumulation of the nitrogenous waste products and imbalances in the body. Bone pain, due to renal osteodystrophy, is a result of the complex interactions among serum calcium, phosphorus, calcitriol, and parathyroid hormone. Normally, low serum calcium stimulates the parathyroid gland to increase its release of parathyroid hormone. Parathyroid hormone acts on the kidney to increase the production of calcitriol. The vitamin acts on the gastrointestinal tract to increase calcium absorption and on the kidney to increase calcium reabsorption from the tubules. Also, calcitriol acts in concert with parathyroid hormone to mobilize calcium from the bone. Parathyroid hormone's action on the renal tubules causes a decrease in phosphorus reabsorption so that the appropriate calcium-phosphorus product is retained in the blood. (See Figure 8-4).

In chronic renal failure, phosphorus retention with the resultant hyperphosphatemia occurs. Serum calcium declines, and because calcitriol is decreased due to the diseased state of the kidney, the normal mechanism for increasing gastrointestinal calcium absorption cannot occur. Parathyroid hormone increases to mobilize calcium from the bone and to decrease phosphorus reabsorption. Compensation occurs in the early stages of renal failure, but ultimately hyperparathyroidism occurs. As renal failure progresses, and the GFR falls to less than 20 ml per minute, the serum phosphorus remains high despite hyperparathyroidism. The result is demineralization of the bone,

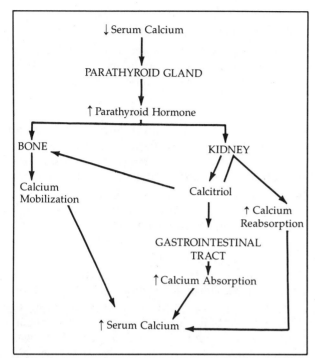

Figure 8-4. The interactions among calcium, parathyroid hormone, and calcitriol.

calcium phosphate deposition in the soft tissue, and progression of renal failure.

In addition to atherosclerosis, other cardiovascular problems may occur in uremic patients. When sodium and fluid retention occur, an increase in blood pressure and edema result. Hyperkalemia is particularly dangerous, as it causes cardiac arrhythmias and cardiac arrest.

Malnutrition and wasting, commonly observed in chronic renal failure, are characterized by decreased body weight, muscle mass, and adipose tissue and low or altered levels of serum proteins and amino acids. A complex problem exists: Malnutrition and wasting caused by inadequate dietary intake are due to anorexia caused by uremic toxins, as well as medications, depression, the catabolic effect of superimposed illness (common in chronic renal failure), endocrine disorders, the impaired metabolic functioning of the kidney, and side effects of the treatment itself (9).

The nurse must be alert to the development of malnutrition and wasting, because the signs of catabolism exacerbate the clinical symptoms of kidney disease and increase the chances of infection. The patient is weighed daily, and changes in status are noted by changes in weight or by calculating relative body weight.

Relative body weight equals observed body weight divided by the standard reference weight times 100% (10). Once patients are on dialysis, dry weight and interdialytic weights are followed. Dry weight is the weight at which patients are free of detectable peripheral edema and have normal blood pressure. Interdialytic weight changes refer to the weight gained between dialyses. Usually, a daily weight gain of one pound between dialyses is caused by fluid retention and provides guidelines for determining fluid intake (4). Changes in muscle mass are determined by monitoring changes in mid-arm circumference. Adipose tissue changes are estimated by skinfold measurements.

In addition to the clinical manifestations already mentioned, patients with chronic renal failure may become disturbed, disoriented, and psychotic as a result of depression and toxicity of accumulated waste products.

TREATMENT OF CHRONIC RENAL FAILURE

Chronic renal failure follows a progressive, downhill course. As renal function declines, different treatment protocols are instituted. Diet therapy is often used to delay dialysis therapy. There eventually comes a point, however, when the kidney function is so deteriorated that further dietary restrictions do not alleviate uremia symptoms, and dialysis or transplantation is critical to survival.

Medication

Medication does not cure chronic renal failure; it is used to deal with the many clinical problems that individuals face. In nondialyzed patients, acidosis is prevented or reduced via protein restriction and the use of alkali supplements. Calcium carbonate is one supplement that may correct mild acidosis and provide the calcium so badly needed by uremic individuals. As acidosis increases in severity, intravenous or oral sodium bicarbonate is administered. Once the patient is on dialysis, acidosis is corrected.

The high serum phosphorus observed in patients with chronic renal failure cannot be reduced via dietary restriction alone. Aluminum carbonate and aluminum hydroxide are phosphate binders used to lower serum phosphorus levels. Currently, controversy exists regarding the role of aluminum in the development of encephalopathy and osteomalacia. In the past, researchers traced these syndromes to aluminum toxicity in individuals on hemodialysis who received dialysate contaminated with high aluminum levels. Once standards for permissable levels of aluminum in dialysate were set, the incidence of dementia and bone disease decreased dramatically (11); however, the syndromes did not disappear (12).

Some researchers believe that the aluminum may enter the body via the digestive tract in individuals with chronic renal failure who must take aluminum-containing phosphate binders (13). Although the gastrointestinal tract provides a formidable barrier to aluminum absorption, it is not effective when exposed to high aluminum loads, as is the case in patients with chronic renal failure who must take the aluminum-containing medications (14). The normal route of excretion of any absorbed aluminum is the kidney. Individuals with compromised renal function would have difficulty excreting aluminum, and this would further add to the possibility of aluminum toxicity.

Vitamin D in the form of calcitriol is another medication given to individuals with chronic renal failure. Vitamin D has the potential for normalizing serum calcium levels, reducing or eliminating bone pain, increasing muscle strength, and decreasing parathyroid hormone (15). Frequent monitoring is required when vitamin D is administered. Hypercalcemia and hyperphosphatemia may result. If sustained hypercalcemia develops, a reversible or permanent decrease in glomerular filtration rate can occur.

Dialysis

Individuals with end-stage renal disease who can no longer remain free of symptoms of uremia through dietary restrictions alone are started on dialysis. This treatment can be maintained indefinitely or used as a temporary measure prior to kidney transplant. Through dialysis, excess nitrogenous waste, water, sodium, and potassium are removed from the body, thereby greatly reducing the symptoms of uremia. However, dialysis does not correct all metabolic problems of chronic renal failure.

The dialysis methods currently available are hemodialysis, chronic intermittent peritoneal dialysis, and chronic ambulatory peritoneal dialysis (CAPD). The number of patients maintained on dialysis has increased since the 1974 and 1979 Medicare and Medicaid legislation, which provided that federal funds could help cover the costs of dialysis. Prior to the legislation, dialysis was not an affordable treatment for all patients, and death was the inevitable result of chronic renal failure. No dialysis procedure is risk-free, however, and the annual mortality rate for dialysis patients is 9%–10% (16).

Hemodialysis. Hemodialysis requires the use of a machine that filters the patient's blood. The blood passes through a dialyzer, which removes wastes and returns the "clean" or dialyzed blood to the patient. The procedure is time-consuming, taking four to six hours to complete, and usually must be repeated three times per week to remove the continuous accumulation of nitrogenous end products, excess electrolytes, and fluid. A restricted diet is followed to avoid wide fluctuations in blood chemistries between dialysis treatments. Some fluctuation is inevitable, however, since the increased blood levels of wastes are decreased during the procedure. It is well recognized that decreasing the degree of fluctuation enhances patient wellbeing and avoids hemodialysis disequilibrium, a condition characterized by seizures during dialysis.

Hemodialysis may be considered to be a catabolic event associated with considerable losses of amino acids and glucose (if glucose-free dialysate is used) (17). Replacement of needed nutrients is difficult because hemodialysis patients frequently experience anorexia, nausea, and vomiting. These circumstances contribute to the development of malnutrition. Anemia, cardiovascular stress, and vascular access problems are also encountered during hemodialysis.

Chronic Intermittent Peritoneal Dialysis. In this type of dialysis, the peritoneal membrane is used as a dialyzer and is bathed in a glucose and electrolyte dialysis solution (dialysate). The solution is placed into the peritoneal cavity, and metabolic wastes pass into the dialysate through the processes of diffusion and osmosis. Usually, two liters of dialysate are placed into the abdominal cavity and removed after 10–12 hours. Like hemodialysis, the procedure must be repeated on a regular basis. Although it is a safe alternative to hemodialysis, chronic intermittent peritoneal dialysis is uncomfortable and time-consuming. Also, protein and amino-acid loss into the dialysate is substantial and must be replaced (18).

Chronic Ambulatory Peritoneal Dialysis (CAPD). This form of dialysis is similar to chronic intermittent peritoneal dialysis, except that dialysis takes place over a 24-hour period. A more constant clearance of waste products, fluid, and electrolytes is achieved through CAPD. Two liters of dialysate are instilled into the peritoneal cavity via an indwelling intraperitoneal catheter and remain there four to six hours at a time (19). Waste products diffuse into the dialysate and fluid removal is regulated by the glucose concentration of the dialysate. After four to six hours, the dialysate is drained by gravity and then new dialysate is installed into the peritoneum.

The advantages of CAPD over other forms of dialysis include better control over blood chemistries and reduction of anemia. Unlike hemodialysis, CAPD requires no machine, is lower in cost, has no vascular access problems, and causes minimal cardiovascular stress. Travel is relatively unrestricted, and minimal dietary restrictions are required (19). The major complication of CAPD is peritonitis, an infection of the peritoneal membrane caused by contamination from an external source (20). Peritonitis increases the permeability of the peritoneum to larger molecules resulting in substantial protein losses. Catabolism with wasting can result, and recurrent peritonitis reduces the individual's defense against disease.

The type of dialysis chosen depends on numerous factors, including the patient's physical state and eligibility for the procedure, ability to accept responsibility for care, and the availability and cost of the procedure.

Transplantation

Renal transplantation is a more permanent treatment of chronic renal failure. When successful, renal transplantation solves the excretory, regulatory, and endocrine problems caused by the diseased kidney. Renal transplant cannot solve the problems associated with atherosclerosis if this condition was present prior to the surgery (21). There is the risk that the disease that caused the patient's kidney to fail initially may also attack the healthy transplanted kidney. The major problems in renal transplantation, however, are the side effects of the immunosuppressive drugs that are used to prevent rejection of the new organ. Possible side effects include catabolism caused by the high dose of glucocorticoids, decreased carbohydrate tolerance or diabetes mellitus, hypokalemia, and decreased red-blood-cell maturation (22). Diet therapy is used to counteract the side effects. As the dose of immunosuppressive drugs is decreased, the dietary restrictions are gradually lifted, until a normal, unrestricted eating pattern is achieved.

Diet

The purposes of nutritional therapy in chronic renal failure are to (a) maintain optimal nutritional status; (b) minimize uremic toxicity; (c) prevent protein catabolism; (d) stimulate patient well-being; (e) retard the progression of renal failure; and (f) postpone the initiation of dialysis (4). In the past, diet therapy in chronic renal failure was the major method for prolonging an individual's life. As kidney function inevitably deteriorated, dietary restrictions increased in severity, until even the most severe restrictions could not keep individuals free of uremic symptoms (16). Dialysis was simply not an affordable alternative for many individuals, and renal transplantation was still an experimental procedure. Uremia eventually resulted in death, which some regarded as welcome relief to the bodily havoc created by the accumulation of toxic waste products.

Today, the picture has changed dramatically. More individuals can be placed on maintenance dialysis because the federal government now shares the burden of the cost. The success rate of kidney transplantation has increased, and the procedure is no longer experimental in nature. Currently, conservative dietary treatment is used until dialysis or transplantation is required.

The exact point at which dialysis should be started is a matter of judgment based on an assessment of the risks versus benefits. Proponents of delaying dialysis until absolutely necessary cite the maintenance of quality of life free of the invasive procedure and the fact that dietary restrictions may retard progression of renal failure and postpone dialysis for about one year (23). Opponents who believe in early dialysis (that is, before the patient is symptomatic) feel that because prolonged protein restrictions can be nutritionally inadequate, wasting can occur. Nutritionally compromised patients are more prone to infection and may not be able to withstand the stresses of dialysis or transplantation (24). Another reason cited in favor of early dialysis is the prophylactic role that early dialysis may play in protecting against the vascular changes of arteriosclerosis (21). Clearly, the patient's physical state must be weighed against the burdens of dialysis.

Once dialysis is started, dietary supervision continues, and restrictions are less severe. Dietary support after renal transplantation is often only temporary and required during the early stages following the surgical procedure.

Because chronic renal failure is a progressive disease, the diet is a dynamic treatment method that must be altered based on the biochemical and clinical status of the patient. For this reason, the discussion of the specifics of the diet is divided into four sections: predialysis, hemodialysis, peritoneal dialysis (including chronic intermittent and chronic ambulatory), and post-transplant. (See Table 8-2 for a summary of dietary recommendations during these stages.)

Predialysis. The major dietary elements of concern for patients with chronic renal failure are protein, kilocalories, sodium, potassium, phosphorus, fluids, and vitamin and mineral supplementation.

Because the end products of protein metabolism are excreted via the urine, protein restrictions are necessary to avoid or reduce uremia. Protein intakes beyond the capabilities of the kidney quickly result in toxic symptoms. As a bench mark, consider that average protein intake in the United States is approximately 100 g, or about twice the RDA of 0.8 g/kg per day. Uremic individuals restricted to 40 g of protein per day have a median survival time of only 150 days (25). You might think that to avoid the accumulation of the metabolic end products of protein metabolism a zero protein diet would be effective. Actually, ingesting too little protein is just as serious as ingesting too much, because the absence of adequate protein results in a negative nitrogen balance. In this state, the body catabolizes muscle tissue, resulting in the formation of nitrogenous waste (refer to Chapter 6 for a discussion of physiologic stress). A delicate balance must be achieved. Ideally, just enough protein should be ingested to replace that which is catabolized, keeping in mind the capabilities of the kidney.

Most physicians agree that initiation of protein restriction depends on the clinical state of the patient. When symptoms of uremia, such as nausea, vomiting, diarrhea, and anorexia appear, protein restriction should be instituted. Sometimes serum (blood) urea nitrogen levels are used as guidelines for when to restrict protein. Many uremic symptoms do not occur until serum urea nitrogen exceeds 90 mg/dl (normal 7–18 mg/dl). However, patients seem to feel better when serum urea nitrogen is less than 60 mg/dl. Therefore, protein restrictions are instituted to maintain serum urea nitrogen to less than 90 mg/dl, and

Table 8-2. SUMMARY OF DIETARY RECOMMENDATIONS IN CHRONIC RENAL FAILURE

NUTRIENT	PREDIALYSIS	HEMODIALYSIS	CHRONIC INTERMITTENT PERITONEAL DIALYSIS	CHRONIC AMBULATORY PERITONEAL DIALYSIS	POST-TRANSPLANT
Protein	15–50 g	1.0–1.2 g/kg	1.2–1.5 g/kg	1.2–1.5 g/kg	1.5–2 g/kg
Calories	35/kg	35/kg	35/kg	35/kg	RDA
Sodium	920–2000 mg	1000–2000 mg	1000–2000 mg	not usually necessary	3–4 g
Potassium	1560–2340 mg	1500–2000 mg	1500–2000 mg	not usually necessary	not restricted
Phosphorus	600–1200 mg	600–1200 mg	600–1200 mg	may or may not be required	not restricted
Fluid	400–600 ml plus urine output	400–500 ml plus urine output (if any)	400–500 ml plus urine output (if any)	not usually necessary	not restricted
Vitamins/ minerals	supplement necessary	supplement necessary	supplement necessary	supplement necessary	supplement necessary

preferably to less than 60 mg/dl (8). Creatinine clearance levels may also be used to determine the initiation of protein restrictions, and clinicians may begin restrictions when creatinine clearance falls below 25 ml per minute (5). (See Table 8-3.)

Before dialysis treatment became a viable option, and if some renal function still existed, protein was restricted to as little as 0.3 g/kg per day. This would be only 21 g of protein for a 70 kg male. At this level, the majority of the protein had to be of high biological value (a complete protein). High-biological-value protein sources are those that provide all essential amino acids. Sources of high-biological-value protein include eggs, milk, meat, fish, and poultry (Table 8-4). Three-fourths of the protein should be of high biological value (26).

The use of essential amino acids as supplements may be necessary when a 40 g protein diet is prescribed in order to meet the body's needs (27); however, they are required when the protein level of the diet is less than 30 g per day (26). In principle, the addition of essential amino acids supplies the uremic patient with the amino-acid building blocks needed without imposing nonessential nitrogenous compounds from nonessential amino acids. The results are improved nitrogen utilization (8) and a slowing in the progression of chronic renal failure (28). When essential amino acids are added to the very low protein diet, the protein intake need not be of high biological value, allowing more variety in the diet and increased palatability. The major drawback of essential-amino-acid supplementation is the number of tablets patients must take (up to 20 per day).

Kilocalories are a critical element in the diet for chronic renal failure. If sufficient kilocalories are

Table 8-3. PROTEIN INTAKES AT VARIOUS LEVELS OF RENAL FUNCTION

CREATININE CLEARANCE (ml per minute)	PROTEIN INTAKE[1] (g per day)
>40	Unrestricted
30–20	50
20–15	40 (+ essential amino acids?)[2]
15–10	30 (+ essential amino acids?)[2]
10–5	15–25 plus essential amino acids

Source: B.T. Burton and G.H. Hirschman, "Current Concepts of Nutritional Therapy in Chronic Renal Failure: An Update." *Journal of the American Dietetic Association* 82 (1983):359–63.

[1]When protein is lost in the urine, the amount lost may be added to the listed protein intake levels.

[2]75% of the total protein should be high biological value (eggs, milk, meat, fish, poultry).

Table 8-4. PROTEIN VALUES OF FOOD GROUPS

HIGH-BIOLOGICAL-VALUE-PROTEIN GROUPS	PROTEIN/SERVING
Meat (includes red meat, fish, poultry, eggs)	7 g/oz
Milk	8 g/cup
LOW-BIOLOGICAL-VALUE-PROTEIN GROUPS	
Bread/starches	3 g/serving (serving examples: 1 slice bread, ½ cup noodles, ½ cup cereal)
Fruit	0.5 g/serving (serving examples: ½ cup juice, ½ cup cut fruit, small apple or orange)
Vegetables	2 g/serving (serving example: ½ cup cooked vegetable)

not supplied, protein will be catabolized for energy, causing a rise in nitrogenous waste products. Because protein is restricted, extra kilocalories must come from carbohydrate sources and fat. Daily kilocalorie needs are approximately 35 kcal per kilogram dry weight (8). Therefore, for a 70 kg male, the total kilocalories needed would be 2450 per day. If the individual is on a 40 g protein diet, 2290 kcal must be provided from fat and carbohydrate (40 g protein times 4 kcal/g = 160 kcal from protein; 2450 − 160 = 2290 kcal).

A simple carbohydrate source is used to make up the kilocalories because complex carbohydrates (breads/starches) supply too much protein of low biological value (see Table 8-4). Some of the simple carbohydrates added to low protein diets are sugar, syrups, jams, hard candies, gum drops, and jelly beans. Commercial carbohydrate supplements are available in the form of high-kilocalorie, high-carbohydate, low-protein beverages. The relationship of the simple carbohydrates to the development of hypertriglyceridemia is being researched, and no definitive answers are yet available. Although expensive, special low-protein food products that are high in carbohydrate have been developed that help provide the necessary kilocalories and add variety to the diet. These low-protein breads, pastas, cereals, and cookies are available by mail order.

Fat intake, because it is kilocalorie dense and low protein (fat contains zero grams of protein per serving) is encouraged to a point. With the recognition that atherosclerosis may be a problem for uremic patients, polyunsaturated fats are emphasized over saturated fats. Because patients are anorectic or have gastrointestinal disturbances, it is often difficult for them to ingest all of the kilocalories needed. Encouragement on the part of the nurse and the family is required.

Sodium and potassium blood values must be monitored carefully, and restrictions must be instituted on an individual basis. Normal serum values for sodium are 136–145 mEq/l and normal serum levels of potassium are 3.5–5.0 mEq/l. If a patient is exhibiting edema and high blood pressure, sodium may be restricted to as little as 920 mg daily.

Vomiting can result in substantial sodium and potassium losses. When patients have low body sodium, approximately 2000 mg sodium are permitted (26). Hyperkalemia must be avoided. High serum potassium results in cardiac arrhythmias and cardiac arrest. Potassium restrictions range from 1560–2340 mg daily, depending on the biochemical and clinical picture of the patient (26). More details on sodium and potassium food sources are included in Chapter 9.

Phosphorus levels increase in chronic renal failure, and in an effort to reduce hyperparathyroidism, phosphorus is restricted to 600–1200 mg daily (9). Because good phosphorus sources are also good protein sources, a protein restriction will result in a decline in phosphorus intake. Dietary intervention is rarely enough to reduce serum phosphorus to 4.5–5.0 mg/dl. Therefore, phosphate binders must be administered.

Fluid intake is based on the amount lost daily in the urine. In addition to the 24-hour urine output, another 400–600 ml is added to account for insensible water loss through the lungs and skin as well as for water lost in the feces (4, 26). The patient is also weighed daily as another measure for calculating fluid loss.

Supplementation with vitamins and minerals is extremely important. Requirements for B vitamins increase during chronic renal failure as a result of insufficient intake and altered metabolism (28–30). Thiamine, riboflavin, niacin, folic acid, and vitamins B_6 and B_{12} are the water-soluble vitamins for which supplements are recommended. Iron deficiency is also observed in chronic renal failure. Heme iron, that iron found in meat, is the well-absorbed iron form. With a restriction in meat intake, iron intake decreases. Iron absorption also declines as a result of the disease itself (31). These two factors plus gastrointestinal blood losses contribute to the development of iron deficiency.

Dietary zinc deficiency is a result of severe restrictions in animal protein. The best sources of zinc are seafood and meat. Cereals, fruits, vegetables, oils, and sugar are poor zinc sources. Zinc status has been related to the function of taste. In chronic renal failure, sour and sweet tastes seem to be affected. Whether zinc is implicated in the taste function of patients with renal disease is unclear (32, 33). From the earlier remarks about calcium metabolism, one can surmise that calcium supplements would be beneficial to increase serum calcium levels. Calcium supplements in conjunction with protein and phosphorus restriction seem to retard the progression of renal disease (29). When given along with vitamin D, calcium can prevent the osteomalacia of chronic renal failure (34).

Hemodialysis. The nutritional objectives in dialysis are to maintain protein and kilocalorie equilibrium, achieve near normal sodium and potassium levels, prevent fluid overload or dehydration, and maintain near normal serum calcium and phosphorus levels (4). Dietary restrictions are designed to prevent widely fluctuating blood chemistries before and after dialysis.

The protein allowance is usually more liberal once dialysis is started. The usual restriction in hemodialysis is 1.0–1.2 g protein per kilogram ideal body weight, with one-half to three-fourths of the protein of high biological value. Essential amino acids may or may not be added to the diet. As in the predialysis patient, kilocalorie needs are high at 35 kcal/kg per day. Carbohydrate and fat intake make up the bulk of kilocalories to preserve lean body mass. Inadequate intake is especially troublesome for patients on hemodialysis because the procedure itself may cause a meal to be omitted or cause nausea and/or vomiting. Sodium is restricted to 1000–2000 mg to prevent fluid retention and hypertension. Because hyperkalemia can be a problem for the dialysis patient, 1500–2000 mg of potassium are permitted daily. Phosphorus restrictions are similar to those for predialysis patients, and phosphate binders are usually given. Fluids are carefully restricted to about 400–500 ml in addition to urine output from the previous 24-hour period (if any). Daily weight gain or loss of approximately one pound between dialyses is expected and should not be exceeded. Hemodialysis causes losses of nonprotein-bound water-soluble vitamins, and a daily supplement is recommended.

Peritoneal Dialysis. Protein losses are greatly increased in peritoneal dialysis, because protein

molecules and amino acids can diffuse across the peritoneal membrane into the dialysate. For individuals using chronic intermittent peritoneal dialysis or chronic ambulatory peritoneal dialysis, rather liberal protein intakes of 1.2–1.5 g/kg per day are recommended. At least half of the protein allowance should be of high biological value.

Kilocalorie requirements are similar to those for patients undergoing hemodialysis. Total kilocalorie allowance should take into account not only the kilocalories provided by the diet, but also kilocalories derived from the concentraiton of glucose in the dialysate. A potentially large uptake of glucose can occur in CAPD, depending on the concentration of glucose in the dialysate. The concentration of glucose in the dialysate is based on the fluid retention of the patient. Problems with fluid retention may cause patients to use highly concentrated dialysate (4.25% glucose) to pull excess fluid from their bodies (36). The net uptake of glucose can range from 50–225 g, depending on the glucose concentration (35). This amounts to about 200–900 kcal per day, just from the dialysate. Patients should try to control fluid retention via sodium or fluid restriction to avoid weight gain.

For patients on chronic intermittent peritoneal dialysis, the sodium, potassium, phosphorus, and fluid restrictions are similar to those for individuals on hemodialysis. Water-soluble vitamin and mineral supplementation are also recommended.

Patients using CAPD do not usually need potassium or sodium restrictions (19). If the individual is changing the dialysate three to four times daily, simply avoiding excessive potassium intake is all that is necessary. Higher numbers of changes result in potassium loss, and intake may need to be increased. Sodium restriction is unnecessary unless fluid retention with resultant weight gain is observed. Even then, only a mild sodium restriction is necessary. Opinions vary with regard to phosphorus. Some researchers do not feel phosphorus restriction is necessary, while others feel that high phosphorus foods should be restricted (19).

The patient using CAPD can drink fluids freely and alter the glucose concentration of the dialysate to compensate. If fluid retention becomes a problem with accompanying weight gain from the high glucose concentrations of the dialysate, a mild fluid restriction may be tried. It is clear that CAPD allows a considerable amount of dietary freedom. Efforts should be made to keep the diet as free as possible.

Post Transplant. After a successful transplant and when the patient begins to eat solid foods, a temporary diet is used. The characteristics of the diet counteract the effects of the drugs used to prevent organ rejection. The diet is high in protein (1.5–2.0 g/kg) due to increased protein needs as a result of the stress of surgery and the catabolic nature of the immunosuppressive drugs. If patients demonstrate carbohydrate intolerance as a result of the high steroid load, carbohydrate may need to be restricted to about 40% of kilocalories. A sodium restriction of three to four grams is often used. Potassium is not restricted and intake is encouraged due to the potassium loss associated with some diuretic and steroid drugs. Folic-acid supplements are required to offset the negative effect on red-blood-cell maturation caused by immunosuppressive drugs. As the dose of the drugs decreases, the diet is liberalized to a regular diet.

NURSING INTERVENTIONS FOR NUTRITIONAL DISORDERS

Work closely with the patient and family, physician, and dietitian to develop a dietary plan to meet the complex changing needs associated with the disease process and the treatment protocols.

Alteration in nutrition; less than body requirements related to:
- anorexia.
- nausea and vomiting.
- altered taste or smell.
- unpalatable food.

- Administer prescribed antiemetic drugs and postpone meals if nausea is a problem.
- Administer frequent mouth care; patient may have a very unpleasant taste in the mouth due to the saturation of metabolic waste products in the bloodstream.
- Serve meals in an attractive manner.
- Encourage the use of dietary supplements as prescribed.

Potential or actual fluid-volume excess due to fluid and electrolyte imbalance related to renal dysfunction.

- Maintain accurate intake and output records.
- Maintain a daily weight record. A weight gain or loss of 0.45 kg (approximately one pound) should be reported to the physician.
- Balance prescribed fluid intake over a 24-hour period.
- Encourage the use of hard candies (sour balls), lemon wedges and/or gum to alleviate thirst and to prevent parotitis (inflammation of the parotid glands). Hard candies will help to increase intake of simple sugars.

Continued

NURSING INTERVENTIONS *(continued)*

Knowledge deficit related to
- **fluid restrictions.**
- **severe dietary restrictions.**

- Emphasize the use of recipes in which meat or other protein of high biological value (a complete protein) can add flavor to or accent a low-protein dish.
- Provide recipes using low-protein products so that the patient and family will not become frustrated with unfamiliar products.
- Help the patient locate a support group in the local community.

Self-care deficit related to fatigue (inability to self-feed).

- Feed the patient as necessary.

SPECIAL PROBLEMS

Children with CRF

A number of metabolic defects of uremia are more pronounced in children than in adults (36). Growth retardation is characteristic in children with chronic renal failure. Children with chronic renal failure are short for their age, but their weight for height is adequate (37). The major factor affecting growth in these children is inadequate kilocalorie intake. Evidence indicates that growth velocity stops at 40 kcal/kg per day. Other factors that may be involved in growth failure include inadequate protein intake and renal osteodystrophy. The restrictive nature of the diet and anorexia caused by uremia often prove to be more than the child can handle. Sensitive, knowledgeable personnel can help parents make the diet as palatable as possible; however, there appears to be no easy solution to the problems faced in this situation.

Dietary Adherence in Renal Patients

The life of individuals with chronic renal failure is filled with numerous regulations. The restrictive nature of the diet and alterations required in lifestyle may cause a considerable amount of psychological stress for the patient and family. A 1970 survey of 201 hemodialysis facilities in the United States indicated a suicide rate in kidney patients 400 times that of the normal population (39). It is not surprising that adherence to the diet is poor. Good dietary compliance is maintained by less than 25% of the renal patients (40). The longer the time on dialysis or diet, the worse the adherence. Patients view the diet as monotonous, unpalatable, difficult to follow, and a major burden.

Efforts have been made to try to identify factors that contribute to the lack of adherence. Characteristics of the patient, such as age, gender, education, socioeconomic status, personality, and knowledge of the diet are not consistently related to compliance (38, 40, 41); neither are characteristics of the illness (length, severity). Characteristics of the relationship between the health professionals and the patient and characteristics of the prescribed regimen may influence adherence. It is essential to build a trusting, honest relationship with the patient. This is necessary but may not be sufficient for adherence. The type of regimen developed is crucial. The simpler you can make the diet to understand and follow, the better. Additionally, the more input a patient has in designing the diet, the more likely the diet will be carried out on a regular basis. Listening closely to patients to understand the problems they face goes a long way in helping people change.

TOPIC OF INTEREST

Keto analogues of essential amino acids have been used in the diets of patients with chronic renal failure. The principle underlying the use of keto analogues is that the transfers between keto analogues and amino acids are reversible. Providing keto analogues of essential amino acids will lower the nitrogen load of the body. Benefits associated with using keto analogues of essential amino acids with mixed low-protein diets include (a) improvement of metabolic abnormalities (42); (b) improvement of nitrogen balance, serum transferrin, and phosphate excess (43); (c) increased variability and palatability in the diet afforded by less reliance on high-biological-value protein (44); and (d) slowing the progression of renal failure (6). Not all scientists are convinced of the benefits of keto analogues. Some researchers believe that not enough data exists to support the use of keto analogues over essential-amino-acid supplements (45). Also, keto analogues are expensive and have a very unpleasant taste.

A unique program for college-aged individuals with CRF began in 1985 at Pennsylvania State University. The Dialysis Unit for Pennsylvania State University Students (DUPSUS) is a dormitory that houses college students with CRF. The goal of DUPSUS is to create a supportive environment in which individuals with CRF can live. Efforts are made to meet medical, social, and psychological needs, making it easier for students to concentrate on earning their degrees. Future plans include the development of a complex that will house a dialysis treatment center, offices for staff, a kitchen, and nutrition center (46).

SPOTLIGHT ON LEARNING

Mr. Smith experienced three episodes of hemodialysis disequilibrium during the past week. His physician informed you that the problem was caused by failure to adhere to his prescribed diet. What action can you take to help Mr. Smith?

Hints:
1. Mr. Smith is depressed and feels that no one understands his situation.
2. The diet was given to him while he was in the hospital. He understands the principles but feels that things are out of his control.

REVIEW QUESTIONS

1. In glomerulonephritis, protein levels are modified on what basis?
   a. urinary output and protein loss
   b. carbohydrate intake
   c. kilocalorie needs
   d. fluid intake

2. What must be adequately provided to reverse the catabolic state in nephrosis?
   a. kilocalories
   b. vitamins
   c. protein
   d. carbohydrate

3. When a patient has renal calculi, it is important to encourage the intake of which of the following?
   a. protein
   b. fluids
   c. fat
   d. carbohydrate

4. Which of the following is not included in the goals of dietary management in acute renal failure?
   a. correct fluid imbalances
   b. prevent breakdown of body tissue
   c. encourage weight loss
   d. correct electrolyte imbalances

5. Choose the biochemical abnormalities that can occur in chronic renal failure.
   a. hypophosphatemia and alkalosis
   b. hypocalcemia, hyperkalemia and increased blood urea nitrogen
   c. decreased blood urea nitrogen and hypokalemia
   d. hyperkalemia and hypophosphatemia

6. In patients with chronic renal failure, when should protein restriction be initiated?
   a. the patient becomes anuric
   b. GFR is 40 ml per minute
   c. dialysis is started
   d. symptoms of uremia appear

7. Which of the following is not a high-biological-value protein source?
   a. bread
   b. milk
   c. fish
   d. meat

8. Which of the following is not restricted for predialysis patients?
   a. sodium
   b. potassium
   c. kilocalories
   d. fluid

9. In chronic ambulatory peritoneal dialysis, the concentration of glucose in the dialysate is based on which of the following?
   a. nitrogen retention
   b. protein catabolism
   c. potassium levels
   d. fluid retention

10. To improve dietary adherence in patients with chronic renal failure, it is best not to do which of the following?
   a. help patients increase their knowledge about the diet
   b. develop a trusting, honest relationship
   c. involve the patient in developing the diet
   d. try to discourage questions concerning the dietary modifications

ACTIVITIES

1. Have a taste testing session. Purchase and prepare low-protein products. Compare these with their regular protein-content counterparts. Judge the products on flavor, color, and consistency.

2. a. Using Table 8-4, calculate a 40 g (for a male) or a 35 g (for a female) protein-restricted diet for yourself with 75% of the protein from high-biological-value sources. How different is this diet compared with your regular diet?
   b. Next, using a kilocalorie chart, try to reach the target of 35 kcal/kg per day while maintaining the protein restriction. You may need to use special low-protein products and carbohydrate supplements.
   c. Add to this diet a sodium restriction of 1000 mg and a potassium restriction of 2000 mg (use tables in Chapter 9 for sodium and potassium content of foods). What problems did you encounter?

3. Invite a dietitian specializing in renal disease to discuss common dietary problems that chronic renal failure patients encounter.

REFERENCES

1. Kopple, J.D. Nutrition, diet and the kidney. In *Modern nutrition in health and disease*, 7th ed., edited by M.E. Shils and V.R. Young. Philadelphia: Lea & Febiger, 1988.
2. Pitts, R.F. *Physiology of the kidney and body fluids*, 3d ed. Chicago: Year Book Medical Publishers, 1974.
3. Robinson, C.H., et al. *Normal and therapeutic nutrition.* New York: Macmillan Publishing Company, 1986.

4. Burton, B.T., and G.H. Hirschman. Current concepts of nutritional therapy in chronic renal failure: An update. *Journal of the American Dietetic Association* 82 (1983):359–63.

5. Burton, B.T. Current concepts of nutrition and diet in diseases of the kidney. I. General principles of dietary management. *Journal of the American Dietetic Association* 65 (1974):623–26.

6. ———. Effect of keto acid diets in chronic renal failure. *Nutrition Reviews* 45 (1987):305–309.

7. DeFronzo, R.A., and A. Alvestrand. Glucose intolerance in uremia: Site and mechanism. *American Journal of Clinical Nutrition* 33 (1980):1438–45.

8. Kopple, J.D. Nutritional therapy in kidney failure. In *Present knowledge in nutrition*, 5th ed., edited by R.E. Olson, et al. Washington, D.C.: The Nutrition Foundation, Inc., 1984.

9. Harvey, K.B., et al. Nutritional assessment and treatment of chronic renal failure. *American Journal of Clinical Nutrition* 33 (1980):1586–97.

10. Blumenkrantz, M.J., et al. Methods for assessing nutritional status of patients with renal failure. *American Journal of Clinical Nutrition* 33 (1980):1567–84.

11. Sedman, A.B., et al. Evidence of aluminum loading in infants receiving intravenous therapy. *New England Journal of Medicine* 312 (1985):1337–43.

12. Sandstead, H.H. Trace elements in uremia and hemodialysis. *American Journal of Clinical Nutrition* 33 (1980):1501–1508.

13. Alfrey, A.C., A. Hegg, and P. Craswell. Metabolism and toxicity of aluminum in renal failure. *American Journal of Clinical Nutrition* 33 (1980):1509–16.

14. Alfrey, A.C. Aluminum intoxication. *New England Journal of Medicine* 310 (1985):1113–15.

15. Massry, S.G. Requirements of vitamin D metabolites in patients with renal disease. *American Journal of Clinical Nutrition* 33 (1980):1530–35.

16. Burton, B.T. Nutritional implications of renal disease. I. Current overview and general principles. *Journal of the American Dietetic Association* 70 (1977): 479–82.

17. Farrell, P.C., and P.W. Hone. Dialysis-induced catabolism. *American Journal of Clinical Nutrition* 33 (1980):1417–22.

18. Grodstein, G.P., M.J. Blumenkrantz, and J.D. Kopple. Nutritional and metabolic response to catabolic stress in uremia. *American Journal of Clinical Nutrition* 33 (1980):1411–16.

19. Bodnar, D.M. Rationale for nutritional requirements for patients on continuous ambulatory peritoneal dialysis. *Journal of the American Dietetic Association* 80 (1982):247–49.

20. Bannister, D.K., et al. Nutritional effects of peritonitis in continuous ambulatory peritoneal dialysis (CAPD) patients. *Journal of the American Dietetic Association* 87 (1987):53–56.

21. Bonomini, V., et al. Atherosclerosis in uremia: A longitudinal study. *American Journal of Clinical Nutrition* 33 (1980):1493–1500.

22. Alplasca, E.C., and M. Rammohan. The effect of prednisone on the levels of serum albumin of 20 patients with renal transplants. *Journal of the American Dietetic Association* 86 (1986):1404–1405.

23. Walser, M. Does diet therapy have a role in the predialysis patient? *American Journal of Clinical Nutrition* 33 (1980):1629–37.

24. Ritz, E., et al. Protein restriction in the conservation management of uremia. *American Journal of Clinical Nutrition* 31 (1978):1703–11.

25. Giordano, G., et al. Modulated nitrogen intake for patients on low-protein diets. *American Journal of Clinical Nutrition* 33 (1980):1638–41.

26. The American Dietetic Association. *Handbook of clinical dietetics.* New Haven and London: Yale University Press, 1981.

27. Alvestrand, A., M. Ahlberg, and J. Bergstrom. Clinical experience with amino acid and keto acid diets. *American Journal of Clinical Nutrition* 33 (1980):1654–59.

28. Piper, C.M. Very-low-protein diets in chronic renal failure: Nutrient content and guidelines for supplementation. *Journal of the American Dietetic Association* 85 (1985):1344–46.

29. Van Duyn, M.A.S. Acceptability of selected low-protein products for use in potential diet therapy for chronic renal failure. *Journal of the American Dietetic Association* 87 (1987):909–14.

30. Swendseid, M.E. Nutritional implications of renal disease. III. Nutritional needs of patients with renal disease. *Journal of the American Dietetic Association* 70 (1977):488–92.

31. Berger, M. Dietary management of children with uremia. *Journal of the American Dietetic Association* 70 (1977):498–505.

32. Burge, J.C., et al. Taste acuity and zinc status in chronic renal disease. *Journal of the American Dietetic Association* 84 (1984):1203–1209.

33. Shapera, M.R., et al. Taste perception of children with chronic renal failure. *Journal of the American Dietetic Association* 86 (1986):1359–65.

34. Machioi, G., et al. Early dietary phosphorus restriction and calcium supplementation in the prevention of renal osteodystrophy. *American Journal of Clinical Nutrition* 33 (1980):1546–54.

35. Bouma, S.F., and J.T. Dwyer. Glucose absorption and weight change in 18 months of continuous ambulatory peritoneal dialysis. *Journal of the American Dietetic Association* 84 (1984):194–97.

36. Chantler, C., et al. Nutritional therapy in children with chronic renal failure. *American Journal of Clinical Nutrition* 33 (1980):1682–89.

37. Spinozzi, N.S., and W.E. Grupe. Nutritional implications of renal disease. IV. Nutritional aspects of chronic renal insufficiency in childhood. *Journal of the American Dietetic Association* 70 (1977):31–37.

38. Blackburn, G.L. Dietary compliance of chronic hemodialysis patients. *Journal of the American Dietetic Association* 70 (1977):31–37.

39. Batterman, C., E. Atcherson, and C. Roy. Restrictions and recreation for patients with chronic renal failure. *Journal of the American Dietetic Association* 83 (1984):333–34.

40. Falciglia, G., et al. Evaluation of an educational program for dialysis patients. *Journal of the American Dietetic Association* 84 (1984):928–30.

41. Dubin, S., and A. Jackson. Automatic calculation for the renal failure diet. *Journal of the American Dietetic Association* 84 (1984):568–71.

42. Schauder, P., et al. Blood levels of branched-chain amino acids and alpha-ketoacids in uremic patients given keto analogues of essential amino acids. *American Journal of Clinical Nutrition* 33 (1980):1660–66.
43. Frohling, P.T., et al. Conservative treatment with ketoacid and amino acid supplemented low-protein diets in chronic renal failure. *American Journal of Clinical Nutrition* 33 (1980):1667–72.
44. Kampf, D., H. Fischer, and M. Kessel. Efficacy of an unselected protein diet (25 g) with minor oral supply of essential amino acids and keto analogues compared with a selective protein diet (40 g) in chronic renal failure. *American Journal of Clinical Nutrition* 33 (1980):1673–77.
45. Giordano, C. Amino acids and keto acids—Advantages and pitfalls. *American Journal of Clinical Nutrition* 33 (1980):1649–53.
46. Sente, M.J. New futures. Revolutionary dialysis program aids student patients. *The Penn Stater* (July/August 1988):11–13 and 54–55.

NUTRITION AND THE PATIENT WITH CARDIOVASCULAR DISEASE

Objectives

After studying this chapter, you will be able to

- describe the development of atherosclerosis.
- list the risk factors for developing atherosclerosis.
- explain the dietary restrictions for hyperlipoproteinemia and the rationale for the restrictions.
- identify dietary sources of cholesterol, saturated fat, polyunsaturated fat, monounsaturated fat, complex carbohydrate, and sodium.
- specify a nutrition plan to decrease dietary intake of total fat, saturated fat, and cholesterol and to increase complex carbohydrate in the diet.
- list the classes of hypertension.
- specify a nutrition plan for decreasing sodium in the diet.
- compare the risk factors with dietary management for a patient with ischemic heart disease.
- describe the rationale for sodium and kilocalorie restriction for a patient with congestive heart failure.
- identify nursing interventions for nutritional disorders associated with selected cardiovascular diseases.

Overview

Today, Americans are bombarded with messages on steps that can be taken to prevent cardiovascular disease. Health reporters on television, medical writers for newspapers, and even advertisers for food products give tips for changing lifestyles, diets, and exercise regimes to reduce the risk of cardiovascular disease. The emphasis on prevention of cardiovascular disease may be one reason for the steady decline in deaths from the disease that has occurred in the past 10 years. Still, cardiovascular disease is responsible for approximately 1 million deaths in the United States per year, making it the leading cause of death in this country and costing an estimated 88.2 billion dollars (1). The major causes of cardiovascular disease are atherosclerosis and hypertension.

ATHEROSCLEROSIS

Atherosclerosis is a slowly progressive disease in which fat accumulates in the wall of the large and medium arteries, causing a partial or total obstruction to the flow of blood (Figure 9-1). Atherosclerosis leads to the development of coronary heart disease. The lesions of atherosclerosis are classified as the fatty streak, the fibrous plaque, and the complicated lesion (2). The fatty streak makes its appearance by about age 10 and is a yellow, focal accumulation of fat (lipid) in the artery wall. The predominant lipid in the fatty streak is cholesterol, but it appears to be cholesterol that was metabolized by the cells in the wall and not from cholesterol in the bloodstream that has settled in the wall. The fatty streak causes no obstruction to the flow of blood and is reversible. Whether or not fatty streaks progress into the more advanced lesions is not known.

The fibrous plaque (living tissue) is the most characteristic lesion of advancing atherosclerosis (2). Unlike the fatty streak, the fibrous plaque grows into the lumen of the artery to cause a narrowing. The lesion consists of a lipid core covered by a whitish fibrous cap. The core contains lipid metabolized by the cells in the artery wall and lipid deposited from the bloodstream.

The third lesion, the complicated lesion, usually occurs during middle age. The complicated lesion is an extension of the fibrous plaque that has enlarged and changed due to hemorrhage, ulceration, and cell death. Plaque buildup can cause the

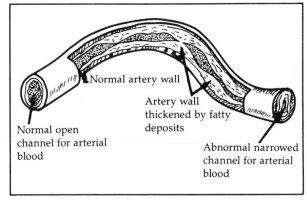

Figure 9-1. Progression of atherosclerosis. (From U.S. Department of Health and Human Services, Public Health Service, National Institutes of Health. Facts about . . . blood cholesterol. NIH Publication No. 86-26-96. Reprinted July 1986.)

artery to become so narrow that blood flow through the vessel is severely hindered, and ischemia of tissues results. Parts of the lesion can break off (from emboli) and interfere with the flow of blood through a vessel. When flow to the heart is blocked (thrombosis), a myocardial infarction (death of localized tissue) occurs; interference with the flow of blood to the brain results in a cerebrovascular accident, and a blockage to the periphery can result in gangrene.

Atherosclerosis can continue for years without symptoms; often, the first symptom is a heart attack or stroke. Because of the devastating consequences of atherosclerosis, extensive research has been conducted to identify the causes of the disease. Unfortunately, the cause of atherosclerosis has remained elusive, although theories do exist. The predominant theory is the endothelial injury hypothesis (3).

A disruption of the endothelium can occur through hemodynamic stresses such as high blood pressure and/or circulating factors such as endotoxins, high levels of carbon monoxide from cigarette smoke, or excessive levels of plasma lipoproteins. Once the endothelium is injured, platelet aggregation, smooth-muscle-cell proliferation, and infiltration of plasma lipid in the arterial wall can occur.

Despite the unknowns about the cause of atherosclerosis, it is known that the disease is universal and that few elderly individuals are free of atherosclerotic lesions (3). The rate of development of atherosclerosis and the extent of lesions, however, are extremely variable and certain risk factors have been identified that play a role in atherosclerosis development.

Risk Factors

Risk factors associated with the development of atherosclerosis development include heredity, gender, diabetes mellitus and hyperglycemia, cigarette smoking, lack of exercise, psychosocial factors, obesity, hypercholesterolemia and elevations of other blood lipids, and hypertension. Obviously, some of the risk factors are impossible for an individual to control. A history of premature coronary heart disease among parents or siblings indicates an increased risk. Males are more susceptible than premenopausal females. Diabetes mellitus is a major risk factor for coronary heart disease, possibly through an acceleration of the atherosclerotic process (3). Dietary management of diabetes is discussed in Chapter 13. Cigarette smoking, lack of exercise, psychosocial factors, obesity, hypercholesterolemia and increases in other blood lipids, and hypertension are considered to be controllable. Health-care providers can help those persons in high-risk categories under-

stand the role of these factors in the development of atherosclerosis.

Smoking appears to promote atherosclerosis by damaging the artery wall and allowing the infiltration of cholesterol. Once the stage is set, more cholesterol attaches to the artery wall and the vessel narrows. Lack of exercise contributes to high serum-lipid levels. It also can be a factor in the promotion of obesity. Aerobic exercises took the United States by storm, and many individuals aged 20-plus began incorporating exercise into their weekly schedules. Unfortunately, while this trend has touched the lives of some adults, it is not universal and has not filtered down to children, many of whom are considered physically unfit (4).

Psychosocial factors, particularly stress, may accelerate atherosclerosis. While stress itself does not seem to be the culprit, the individual response to stress appears to be more important. Currently, the relationship between stress and atherosclerosis is still unclear (5).

Thirty-four million adults in the United States are considered obese, making obesity a prevalent, national problem (6). It has been demonstrated that among persons 30% above their average weight, the risk for coronary heart disease is 44% greater for males and 34% greater for females than for similar persons of average weight (7). The actual mechanism through which obesity increases coronary heart disease is not known; however, it is clear that obesity raises blood pressure and negatively affects plasma lipoproteins. The metabolic problems, methods for identifying, and current treatments for obesity are discussed in Chapter 11.

Hypertension is considered both a risk factor for atherosclerosis and a problem by itself. Details on hypertension are discussed later in this chapter.

Hyperlipoproteinemia refers to elevated lipoproteins in the blood. Lipoproteins are the lipid-protein complexes (Table 9-1) used for transporting lipids (fats) throughout the body.

Normal Lipoprotein Metabolism. During the digestive process, dietary triglycerides are metabolized in the intestine. The triglycerides are chemically altered (hydrolyzed) and packaged into chylomicrons consisting of a lipid core with a

Table 9-1. LIPOPROTEIN CLASSES

LIPOPROTEIN	CHEMICAL COMPOSITION
Chylomicron (lowest density)	triglyceride 85% cholesterol ester 3% unesterified cholesterol 1% protein 2% phospholipid 9%
VLDL (very low density)	triglyceride 50% cholesterol ester 12% unesterified cholesterol 7% protein 10% phospholipid 18%
LDL (low density)	triglyceride 10% cholesterol ester 37% unesterified cholesterol 8% protein 23% phospholipid 20%
HDL (high density)	triglyceride 4% cholesterol ester 15% unesterified cholesterol 2% protein 55% phospholipid 24%

(Adapted from P.M. Kris-Etherton and T.D. Etherton, "The Role of Lipoproteins in Lipid Metabolism of Meat Animals." *Journal of Animal Science* 55(1982):804–17. Used with permission.)

protein exterior to travel through the lymph system and into the bloodstream. Chylomicrons transport the fat of intestinal origin (primarily triglycerides) to sites of utilization and storage throughout the body. After the body cells have at least partially emptied the chylomicrons, chylomicron remnants remain and are taken up by the liver (8). (See Figure 9-2). Chylomicrons are usually cleared from the plasma after a 12- to 14-hour fast (9).

Very low density lipoproteins (VLDL) originate primarily in the liver and also in the small intestine. They differ from chylomicrons in that the triglyceride they carry is that of endogenous rather than dietary origin. VLDL also transport some cholesterol but as shown in Table 9-1, they account for only a small amount of plasma cholesterol.

VLDL transport lipids to peripheral tissues (adipose, heart and skeletal muscle), rapidly undergo lipolysis and ultimately low density lipoproteins (LDL) are formed in the liver. LDL are the major carriers of cholesterol in the blood. LDL bind to target cells via specific membrane receptors and are able to enter the cell body. Once inside the cell, the cholesterol in the LDL regulates cellular cholesterol synthesis and also LDL membrane receptor synthesis, thus regulating subsequent cellular LDL uptake (8). In the United States, LDL cholesterol levels begin to rise after adolescence and continue increasing until about age 50.

High density lipoproteins (HDL) have been dubbed "the good cholesterol." This small group of lipoproteins originates in the liver and intestine

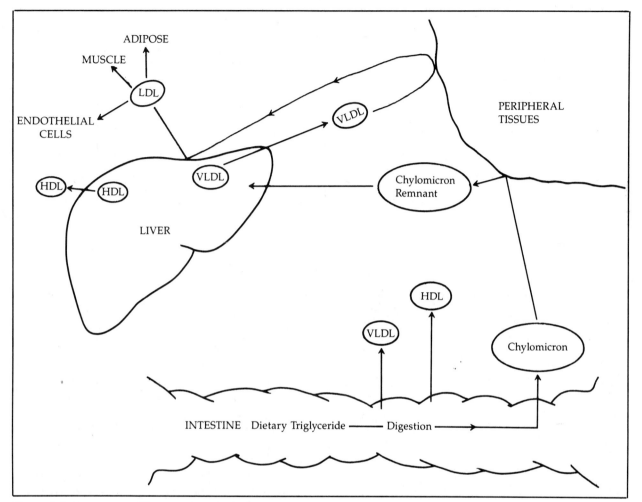

Figure 9-2. Summary of lipoprotein metabolism.

and removes cholesterol from VLDL, chylomicrons, and possibly from tissues, including the arterial wall (9). Individuals with low HDL levels have an increased risk of coronary heart disease; conversely, high HDL levels may have a protective effect on the body, with a lower incidence of heart disease. Aerobic exercise appears to increase HDL levels.

Altered Lipoprotein Metabolism. The concentration and ratios of the lipoproteins provide important information. Lipoprotein abnormalities are based on direct measurement of lipoproteins (Table 9-2).

Elevated chylomicrons indicate an inability to clear dietary triglycerides from the plasma. It is rare, nearly always familial, and associated with pain after the ingestion of dietary fat.

Severe coronary heart disease results from elevated LDL (hypercholesterolemia) even in the absence of other risk factors. A large body of epidemiological research, animal studies, and multiple clinical trials have established the role of hypercholesterolemia in the development of coronary heart disease. Results of these studies demonstrated that serum cholesterol levels greater than 200 mg/dl are associated with an increased risk of

Table 9-2. THE HYPERLIPOPROTEINEMIAS

LIPOPROTEIN PROFILE	MAJOR LIPID ABNORMALITY
↑Chylomicrons (rare)	↑↑triglycerides
↑LDL	↑↑cholesterol
↑LDL, ↑VLDL	↑cholesterol, ↑triglycerides
↑VLDL, abnormal LDL (rare)	↑triglycerides, ↑cholesterol
↑VLDL	↑triglycerides
↑Chylomicrons, ↑VLDL (rare)	↑↑triglycerides

Source: Department of Health, Education, and Welfare, *The Dietary Management of Hyperlipoproteinemia.* DHEW Pub. No. (NIH) 78-110, 1978.

developing premature coronary heart disease (1). Levels in this range represent about one-half of the United States population.

Elevated LDL (hypercholesterolemia) can be the result of a genetic abnormality or induced by dietary and lifestyle factors. Children with inherited severe hypercholesterolemia lack the cellular receptors that remove LDL from the blood. Because LDL internalization does not occur, there is no regulation of cholesterol synthesis by the cells, and LDL levels in the blood are extremely high. These children develop severe coronary heart disease, and death may even occur in childhood. Partial deficiencies of functioning LDL receptors induced by diet or life-style factors appear to result in less severe hypercholesterolemia than that seen with the genetic abnormality.

Elevated VLDL (hypertriglyceridemia) is often secondary to other clinical disorders. The most common reason for elevated triglycerides is obesity (10). Diabetes and renal disease are other clinical disorders associated with increased triglycerides. Management of the underlying clinical conditions generally results in a lowering of VLDL levels.

Acute physiological stress (burn, for example) and some medications may also cause elevated triglycerides. Finally, increased levels of VLDL may occur as a result of heredity.

A lipid profile of the patient will clearly show the type of lipoprotein abnormality that needs to be corrected. Total cholesterol measurement can be completed quickly, because no dietary restrictions are required for the test. It should be recognized that the test is really just a screening tool, since the total cholesterol value includes the cholesterol contained in the VLDL, LDL, and HDL components. Individuals with high levels of total cholesterol (>240 mg/dl) or borderline high levels (200–239 mg/dl) who also have two risk factors or diagnosed cardiovascular disease should have an LDL test. (See Table 9-3). The more specific, expensive and difficult LDL tests should take place after the patient has had no solid food for 12 hours. The LDL test will confirm whether or not the total cholesterol elevation is a result of increased LDL.

A blood-glucose test may indicate the presence of diabetes. Guidelines for assessing abnormal glucose levels are detailed in Chapter 13.

Table 9-3. TOTAL CHOLESTEROL AND LDL GUIDELINES FOR ADULTS AGED 21 AND OLDER

TOTAL CHOLESTEROL	
Desirable	<200 mg/dl
Borderline–high	200-239 mg/dl
High	≥240 mg/dl
LDL LEVELS	
Desirable	<130 mg/dl
Borderline–high risk	130-159 mg/dl
High risk	≥160 mg/dl

Source: National Cholesterol Education Program, Report of the Expert Panel on Detection, Evaluation, and Treatment of High Blood Cholesterol in Adults. NIH Publication No. 88-2925, January 1988.

A discussion of the patient's life-style enables the nurse to assess for the presence of other risk factors: heredity, smoking, lack of exercise, and stress. A dietary history should provide information on usual dietary intakes of cholesterol and saturated fat. The nurse is in a unique position to work with other health professionals to develop a dietary regimen that can help to meet the patients' needs.

Diet

Recently, the National Institutes of Health and the American Heart Association approached the treatment of hyperlipidemia in a unified way (11). Rather than prescribing different dietary treatments for each type of hyperlipoproteinemia, a single approach is used, because research has demonstrated that most elevations in plasma cholesterol and/or triglycerides respond favorably to the same types of dietary restrictions. The unified approach involves dietary reductions in total fat, saturated fat, and cholesterol. Decreases in total dietary fat reduce LDL and chylomicrons, reductions in saturated fat reduce LDL, and decreases in dietary cholesterol decrease LDL and VLDL. If the individual is overweight, caloric restriction is add-ed to the dietary modifications. Weight loss itself usually results in reductions of VLDL and LDL.

Dietary modifications for hyperlipoproteinemia can result in a substantial lowering of serum cholesterol by 10%–15% (12). (See Table 9-4). Patients are first instructed to follow the Step-One Diet. Serum total cholesterol level should be measured after the patient adheres to the diet for four to six weeks and again at three months. If a response to diet therapy is not obtained on the more liberal diet, patients are counselled on the Step-Two Diet in which dietary intake of saturated fat and cholesterol are reduced even further. The effectiveness of the Step-Two Diet is assessed after the patient follows it for three months. If serum cholesterol is not lowered, drug therapy should be considered (13).

How does a patient begin to make changes in food selection to modify fat and cholesterol intake and to increase complex carbohydrate intake? A basic understanding of the various types of fat and carbohydrate in the diet is an essential step in learning how to modify the diet. (See Table 9-5).

Saturated Fat. Numerous studies have demonstrated that intake of saturated fat tends to increase blood cholesterol. Saturated fat is primarily found in animal sources, with the exception of palm and

Table 9-4. DIETARY MODIFICATIONS FOR HYPERLIPOPROTEINEMIA

DIET	INDICATIONS FOR USE	DIETARY COMPONENTS
Step-One Diet	Initial step in treatment of adults with borderline-high cholesterol, borderline-high risk, and high risk LDL cholesterol. Note: This diet is very similar to the American Heart Association's dietary modifications recommended for healthy adults.	**Total kilocalories:** to achieve and maintain desirable weight **Total fat:** less than 30% of total kilocalories **Saturated fat:** less than 10% of total kilocalories **Polyunsaturated fat:** up to 10% of total kilocalories **Monounsaturated fat:** 10%-15% of total kilocalories **Cholesterol:** less than 300 mg per day **Protein:** 10%-20% of total kilocalories **Carbohydrate:** 50%-60% of total kilocalories, emphasizing complex carbohydrates
Step-Two Diet	Insufficient response to Step-One Diet.	**Total kilocalories:** to achieve and maintain desirable weight **Total fat:** less than 30% of total kilocalories **Saturated fat:** less than 7% of total kilocalories **Polyunsaturated fat:** up to 10% of total kilocalories **Monounsaturated fat:** 10%-15% of total kilocalories **Cholesterol:** less than 200 mg per day. **Protein:** 10%-20% of kilocalories **Carbohydrate:** 50%-60% of total kilocalories, emphasizing complex carbohydrates

Source: National Cholesterol Education Program, Report of the Expert Panel on Detection, Evaluation and Treatment of High Blood Cholesterol in Adults. NIH Publication No. 88-2925, January 1988.

Table 9-5. FOOD SOURCES OF FATS, CHOLESTEROL, AND COMPLEX CARBOHYDRATES

SATURATED FAT	
Meat Products	Red meats: visible fat and marbling; prime-grade meats are heavily marbled and therefore, highest in fat content Processed meats: frankfurters, luncheon meats (corned beef, salami, bologna, bacon, sausage) Fowl: most fat is located directly beneath the skin in chicken and turkey; duck and goose are considered high fat throughout
Milk Products	Whole milk and whole-milk products (cheese, whole-milk yogurt, cream, ice cream, cream sauces, cheese sauces)
Fats/Oils	Butter, lard, meat fat, coconut oil, palm kernel oil, completely hydrogenated shortening and margarine.
POLYUNSATURATED FAT	
Oils	Safflower, walnut, sunflower, corn, soybean, cottonseed, sesame, mustard seed
Fish	Salmon, mackerel, herring, sardines, sablefish, lake, rainbow and sea trout, fresh tuna, whitefish, halibut, perch, bass, smelt
MONOUNSATURATED FAT	
Oils	Olive oil, peanut oil, canola oil
Other Foods	Avocado, olives, peanuts
CHOLESTEROL	
Meat/Poultry/ Fish Products	All meat, poultry, and fish contain cholesterol; organ meats (liver, kidney, brain, heart) and egg yolks are highest sources; shrimp and lobster are particularly high in cholesterol, other shellfish are roughly equivalent to meat in cholesterol content
Milk Products	All milk products contain cholesterol
Fats	Butter
COMPLEX CARBOHYDRATES	
Legumes	Dried beans, peas, and lentils
Grains	Cereals (whole-grain cereals add fiber), pastas, and breads (whole-grain breads add fiber)
Fruits/Vegetables	All fruits and vegetables

coconut oils. Other vegetable fats are unsaturated; however, they can be converted to partially saturated fats through the process of hydrogenation. Saturated fats are usually solid at room temperature.

Polyunsaturated Fat. Studies show that polyunsaturated fats decrease serum cholesterol. Because only a small amount of data exists on the long-term use of diets high in polyunsaturates, the recommendation calls for polyunsaturated fats to make up less than 10% of the kilocalories from fat.

Polyunsaturated fats are found in high amounts in vegetable oils and are liquid at room temperature. Fish also contain fat that is mostly polyunsaturated. Fish oils in particular contain a unique kind of polyunsaturated fat called omega-3 fatty acids (polyunsaturated fats from vegetable sources are primarily omega-6 fatty acids). Preliminary work indicates that fish oils significantly lower plasma triglycerides; however, data is not clear regarding the effect on serum cholesterol (14). Most nutritionists recommend eating fish two or three times per week rather than relying on fish oil supplements, because little is known about the long-term safety of the fish oil capsules. The optimal and safe dose is unknown, and the purity of the fish oil in the capsules has been questioned. Fattier fish such as salmon, albacore tuna, mackerel, sardines, and herring contain the largest amount of omega-3 fatty acids. The leaner fish, such as cod, flounder, and haddock also contain omega-3 fatty acids, but in smaller concentrations.

Monounsaturated Fat. Monounsaturated fats are obtained from vegetable sources. Long considered "neutral fats," recent evidence indicates that they may lower serum cholesterol (15, 16). More emphasis has been placed on including monounsaturated fats in the diet within the total fat constraints due to their beneficial effects and in an effort to avoid an excessive intake of polyunsaturated fats. Excessive intake of polyunsaturated fats has been linked to carcinogenesis in animals (17) and alteration of the composition of cell membranes with unknown consequences (18). Rich in monounsaturated fat are olive oil, peanut oil, and canola oil.

Cholesterol. Dietary cholesterol increases serum cholesterol, but to a lesser extent than saturated fat. Cholesterol is found only in foods of animal origin. Foods high in cholesterol are often rich sources of saturated fat, with a few exceptions. Some foods, such as shrimp and lobster are high in cholesterol but very low in saturated fat. On the other hand, some breakfast cereals and snack crackers, while containing no cholesterol can contain substantial amounts of saturated fat. Label reading on packaged food is, therefore, essential for individuals working to reduce their serum cholesterol. Examples of ingredient lists from food labels, with problem ingredients identified, are shown in Figure 9-3.

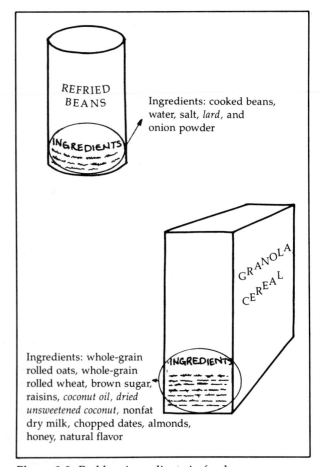

Figure 9-3. Problem ingredients in foods.

Complex Carbohydrates. Found in fruits, vegetables, and grains, complex carbohydrates add fiber to the diet. Some types of fiber, such as pectin and oat bran, have been found to decrease blood cholesterol. Other types of fiber, such as bran from whole-grain cereals and breads, maintain the healthy functioning of the gastrointestinal tract. In the United States, carbohydrates account for 40%–45% of the kilocalories in the diet, and a large portion is made up of simple, refined sugars.

Drug Therapy and Other Treatment Modalities

If the patient does not show lower lipid levels as a result of dietary intervention, drug therapy may be necessary. Clofibrate (Atromid-S), gemfibrozil (Lopid) and nicotinic acid are used to decrease triglyceride levels. Unfortunately, clofibrate and gemfibrozil increase LDL levels as a side effect, so their usefulness has been questioned. Side effects observed in nicotinic acid therapy include flushing of the face, hyperglycemia, and hyperuricemia. Cholestyramine (Questran), colestipol (Colestid), nicotinic acid, lovastatin (Mevacor), and probucol (Lorelco) are used to decrease blood-cholesterol levels.

Severe atherosclerosis of the coronary arteries is sometimes treated by surgical intervention, even though surgery does not reverse the process of atherosclerosis. Depending on the patient and the degree of blockage in the coronary artery (or arteries), the physician may choose to do a coronary artery bypass graft, sometimes called a "jump-graft," in order to increase the blood flow to the myocardial muscle.

If one coronary artery is blocked, percutaneous transluminal coronary angioplasty may be performed in order to dilate the artery. For some patients, the physician may choose to create a larger arterial channel by destroying the atheroma by means of a laser.

POSSIBLE NURSING DIAGNOSES

Potential alteration in nutrition; greater than body requirements related to increased intake of lipids.

Potential alteration in nutrition; less than body requirements related to decrease in lipid intake.

Knowledge deficit related to
- risk factors associated with dietary intake of lipids.
- potential complications associated with disease process.

Potential noncompliance with dietary regimen related to denial of disease state.

NURSING INTERVENTIONS FOR NUTRITIONAL DISORDERS

Work closely with the patient, dietitian, and physician to develop a diet plan that will help to reduce blood lipids.

Potential alteration in nutrition; greater than body requirements related to increased intake of lipids.

- Instruct patients in cooking methods that decrease total intake of fat. These include broiling, boiling, steaming, or microwaving foods instead of frying them. If foods are sauteed, only a small amount of monounsaturated or polyunsaturated fat should be used.
- Teach the patient how to choose lean cuts of red meat. The leaner cuts are usually from the part of the animal that is heavily exercised. All visible fat should be trimmed and discarded before cooking.

    Lean beef cuts: round steak, sirloin tip roast, rolled rump, flank steak.

    Lean lamb cuts: leg of lamb, rolled leg of lamb.

    Lean pork cuts: rolled fresh leg of ham, canned ham (caution: high in sodium), smoked ham (shank, butt, center slice— caution: high in sodium).

- Counsel patients to remove the skin from chicken and turkey before cooking, since the majority of the fat in poultry is located right beneath the skin.
- Encourage the inclusion of more fish in the individual's diet. This will result in a lower saturated-fat intake. All kinds of shellfish can be included with the exception of shrimp and lobster, which should be limited to special occasions.

- Instruct the patients to limit egg intake to two per week or less, depending on the cholesterol restriction. Many patients are shocked when they learn that one egg yolk contains more than 200 mg of cholesterol.
- Introduce patients to low-fat cheeses (labeled as containing no more than two grams of fat per ounce), for example, low-fat cottage cheese, farmers cheese, and ricotta cheese made with part skim milk. Numerous low-fat, low-cholesterol cheeses have been introduced to the market, and your patients may be willing to try them.
- Encourage the patient to drink, cook, and bake with skim or low-fat (1% fat) milk. If the patients currently use whole milk, have them try to switch to lower-fat milk in stages, first to 2%-fat milk, then to 1%-fat milk, and finally to skim milk.

Potential alteration in nutrition; less than body requirements related to decrease in lipid intake.

- Suggest ways to increase complex carbohydrate intake through the use of whole-grain breads and cereals; raw fruits and vegetables can be eaten as snacks and at mealtimes.
- Encourage the patient to learn to use meatless equivalents. Excellent vegetarian cookbooks include *Diet for a Small Planet* and *Laurel's Kitchen,* available in local bookstores.
- Encourage the use of low-fat, low-cholesterol snacks, such as fresh fruit, popcorn (no butter), rice cakes, animal cookies, pretzels, and crispbreads such as

Continued

NURSING INTERVENTIONS *(continued)*

melba toast and rye crisp. Low-fat plain yogurt can be used as a base for dips instead of sour cream or mayonnaise to substantially reduce fat intake.

Knowledge deficit related to
- **risk factors associated with dietary intake of lipids.**
- **potential complications associated with disease process.**

- Teach the patient how to read food labels. Ingredients are listed in descending order by weight, with the ingredient in highest quantity listed first and the ingredient in least quantity listed last. Coconut and palm kernel oils and ingredients such as cream and butter should be low on the list (the sixth ingredient or lower). Patients can double-check the amount of fats added by reading the nutrition label if it is available. Instruct the patient to try to choose those items with no more than two grams of fat per serving. Many surprises await the new label reader: granola-type cereals often contain coconut and coconut oils; many nondairy cream substitutes contain a high amount of coconut oil; snack crackers can be high in fat; muffin, pancake, and biscuit mixes may contain coconut and/or palm kernel oils high on the ingredient list.

Potential noncompliance with dietary regimen related to denial of disease state.

- Caution the patient to avoid making too many changes at once. Change introduced gradually is likely to be more long lasting. Those things that seem easiest to change should be attacked first, and once the patient achieves success, difficult changes can be tried.
- Teach the patient how to keep dietary progress records. It is much easier to note problem areas and obstacles and measure success with written notes.
- Encourage the patient to follow an exercise regimen (as prescribed) concurrently with diet modifications.

HYPERTENSION

Hypertension (high blood pressure) is not only a risk factor for cardiovascular disease through its promotion of atherosclerosis, but it is also the major cause of congestive heart failure in the United States (19). It is also implicated in eye damage, stroke, and renal failure. Recent estimates indicate that of adults in the United States aged 18–74, high blood pressure is found in 33% of white males, 38% of black males, 25% of white females, and 39% of black females (20). Although difficult to believe, the cause of hypertension cannot be determined in 95% or more of the millions of individuals with the disorder. Hypertension of unknown cause is referred to as essential or primary hypertension. In the remaining 5% or less of the cases, the hypertension is a direct result of renal problems, endocrine disorders or tumors, or toxemia of pregnancy, and is referred to as secondary hypertension.

Even with mild hypertension (see Table 9–6 for classification of blood pressure), cardiovascular-disease risk is twice that of normotensive individuals, making treatment warranted. It should be noted that even in severe hypertension, symptoms are usually absent.

Dietary management of hypertension is considered to be a reasonable initial approach, particularly in young individuals with mild hypertension and no other cardiovascular-risk factors. Even

Table 9-6. CLASSIFICATION OF BLOOD PRESSURE

CLASS	DIASTOLIC BLOOD PRESSURE mm Hg
Normal	<85
High normal	85–89
Mild	90–104
Moderate	105–114
Severe	≥115
	SYSTOLIC BLOOD PRESSURE (when diastolic blood pressure <90 mm Hg) mm Hg
Normal	<140
Borderline isolated systolic hypertension	140–159
Isolated systolic hypertension	≥160

Source: Joint National Committee on Detection, Evaluation, and Treatment of High Blood Pressure, "1988 Report."

when drug therapy is used to treat hypertension, dietary modification can enhance the effectiveness of the drugs and reduce drug dosage, thereby lessening some of the drug side effects. In recent years, much effort has been devoted to researching dietary factors that may influence hypertension.

Diet

The theory that manipulating a single dietary factor would have a universal effect on blood pressure has long been discredited. Some nutrients affect blood pressure more than others, but even then, the benefits are often observed in only susceptible individuals. Currently, work in the area of

nutrition and hypertension is focused on fiber, fat, calcium, obesity, alcohol, potassium, and sodium.

Fiber. The idea that plant fiber might be linked to blood pressure stems from the epidemiological observation that more industrialized societies, with their low-fiber diets, have a higher prevalence of hypertension than nonindustrialized societies, with their high-fiber diets. Additionally, vegetarians consistently demonstrate lower blood pressure than matched control groups (21). Mechanisms through which fiber may exert an influence on blood pressure include its effect on intestinal transit times (which may alter neural signals), nutrient absorption, gastrointestinal and hormone responses, and electrolyte excretion. Because the specific role of fiber in blood-pressure regulation has not been critically evaluated through controlled research, specific recommendations on the fiber intake of individuals with high blood pressure have not been made. A prudent approach would be to ensure that fiber is included in the diet through the frequent use of whole-grain breads and cereals and fruits and vegetables.

Fat. Several epidemiological, clinical, and animal studies suggest that polyunsaturated fats lower blood pressure and that saturated fats raise blood-pressure levels (22). The exact mechanism through which fat exerts its effect has not been identified, and the data must still be considered preliminary. The general recommendation from the American Heart Association to reduce total fat and saturated fat in the diet is the most prudent advice to follow until more work is completed on the role of fat in hypertension.

Calcium. Retrospective and epidemiological reports indicate that a low-calcium intake is associated with an increased risk of hypertension. Animal studies have shed some light on the possible role of calcium in the development of high blood pressure. Some evidence exists to support a cellular defect in calcium metabolism in the spontaneously hypertensive rat (23). It has been proposed that a similar defect is present in some individuals with hypertension. The current hypothesis is that dietary calcium corrects the underlying cellular calcium defect and alters vascular smooth muscle to make it less reactive. Further research is needed to clarify calcium's role in the control of hypertension before specific recommendations can be made. Currently, nutritionists recommend that calcium-rich foods such as skim or low-fat milk and yogurt, as well as calcium-rich leafy greens such as collards, kale, mustard, and turnip greens, be included in the diet. Calcium supplements are not generally prescribed.

Obesity. The relationship between weight and hypertension is well established, and the association has been noted in most societies, whether industrialized or not (7). Large clinical trials, such as the Hypertension Detection and Follow-up Program (HDFP) have clearly demonstrated a greater frequency of hypertension among obese individu-

als, and findings from large prospective studies, such as the Framingham Heart Study, support the positive effect that weight reduction has on blood pressure. The true mechanism through which obesity increases blood pressure is not known; however, several physiologic changes occur in obesity that can exert an influence on blood pressure. Obese individuals have an increased cardiac output, higher body sodium due to hyperinsulinemia or abnormal aldosterone and renin relationships, and neuroendocrine abnormalities (24). Prevention and control of obesity is considered an essential step in programs developed to prevent and treat hypertension. Weight reduction is discussed in detail in Chapter 15.

Alcohol. A close relationship exists between the amount of alcohol consumed and the level of blood pressure, independent of age and obesity. Two or fewer drinks per day may be associated with no ill effects on blood pressure (25); however, there is a significant increase in the incidence of hypertension in individuals consuming more than three to four drinks daily (26). Due to the numerous negative aspects related to alcohol consumption in the United States, the American Heart Association recommends that daily kilocalorie intake from alcoholic beverages be limited to 15% of total kilocalories.

Using the figures in Table 9–7, an individual who consumes a total of 1500 kcal in his or her daily diet would be limited to approximately one-and-a-half 12-ounce beers, or two-and-a-half glasses of table wine, or approximately two drinks made with one-and-a-half ounces of gin, rum, vodka, or whiskey. As also demonstrated in the table, alcohol is a significant source of kilocalories. However, the kilocalories are considered "empty," since alcohol is practically devoid of nutrients.

In view of the positive association between obesity and hypertension, and the effect of alcohol raising blood pressure, a discussion of alcohol intake is clearly warranted when counseling individuals who have hypertension. Advise individuals who drink alcohol to reduce or eliminate alcohol from their diets. For the problem drinker, a referral to a support group such as Alcoholics Anonymous may be suggested.

Table 9-7. KILOCALORIES AND ALCOHOL CONTENT OF BEVERAGES

BEVERAGE	AMOUNT (fluid ounces)	KILOCALORIES	ALCOHOL (grams)
Beer	12	151	13
Gin, rum, vodka, whiskey			
80-proof	1½	97	13.9
90-proof	1½	110	15.9
100-proof	1½	124	17.9
Wines			
Dessert*	3½	141	15.8
Table**	3½	87	10.1

Source: Adams, C.F. *Nutritive value of American foods in common units.* Agriculture handbook no. 456. Washington, D.C.: U.S. Department of Agriculture, Agricultural Research Service, 1975.

*apple muscatel, sherries, port, Tokay, aperitif wines, vermouth
**burgundy, cabernet, chablis, champagnes, chianti, claret, Rhine wines, rosé, sauternes

Potassium. Although a high potassium intake (4680-6825 mg daily) has been found to modestly decrease blood pressure in some individuals with hypertension, the effect is extremely variable (27). Potassium's beneficial effect may more likely be linked to the ratio of sodium to potassium rather than to the absolute level of potassium in the diet (28), with low-sodium, high-potassium diets showing more positive results. Potassium appears to exert its influence by inhibiting sodium reabsorption in the kidney, decreasing plasma-renin activity and altering the neurogenic components of blood-pressure regulation. In view of the preliminary nature of the data, it is recommended that patients ensure that they include rich sources of potassium in their diets (Table 9–8) rather than taking potassium supplements. An exception to this occurs if patients are taking diuretics, which deplete both sodium and potassium from the body. In this instance, the physician may recommend a potassium supplement in addition to an increased intake of high-potassium foods. Salt substitutes often contain high amounts of potassium, and patients should check with their physicians before using these.

Sodium. The relationship of sodium to blood pressure has a long history. Despite an enormous amount of research about sodium's role in the development and treatment of hypertension, controversy continues. Advocates cite the following as evidence of a causal relationship between excess dietary sodium and hypertension: Dietary sodium restriction often results in a decrease in blood pressure; diuretics effective in the treatment of hypertension decrease body sodium and reduce the volume of extracellular fluid; sodium-sensitive individuals fed sodium show an increase in blood pressure; high-sodium intakes are associated with an increased prevalence of hypertension in population studies; and animal models of hypertension show an extreme sensitivity to dietary manipulations of sodium (29). Others believe that rather than making blanket recommendations that all persons reduce their sodium intake to prevent hypertension, sodium restriction should be applied only to individuals with hypertension in whom effectiveness of sodium restriction has been established (30).

It is clear that not everyone who has a high-sodium intake will develop hypertension and that

Table 9-8. POTASSIUM IN FOODS

FOOD GROUP	SERVING SIZE	POTASSIUM (mg)
Meat, fish, poultry	2 oz.	200–300
Milk	1 cup	350
Ice cream	½ cup	130
Cheese	2 oz.	50
Grain		
Breads	1 slice	25–50
Cereals	1 cup	25
Noodles	1 cup	75
Vegetables*		
Cucumber, raw	7 slices	41
Beans, green, canned	½ cup	59
Onions, green	2 medium	78
Lettuce	1 cup	99
Mushrooms, raw	½ cup	128
Peas, green, cooked	½ cup	157
Celery, raw	3 stalks	170
Okra, cooked	5 pods	170
Potatoes, french fries	10	199
Cauliflower, cooked	½ cup	200
Broccoli, cooked	½ cup	203
Carrots, raw	1 medium	231
Collards, cooked	½ cup	249
Pumpkin, canned	½ cup	251
Squash, summer, cooked	½ cup	257
Beets, cooked	½ cup	265
Spinach, cooked	½ cup	292
Kale, frozen	3.3 oz.	313
Tomatoes, cooked	½ cup	344
Corn, cooked	1 ear	364
Beans, lima, frozen	½ cup	394
Brussels sprouts, cooked	5 medium	408
Chard, cooked	½ cup	456
Sweet potatoes, baked	1 medium	545
Potatoes, baked	1 medium	587
Beet greens, cooked	½ cup	653
Fruits**		
Blueberries, fresh	½ cup	58
Plum, 1-inch diameter	2	60

Continued

Table 9-8. POTASSIUM IN FOODS (continued)

FOOD GROUP	SERVING SIZE	POTASSIUM (mg)
Raisins	1 tbs	69
Grapes, seedless	10	87
Prunes	2 medium	90
Applesauce, canned, unsweetened	½ cup	95
Figs	1 medium	97
Pineapple, canned, heavy syrup	½ cup	122
Cherries, sweet	10	129
Grapefruit	½	132
Apple, 3-inch diameter	1	182
Peach, 2½-inch diameter	1	202
Pears, bartlett	1	213
Strawberries, whole	1 cup	244
Orange	1	263
Apricots	3	301
Cantaloupe	¼ melon	341
Orange juice, from frozen concentrate	6 fluid ounces	378
Watermelon	1/16 melon	426
Banana	1 medium	440

Salt substitutes
NoSalt
  (Norcliff Thayer, Inc.)
Morton Lite Salt
  (Morton Thiokol, Inc.)
	¼ teaspoon
	
	½ teaspoon
		625
		
		733

Sources: *A.C. Marsh and P.C. Koons, "The Sodium and Potassium Content of Selected Vegetables," *Journal of the American Dietetic Association* 83(1983):24–27.

**Adams, C.F. *Nutritive value of American foods in common units.* Agriculture handbook no. 456. Washington, D.C.: U.S. Department of Agriculture, Agricultural Research Service, 1975.

not all individuals with hypertension will benefit from sodium restriction only; however, the fact is that, in the United States, individuals consume much more sodium than is necessary. The Estimated Minimum Requirement for adults established by the Food and Nutrition Board of the National Academy of Sciences is 500 mg daily. Present consumption in the United States is estimated at four to six grams per day (31), well above physiological needs.

Additionally, one cannot predict with certainty who will and who will not develop hypertension, and preventive means that have no side effects, such as a decrease in sodium intake, are prudent measures. To this end, the American Heart Association has recommended that as a preventive measure, individuals consume no more than 3000 mg of sodium per day. Furthermore, while sodium restriction alone may benefit only one-third to one-half of those with hypertension, it is a rational initial approach to treatment of uncomplicated mild hypertension, especially when the side effects of drugs used to treat hypertension are considered. Finally, in persons with moderate and severe hypertension, sodium restriction has been found to enhance the action of antihypertensive drugs.

The concept that sodium restriction must be severe to have beneficial effects in the treatment of hypertension is no longer accepted (32). A modest sodium restriction in the range of 1400-2000 mg is considered appropriate in the management of the disease (33, 34). In order to restrict sodium intake, patients must understand where dietary sodium is found.

There are three sources of sodium in the American diet: the sodium in the form of salt added to food during cooking or at the table; sodium naturally occurring in food; and sodium added to food during commercial processing. Although each source contributes to total intake, individual addition of table salt is minor as a result of the growing awareness of the sodium-hypertension connection. To follow the American Heart Association

guidelines for prevention purposes, a relatively simple way to decrease sodium intake would be reduce the intake of convenience foods high in sodium content, do without the salt shaker at the table, and forgo the addition of salt during cooking. Salt is sodium chloride, and sodium makes up about 40% of the compound. A handy measure to remember is that one teaspoon of *salt* contains 2000 mg of *sodium*.

Foods of animal origin such as meat, fish, poultry, eggs, and milk generally contain more *natural* sodium than foods of vegetable origin, as shown in Table 9–9. As indicated in the table, the natural sodium in unprocessed foods (other than cheese) is considered to be low, and while dietary restrictions of sodium may eliminate a few foods, no major food group is ever eliminated completely.

Sodium in processed foods is added to preserve or flavor foods. Salt is the major source of sodium

Table 9-9. NATURAL SODIUM IN FOODS

FOOD SOURCE	SODIUM CONTENT
Animal Origin	
Meat, poultry, fish	45-75 mg per 3 oz. serving
Eggs	60 mg each
Milk	125 mg per cup
Natural cheeses	75-300 mg per oz.
Plant Origin	
Fruit (fresh, frozen, canned)	Less than 10 mg per ½ cup
Vegetables (fresh or frozen, no salt used in cooking)	35 mg or less per ½ cup
Cooked cereal (not instant), pasta, rice (unsalted)	Less than 5 mg per ½ cup

Source: U.S. Department of Agriculture, *Food News* (Summer 1986).

in commercially processed foods, although other compounds added to food also contain sodium. Baking soda (sodium bicarbonate), monosodium glutamate, disodium inosinate, disodium guanylate (flavor enhancers), sodium propionate (mold inhibitor), sodium benzoate, sodium sulfite (preservatives), and sodium nitrite (curing agent for meat), are some examples of sodium compounds used in processing foods. Listed in Table 9–10 are the sodium contents of some representative foods in their natural state and once they are processed. Note how quickly the sodium escalates in some of the processed foods. For example, regular hot cereals contain just five milligrams or less of sodium per one-half cup serving. This jumps to 100-360 mg of sodium per serving if it is quick cooking or a cold cereal. Convenience foods such as canned and frozen entrees can also be high in sodium, and the label should be checked for sodium content. Condiments, such as soy sauce, mustard, chili sauce, and tartar sauce also add sodium to the diet, and use may need to be moderated.

Processing low-sodium foods has been a dilemma for food manufacturers. Although consumers express a desire for more low-sodium products, their behavior indicates the opposite (35). Low-sodium products do not sell as well as unmodified products for three possible reasons. Low-sodium items are sometimes more expensive than full-sodium products. Consumers frequently equate low sodium with low flavor, and either do not buy the products or buy them just once before deeming them unacceptable. Also, consumers are accustomed to higher levels of salt in foods and their taste buds have not adjusted to a lower-sodium content.

There is evidence to support a delayed response in taste changes as a result of dietary sodium reductions. A moderate decrease in dietary sodium for a duration of about two months or longer is followed by a taste change. Foods that used to be judged as tasteless due to a low level of salt begin to taste just right, and foods judged to be the most pleasant are those with a lower salt concentration (36, 37). To accommodate a slower pace of taste changes, manufacturers have begun to reduce so-

dium in foods gradually. For example, instead of introducing "unsalted" snack crackers, snack crackers with 75% less sodium are now available. Perhaps a reduction of sodium in stages will prove to be more acceptable.

Regulations have recently been issued by the FDA for sodium labeling of foods under its jurisdiction. FDA-regulated foods that are nutritionally labeled must now also list sodium content. Additionally, guidelines for sodium-label claims were issued. For a food to be labeled "sodium free," it must contain less than five milligrams of sodium per serving. To be considered "very low sodium," the food must contain 35 mg or less sodium per serving. "Low sodium" foods can contain 140 mg or less per serving. Reduced-sodium foods must have a 75% reduction of sodium compared with the regular item. The terms "unsalted," "no salt added," or "without added salt" may be used only if no salt was added during processing and the food for which it substitutes is normally processed with salt. When the claims described above are used on food labels, sodium content must be listed even in the absence of other nutrition labeling.

Another important source of sodium intake is the sodium content of the water. Sodium levels may be obtained from the municipal water company. Persons who live in areas of the country where water is extremely hard sometimes install water softeners. Softened water can add appreciable amounts of sodium to the diet, and the amount should be checked. Installing the water-softening system to bypass faucets used for drinking and cooking or attaching it only to the hot water lines are methods that help to avoid the extra sodium load resulting from the installation of some water-softening systems.

Drugs

Diuretics and beta blockers are used when dietary intervention fails or in conjunction with diet therapy. An increase in serum triglycerides and cholesterol may occur as side effects of the medications, and modification of fat and cholesterol intake is often required.

Table 9-10. SODIUM IN FOODS

PRODUCT	SERVING SIZE	SODIUM CONTENT (mg)
Fruits and fruit juices fresh, frozen, or canned	½ cup	8

Vegetables
  fresh, frozen
  canned, or with sauce
	½ cup
	½ cup
		35 or less
		140–160

Pasta, unsalted	½ cup	5 or less

Hot cereals
  regular
  instant
	½ cup
	½ cup
		5 or less
		100–360

Cold cereals	1 oz.	100–360
Bread	1 slice	110–150
Crackers	2 or 3	110–150
Milk, plain	1 cup	125

Cheese
  natural
  processed
  creamed/low fat cottage cheese
	1 oz.
	1 oz.
	½ cup
		75–300
		350–450
		450

Eggs	1	60

Meat
  fresh
  sausage
  luncheon meats
  frankfurters
  bacon, cooked
  ham
	1 oz.
	1 oz.
	1 oz.
	1 oz.
	1 slice
	1 oz.
		15–25
		250–450
		250–450
		250–450
		65–170
		250–450

Poultry
  fresh
  canned
	1 oz.
	1 oz.
		15–25
		90–150

Fish
  fin
  canned
	1 oz.
	1 oz.
		15–25
		90–150

Continued

Table 9-10. SODIUM IN FOODS *(continued)*

PRODUCT	SERVING SIZE	SODIUM CONTENT (mg)
Convenience Foods		
pot pies	8 oz.	800–1400
ravioli, canned	8 oz.	800–1400
pizza	2–3 slices	800–1400
soups (canned, dehydrated)	1 cup	800–1300
Desserts		
ice cream, ice milk, sherbet	½ cup	35–80
cookies	1	5–50
frozen fruit pies	1 small slice	180
cake, unfrosted	1 small slide	130–310
candy	1 oz.	2–80
Sweets, Sweet Drinks		
sugar, syrups, jams, jellies	1 tbs	20 or less
sodas, fruit-flavored drinks	8 oz.	0–80
Snacks		
nuts, unsalted	1 oz.	5
nuts, salted	1 oz.	150–300
popcorn, unsalted	1 oz.	5
caramel corn	1 oz.	150–300
potato chips	14 chips	150–300
corn chips	14 chips	150–300
Sauces, seasonings, and specialty foods		
soy sauce	1 tbs	1,000
catsup, steak sauce		
tartar sauce, chili sauce, mustard	1 tbs	125–275
Pickles, olives		
dill	1 average	928
small sweet	1 average	128
pickle relish	1 tbs	100–125
olives, black	3	100–125
Butter, cream, oils		
unsalted butter, margarine	1 tsp	1
salted butter, margarine	1 tsp	45
creams, including sour cream	1 tbs	6
powdered, imitation creams	1 tbs	12
vegetable oil	1 tbs	0
prepared salad dressing	1 tbs	100–250

Source: U.S. Department of Agriculture, *Food News* (Summer 1986).

POSSIBLE NURSING DIAGNOSES

Potential alteration in nutrition; greater than body requirements related to increased intake of lipids and sodium.

Alteration in nutrition; less than body requirements related to decreased intake of lipids and sodium.

Knowledge deficit related to risk factors associated with dietary intake of lipids and sodium.

Potential noncompliance with dietary regimen related to denial of disease state.

NURSING INTERVENTIONS FOR NUTRITIONAL DISORDERS

Work closely with patient, dietitian, and physician to develop a dietary plan that will help reduce blood pressure.

Potential alteration in nutrition; greater than body requirements related to increased intake of lipids and sodium.

- Encourage patients to decrease sodium in stages, if going "cold turkey" seems too difficult. First, reduce the amount of salt used in cooking and then eliminate it totally. Next, decrease salt added at the table (suggest that they taste the food before adding salt). Then, decrease the number of foods they salt until they can eat most foods without adding salt. Elimination of salt in cooking and at the table reduces intake by about one-third.

Alteration in nutrition; less than body requirements related to decreased intake of lipids and sodium.

- Encourage the inclusion of calcium-, potassium-, and fiber-rich foods in the diet.
- Caution patients on sodium-restricted diets to be very careful during periods of extreme heat and following vomiting and/or diarrhea. They should consult the physician if they recognize symptoms associated with loss of electrolytes, such as weakness, abdominal cramps, lethargy, and decreased urinary output.

(Refer to Nursing Interventions listed in the section on atherosclerosis in this chapter.)

Continued

NURSING INTERVENTIONS *(continued)*

Knowledge deficit related to risk factors associated with dietary intake of lipids and sodium.

- Providing the patient with information about labeling can be of practical benefit once a patient is discharged. If a food item does not carry nutritional labeling, sodium content can still be estimated. Because ingredients must be listed on the label in descending order by weight, those foods that list salt or sodium near the top of the list contain more sodium than those foods with these ingredients listed further down the list. Also, by law, the name and address of the food manufacturer must be listed on the label. Patients should consider writing to the manufacturer for the sodium information.
- Instruct the patient who may be limited to 2000 mg (2 g) of sodium per day to consume 650 mg or less per meal (three-meals-per-day pattern). Avoid foods with excessive amounts of sodium, such as processed meats and most canned vegetables.
- Instruct the patient who may be traveling or socializing to adjust sodium intake. If a high-sodium food is eaten at one meal, reduce intake at the next meal. Major airlines accommodate low-sodium diets if given advance notice.
- Instruct patients that the intake of convenience foods may have to be restricted. Processed meats, canned entrees, and frozen dinners may be too high in sodium to include on a regular basis.
- Recommend moderating alcohol intake, if appropriate.
- Remind the patient to maintain optimal weight.

Potential noncompliance with dietary regimen related to denial of disease state.

(Refer to Nursing Interventions listed in the section on atherosclerosis in this chapter.)

ISCHEMIC HEART DISEASE (MYOCARDIAL INFARCTION)

Ischemic heart disease occurs when the metabolic demands of the heart muscle cannot be supplied by the coronary blood flow. Myocardial infarction is a type of ischemic heart disease. The oxygen demand of the heart muscle exceeds the supply, consequently necrosis (death of living tissue) of a portion of the heart muscle can result. Since atherosclerosis (discussed earlier in this chapter) is a major cause, the coronary arteries become obstructed as a result of thrombi that attach to the fibrous plaque. Coronary artery spasm may also be a cause of coronary artery disease.

Risk factors for ischemic heart disease are very similar to those for atherosclerosis: increased blood cholesterol, hypertension, cigarette smoking, diabetes mellitus, psychosocial factors, and a family history of coronary heart disease.

Patients with ischemic heart disease due to atherosclerosis will frequently suffer from angina pectoris (chest pain that may radiate up the neck and/or down the left arm) as a result of decreased blood supply to the cardiac muscle. Angina pectoris may occur during periods of physical stress (e.g., following meals or increased physical activity) or be associated with psychological stressors. Anginal pain can serve as a warning signal to the patient. Severe, crushing-type chest pain is frequently associated with myocardial infarction. Prompt medical treatment is essential, or death may result from complications.

Treatment protocols are designed to reduce the amount of damage to the myocardial muscle by reducing the work load of the heart. Rest, both physical and psychological, are essential. Initial treatment during the acute phase will usually begin in the coronary-care unit.

Dietary management may involve a progressive regimen. Initially, careful administration of intravenous fluids is required in order to prevent fluid overload for the damaged heart and prevent pulmonary edema. Oral feedings generally begin with clear liquids for one to two days and progress to full liquids, then to soft food, and, ultimately, to a diet restricted in kilocalories, fat, cholesterol, and sodium (if prescribed). Six smaller feedings per day create less stress on the heart. Some persons may progress to a regular diet with minimal modifications; other persons will need to adhere to a strict regimen of reduced kilocalories and restricted cholesterol, saturated fats, and sodium. A discussion of these modifications is included in the sections on atherosclerosis (lipid restriction) and hypertension (sodium restriction) in this chapter.

POSSIBLE NURSING DIAGNOSES

Knowledge deficit related to risk factors associated with dietary intake of lipids.

Potential alteration in bowel elimination; constipation related to
- bed rest.
- life-style.
- medications.

Potential noncompliance with dietary regimen related to
- denial of disease process.
- dietary intake of lipids and cholesterol.

NURSING INTERVENTIONS
FOR NUTRITIONAL DISORDERS

Work closely with the patient, dietitian, and physician to develop a dietary regimen that will create less burden on the damaged heart muscle and that will be acceptable to the patient.

Knowledge deficit related to risk factors associated with dietary intake of lipids.

- Instruct the patient to:
    limit caffeine-containing beverages (coffee, tea, colas, hot chocolate) that act as stimulants (decaffeinated beverages are readily available and should be substituted in lieu of caffeine-containing beverages);

    consume foods and liquids at moderate temperature (avoid extremes) in order to prevent potential cardiac arrhythmias.
(Refer to "Nursing Interventions" pertaining to atherosclerosis and hypertension for additional information related to lipid and sodium restriction.)

Continued

NURSING INTERVENTIONS (continued)

Potential alteration in bowel elimination; constipation related to
- bed rest.
- life-style.
- medications.

- Encourage the patient to consume high fiber foods and drink adequate fluids to prevent constipation.

Potential noncompliance with dietary regimen related to
- denial of disease process.
- dietary intake of lipids and cholesterol.

- Encourage the patient to adhere to the altered dietary regimen to prevent complications such as congestive heart failure.

(Refer to "Nursing Interventions" pertaining to atherosclerosis and hypertension for additional information.)

CONGESTIVE HEART FAILURE

Congestive heart failure occurs when the heart muscle is unable to pump the blood needed to supply the cellular needs of the body. A series of events occurs as cardiac output is decreased: (1) vascular congestion leads to pulmonary fluid retention and can lead to pulmonary edema, and (2) decreased blood flow to the kidney results in sodium retention and subsequent retention of fluids throughout the body.

The heart attempts to compensate for the inadequate pumping action by increasing the size of the ventricular muscle. The hypertrophied muscle requires a greater oxygen supply. The atherosclerosis that is undoubtedly present further compounds the problem, because the blood flow to the heart muscle is diminished.

The work load of the heart must be relieved by a combination of therapeutic protocols. These include bed rest, drugs (diuretics to reduce edema and digitalis preparations to strengthen the force of the cardiac contraction), and diet therapy. If these protocols are not successful, cardiac failure and death will result.

Dietary management aims to control edema through the use of sodium-restricted diets and avoidance of cardiac stimulants such as caffeine-containing beverages and foods. Weight control may be indicated because kilocalorie expenditure is diminished due to physical inactivity associated with the disease process. (Refer to the section on sodium-restricted diets in this chapter.)

POSSIBLE NURSING DIAGNOSES

Alteration in body requirements related to
- nausea.
- anorexia related to fatigue and/or vascular congestion of the gastrointestinal tract.

Potential fluid-volume excess related to ineffective pumping action of the heart and compensatory mechanisms of the kidney.

Knowledge deficit related to the management of a sodium-restricted diet.

Potential noncompliance related to the unpalatable, restricted sodium diet.

Potential self-care deficit related to inability to prepare diet related to dyspnea and inadequate oxygen supply.

NURSING INTERVENTIONS FOR NUTRITIONAL DISORDERS

Work closely with the patient, physician, and dietitian to develop a dietary plan that will reduce the work load of the heart and that will be acceptable to the patient.

Alteration in body requirements related to
* nausea.
* anorexia related to fatigue and/or vascular congestion of the gastrointestinal tract.

Potential fluid volume excess related to ineffective pumping action of the heart and compensatory mechanisms of the kidney.

Knowledge deficit related to the management of a sodium-restricted diet.

Potential noncompliance related to the unpalatable, restricted sodium diet.

(Refer to "Nursing Interventions" related to sodium restriction discussed in the section on hypertension in this chapter.)

Potential self-care deficit related to inability to prepare diet related to dyspnea and inadequate oxygen supply.

* Recall that patients with congestive heart failure may tire easily and may frequently complain of anorexia related to edema.

TOPIC OF INTEREST

Obviously, many Americans could improve their dietary habits. Currently, total fat intake is nearly 40% of kilocalories with 15%-20% of kilocalories from saturated fats. The majority of Americans consume 400-500 mg of cholesterol daily. Carbohydrate consumption is a low 40%-45% of caloric intake. To help consumers quickly locate cholesterol-free foods and foods low or reduced in cholesterol, the FDA has proposed specific language that food manufacturers could use on their food packages. Under the proposed legislation, "cholesterol free" would be used if the cholesterol content of the food is less than two milligrams per serving. "Low cholesterol" would be reserved for products with less than 20 mg per serving. "Cholesterol reduced" would describe products that have been reformulated so that the cholesterol content has been reduced by least 75% from the original product. If the manufacturer states the cholesterol content, the label would also have to include the amounts of polyunsaturated and saturated fatty acids, unless the product contained less than 10% fat or less than two grams of fat per serving. Cholesterol labeling would also trigger full nutritional labeling. The proposal has not yet been adopted.

On the educational front, the National Heart, Lung, and Blood Institute launched the National Cholesterol Education Program (NCEP), a nationwide effort aimed at high blood-cholesterol levels. The goals of the NCEP are to increase awareness of the importance of decreasing elevated blood-cholesterol levels and to provide information and skills necessary to use dietary changes and drugs for achieving a lowering of blood cholesterol. Representatives from major medical and health professional organizations, voluntary health organizations, community programs, and federal agencies make up the program's coordinating committee, a source of guidance to the program. The NCEP goals will be realized through physician education, television commercials, and health-care associations.

SPOTLIGHT ON LEARNING

Your patient feels that he can decrease the total fat, saturated fat, and cholesterol in his diet when he or his wife does the cooking. He worries about his travel schedule, however. He asks you, "What can I do when I have to eat out?"

Here are some suggestions that he can try:

- Choose a consomme or vegetable soup rather than cream soups.
- Choose meat, fish, or poultry that is steamed, broiled, roasted, or poached. If eating pasta, try a red sauce rather than a cream sauce.
- Steer clear of vegetables in cream or cheese sauces, and opt instead for steamed, boiled, or baked vegetables.
- Choose whole-grain breads in the bread basket to increase complex carbohydrate and fiber intake (use no butter or one-half pat instead of the entire amount).
- Ask for sherbet, fruit ices, gelatin, angel food cake, or fruit for dessert.

A patient who has always salted food says to you: "I can't cook without salt. I don't know what else to use to make foods taste good." You can recommend that the person begin to try using herbs and spices to season foods. In the chart below, herbs that enhance the flavors of particular foods are listed, and recipes for herb blends to use in place of salt are given.

Food	Flavor Enhancers
Soups	bay, chervil, tarragon, marjoram, parsley, savory, rosemary
Poultry	garlic, oregano, rosemary, savory, sage
Beef	bay, chives, cloves, cumin, garlic, hot pepper, marjoram, rosemary, savory
Lamb	garlic, marjoram, oregano, rosemary, thyme
Pork	coriander, cumin, garlic, ginger, hot pepper, pepper sage, savory, thyme
Fish	chervil, dill, fennel, tarragon, garlic, parsley, thyme

Vegetables   basil, burnet, chervil, chives, dill, tarragon, marjoram, mint, parsley, pepper, thyme

Salads   basil, borage, burnet, chives, tarragon, garlic, chives, parsley, herb and regular vinegars.

Recipes for Herb Blends

Saltless Surprise   2 tsp garlic powder and 1 tsp each of basil, oregano, and powdered lemon rind. Put ingredients into a food processor and mix well. Store in glass container, label, and add rice to prevent caking.

Spicy Saltless Seasoning   1 tsp each of cloves, pepper and coriander seed (crushed), 2 tsp paprika, and 1 tbs rosemary. Mix ingredients in a food processor. Store in airtight container.

From H.H. Shimizu, "Do Yourself a Flavor," *FDA Consumer* (April 1984). HHS Publication No. (FDA) 84-2912.

REVIEW QUESTIONS

1. Which of the following is considered to be a lesion of atherosclerosis?
   a. fibrous plaque
   b. VLDL
   c. hypercholesterolemia
   d. endothelial injury

2. Which of the following food selections indicates that the patient understands a low-cholesterol food?
   a. sauteed shrimp
   b. broiled chicken
   c. braised liver
   d. egg salad

3. Which of the following lipoproteins is the major carrier of cholesterol?
   a. chylomicron
   b. VLDL
   c. HDL
   d. LDL

4. Which of the following is a saturated fat source?
   a. coconut oil
   b. olive oil
   c. safflower oil
   d. peanut oil

5. To reduce saturated fat in the diet, a patient should choose which of the following menu selections?
   a. baked chicken, broccoli, tossed salad with vinaigrette dressing
   b. spare ribs, sauerkraut, mashed potatoes, apple pie
   c. liver and onions, scalloped potatoes with cheese, sliced tomatoes with French dressing
   d. hamburger, corn on the cob, tomato slices, ice cream

6. Which of the following is not a complex carbohydrate?
   a. grains
   b. legumes
   c. vegetables
   d. poultry

7. Which of the following snack choices indicates that the person understands low-sodium foods?
   a. swiss cheese and crackers
   b. peanut butter on celery
   c. chilled grapefruit sections
   d. fresh vegetables and dip

8. Which of the following dietary factors is not thought to increase blood pressure?
   a. high-sodium intake
   b. high-alcohol intake
   c. high-potassium intake
   d. low-calcium intake

9. How are ingredients listed on food labels?
   a. in ascending order by weight
   b. in descending order by weight
   c. in ascending order by volume
   d. in descending order by volume

10. What does "low sodium" on a food label mean?
   a. the product contains less than 5 mg sodium per serving
   b. the product contains 35 mg or less sodium per serving
   c. the product contains 140 mg or less sodium per serving
   d. the product has a 75% reduction in sodium compared with the regular item

ACTIVITIES

1. Obtain menus from local restaurants. Choose appetizers, salads, entrees, and desserts that are low in fat, saturated fat, and cholesterol. If you had to watch sodium intake as well as fat and cholesterol, what foods would be appropriate?

2. Bring in to class labels from foods and decide whether the foods would be appropriate on a low-cholesterol, low-fat, low-saturated-fat diet. Include cereals, cookies, snack crackers, frozen desserts, and frozen entrees. Evaluate the sodium content of the foods.

3. Check the grocery store for fat-, cholesterol-, and sodium-modified foods. If possible, purchase them and have a taste-testing session.

4. Recall and record what you ate during the past 24 hours. What source of food or type of food preparation added the most total fat to your diet? What source of food or type of food preparation added the most saturated fat to your diet? Which foods added the most cholesterol? Which foods added the most sodium?

5. Interview someone who is following a sodium- or fat-restricted diet for cardiovascular disease. Ask him or her what difficulties are faced when trying to follow the diet. If the person has been following a sodium-restricted diet, find out whether any taste changes have occurred.

6. If you use salt at the table, try doing without it for one meal. How did the food taste? Which foods tasted fine without added salt?

7. Modify the following menu to decrease total fat, saturated fat, and cholesterol and increase complex carbohydrates:

Breakfast:
2 eggs fried in 1 tsp butter
2 slices bacon
½ cup hash brown potatoes fried in bacon fat
2 slices white toast with 2 tsp butter
1 glass whole milk

Lunch:
sandwich consisting of 2 slices salami, 2 slices American cheese, 1 tsp mayonnaise, 1 Kaiser roll
milkshake

Dinner:
8 ounce T-bone steak
½ cup mashed potatoes made with whole milk and butter
½ cup broccoli with cheese sauce
1 slice coconut cream pie
coffee with cream

Snack:
cheese and crackers

8. Now try to decrease the sodium content of the above menu.

REFERENCES

1. American Heart Association. *1989 heart facts.* Dallas: The American Heart Association, 1988.
2. Ross, R., and J.A. Glomset. The pathology of atherosclerosis. *New England Journal of Medicine* 295(1976):369–77.
3. Grundy, S.M. Atherosclerosis: pathology, pathogenesis, and role of risk factors. In *Disease a month,* vol. 24, no. 9. Chicago: Yearbook Medical Publishers, Inc., 1983.
4. Brandt, E.N., and J.M. McGinnis. National children and youth fitness study: Its contribution to our national objectives. *Public Health Reports* 100(1985):1–3.
5. American Heart Association. Report of the committee on stress, strain and heart disease. *Circulation* 55(1977):825A–831A.
6. U.S. Department of Health and Human Services, Public Health Service, National Institutes of Health, Office of Medical Applications of Research. Health implications of obesity. *Consensus Development Conference Statement* vol. 5, no. 9 (1985).
7. Havlik, R.J., et al. Weight and hypertension. *Annals of Internal Medicine* 98, Part 2(1983):855–59.
8. Kris-Etherton, P.M., and T. Etherton. The role of lipoproteins in lipid metabolism of meat animals. *Journal of Animal Science* 55(1982):804–17.
9. Levy, R.I. Cholesterol screening—When, why, and how. In *Cholesterol and coronary disease—Reducing the risk,* Volume 1, No. 1. New York: Science and Medicine, 1986.
10. U.S. Department of Health and Human Services, Public Health Service, National Institutes of Health, Office of Medical Applications of Research. Treatment of hypertriglyceridemia. *Consensus Development Conference Summary* vol. 4, no. 8.
11. American Heart Association. *Counseling the patient with hyperlipidemia.* Dallas: American Heart Association, 1984.
12. Ernst, N.D., and J. Cleeman. Reducing high blood cholesterol levels: Recommendations from the National Cholesterol Education Program. *Journal of Nutrition Education* 20(1988):23–29.
13. National Cholesterol Education Program. *Report of the expert panel on detection, evaluation, and treatment of high blood cholesterol in adults.* NIH Publication No. 88-2925. January 1988.
14. Herold, P.M., and J.E. Kinsella. Fish oil consumption and decreased risk of cardiovascular disease: A comparison of findings from animal and human feeding trials. *American Journal of Clinical Nutrition* 43(1986):566–98.
15. Grundy, S.M. Comparison of monounsaturated fatty acids and carbohydrates for lowering plasma cholesterol. *New England Journal of Medicine* 314(1986):745–48.
16. Mattson, F.H., and S.M. Grundy. Comparison of effects of dietary saturated, monounsaturated, and polyunsaturated fatty acids on plasma lipids and lipoproteins in man. *Journal of Lipid Research* 26(1985):194–202.
17. Gammal, E.B., K.K. Carroll, and E.R. Plunkett. Effects of dietary fat on mammary carcinogenesis by 7,12-dimethylbenz(alpha)anthracene in rats. *Cancer Research* 27(1967):1737–42.

18. King, M.E., and A.A. Spector. Effect of specific fatty acyl enrichment on membrane physical properties detected with a spin label probe. *Journal of Biological Chemistry* 253(1978):6493–6501.

19. Frolich, E.D. Mechanisms contributing to high blood pressure. *Annals of Internal Medicine* 98, Part 2(1983):709–14.

20. American Heart Association. *High blood pressure fact sheet.* Dallas: The American Heart Association, 1986.

21. Anderson, J.W. Plant fiber and blood pressure. *Annals of Internal Medicine* 98, Part 2(1983):842–46.

22. Smith-Barbaro, P.A., and G.J. Pucak. Dietary fat and blood pressure. *Annals of Internal Medicine* 98, Part 2(1983):828–31.

23. Wegener, L.L., and D.A. McCarron. Dietary calcium: an assessment of its protective action in humans and experimental hypertension. *Food Technology* 12(1986):93–95.

24. Dustan, H.P. Mechanisms of hypertension associated with obesity. *Annals of Internal Medicine* 98, Part 2(1983):860–64.

25. Friedman, G.D., A.L. Klatsky, and A.B. Siegelaub. Alcohol intake and hypertension. *Annals of Internal Medicine* 98, Part 2(1983):846–49.

26. American Heart Association, Nutrition Committee Position Statement. *Dietary guidelines for healthy American adults,* 1986.

27. Tannen, R.L. Effects of potassium on blood pressure control. *Annals of Internal Medicine* 98, Part 2(1983):773–80.

28. Weaver, C.M., and G.H. Evans. Nutrient interactions and hypertension. *Food Technology* 12(1986):99–101.

29. Porter, G.A. Chronology of the sodium hypothesis and hypertension. *Annals of Internal Medicine* 98, Part 2(1983):720–23.

30. Laragh, J.H., and M.S. Pecker. Dietary sodium and essential hypertension: Some myths, hopes, truths. *Annals of Internal Medicine* 98, Part 2(1983):735–43.

31. U.S. Department of Health and Human Services, Public Health Service. *The Surgeon General's report on nutrition and health. Summary and recommendations, 1988.* DHHS (PHS) Publication No. 88-50211.

32. Hunt, J.C. Sodium intake and hypertension: A cause for concern. *Annals of Internal Medicine* 98, Part 2(1983):724–28.

33. Tobian, L. Human essential hypertension: Implications of animal studies. *Annals of Internal Medicine* 98, Part 2(1983):729–34.

34. U.S. Department of Health and Human Services, Public Health Service, National Institutes of Health. *The 1980 report of the joint national committee on detection, evaluation, and treatment of high blood pressure.* NIH Publication No. 81-1088, 1980.

35. Dunaif, G.E., and C. Khoo. Developing low and reduced sodium products: An industrial perspective. *Food Technology* 12(1986):105–107.

36. Beauchamp, G.K., M. Bertino, and K. Engelman. Modification of salt taste. *Annals of Internal Medicine* 98, Part 2(1983):763–69.

37. Blais, C.A., et al. Effect of dietary sodium restriction on taste responses to sodium chloride: A longitudinal study. *American Journal of Clinical Nutrition* 44(1986):232–43.

CHAPTER
10

NUTRITION AND THE PATIENT WITH BLOOD DISORDERS

Objectives

After studying this chapter, you will be able to
- describe the metabolic changes associated with a decreased number of red blood cells and/or a supply of hemoglobin that is insufficient to meet the oxygen needs of the body.
- differentiate among the nutritional needs for a patient suffering from anemia related to inadequate production of red blood cells; excessive destruction of red blood cells and/or hemoglobin; and a decrease in the number of red blood cells.
- describe dietary management for patients with selected types of anemia.
- identify nursing interventions for nutritional disorders associated with selected types of anemia.

250

Overview

Anemia is a condition (not a primary disease) that is characterized by either a decreased number of circulating red blood cells or a supply of hemoglobin that is insufficient to meet the required oxygen needs of the body or a combination of both factors. Since anemia is always secondary to some other pathological phenomenon, the whole body is affected when the person suffers from some form of anemia. The discussion in this chapter focuses on the nutritional implications for the selected types of anemia listed in Table 10-1.

Table 10-1. TYPES AND CAUSES OF ANEMIA

TYPE	CAUSE
Nutritional Deficiency Iron Vitamin B_{12} Folic acid (folate)	Inadequate production of red blood cells
Aplastic	Bone marrow failure
Hemolytic Sickle cell	Destruction of red blood cells
Blood Loss Acute/hemorrhagic Chronic	Loss of red blood cells
Chronic disease	Infection: shortened life of red blood cell Cirrhosis of the Liver; defective utilization of iron Azotemia: decreased production of erythropoietin Cancer: malfunction of bone marrow

Sources:

J.D. Crapo, M.A. Hamilton, and S. Edgman, *Medicine and Pediatrics in One Book* (St. Louis: Hanley Belfus, Inc., The C.V. Mosby Company, 1988), 280.

B.L. Bullock, and P.P. Rosendahl, *Pathophysiology: Adaptations and Alterations in Function*, 2d ed. (Glenview: Scott, Foresman and Company, 1988), 223.

M.A. Krupp, M.J. Chatton, and L.M. Tierney, *Current Medical Diagnoses and Treatment 1986* (Los Altos: Lange Medical Publications, 1986) 324–26.

POSSIBLE NURSING DIAGNOSES

Activity intolerance related to inadequate oxygen supply secondary to a decreased number of red blood cells or inadequate hemoglobin concentration.

Potential for injury, bleeding tendency secondary to an abnormal blood profile.

Potential alteration in bowel elimination, constipation, or diarrhea, secondary to gastric mucosal atrophy and/or drug-replacement therapy.

Potential alteration in nutrition; less than body requirements related to lack of interest in food secondary to sore, inflamed mouth.

Knowledge deficit related to
- nutritional requirements and food choices.
- hazards of decreased blood count and/or hemoglobin levels.
- hereditary factors (pernicious anemia and sickle cell disease).

Noncompliance related to diet and/or drug therapy.

Potential fluid-volume deficit related to decreased oral intake (sickle cell disease).

Potential alteration in tissue perfusion related to viscosity of blood and occlusion of blood flow (microcirculation) (sickle cell disease).

Potential alteration in comfort; pain related to vascular occlusion (sickle cell disease).

NUTRITIONAL ANEMIAS

Nutritional anemias can result from insufficient intake of protein (amino acids); vitamins, especially B_{12}, C, and folic acid; or minerals, particularly iron. The depressed production of red blood cells can result from inadequate intake and/or utilization, malabsorption, or increased bodily need for the substances. Iron deficiency, folic-acid deficiency, and vitamin-B_{12} deficiency, including pernicious anemia, are discussed in this section.

Iron Deficiency Anemia

The most common form of anemia in this country, iron-deficiency anemia, is characterized by reduced hemoglobin production. Microscopic ex-amination of the blood reveals that the red blood cells are microcytic (smaller in size) and hypochromic (pale in color with a decreased hemoglobin level). Iron is an essential mineral that is present in the body as the heme portion of hemoglobin, as part of myoglobin, and as part of tissue enzymes. It is stored in the liver, spleen, and bone marrow in the form of ferritin and hemosiderin.

Iron that is available for use in the body is derived from several sources. Red blood cells are recycled by the reticuloendothelial system (liver and spleen), and heme is broken down to yield the available iron to be reused. Exogenous sources of iron are available through foods in both the heme and nonheme forms. Heme iron, which is found in animal tissues (fish, poultry, and meat) is better absorbed; the nonheme iron compounds are found in fruits and vegetables (refer to Chapter 2 for a discussion of iron sources).

Approximately 1.8 mg of iron must be absorbed daily in order to meet the needs of those persons in the high-risk groups (1). The way the body uses the iron that is ingested is a complex process. Iron is absorbed from the intestinal wall (proximal duodenum), in the ferrous state, and only in relation to the body's need. Absorption is also affected by the level of acid in the intestinal lumen and by the food mixture that is consumed. For example, meats and vegetables eaten together enhance the absorption of iron from the vegetable (nonheme compounds). Generally, foods high in ascorbic acid enhance the absorption of nonheme iron.

The type of cooking utensil may affect the amount of iron available for absorption. The use of iron cookware (non-Teflon coated) may increase the iron content of the foods prepared in that type of utensil (2). Because of technological advances in methods of cooking (cast iron on the hearth evolving to glassware and ceramics in the microwave), people need to be more aware of food choices in increasing the amount of available iron in the diet.

Food combinations can also negatively affect the amount of nonheme iron that is absorbed. Tannic acid, found in tea and coffee, certain food preservatives (EDTA, added to some processed fruits, vegetables, mayonnaise, and condiments), and antacid preparations can inhibit the absorption of nonheme iron. Research continues to be conducted to determine the actual impact on absorption (3).

The incidence of iron-deficiency anemia involves a wide spectrum of the population. Iron-deficiency anemia is most often associated with blood loss, but the risk is also higher in certain age groups. It is prevalent among infants because of their rapidly expanding blood volume. Adolescents are frequently affected because their dietary intake is insufficient to meet the demands made by rapid growth and, for girls, the onset of menses. Pregnancy causes additional demands on the available iron supply, as does heavy menstrual flow for women of childbearing age. The elderly are also

prone to developing iron-deficiency anemia because of inadequacies in the diet and/or undetected blood loss. Persons with low incomes can be at risk if they are unable to purchase the proper foods (4).

Symptoms of iron-deficiency anemia are frequently nonspecific; the patient may complain of fatigue, dyspnea, weakness, or anorexia. Characteristic signs may include pallor, tachycardia, stomatitis, and brittle hair and nails.

Treatment involves detecting and correcting the source of blood loss, if appropriate, or determining other causes of the deficiency. Oral and parenteral doses of iron may be prescribed. Some foods are good sources of iron. Liver is the best source, but meats, legumes, green vegetables such as broccoli, collards, and green beans, fruits such as figs, dried apricots and dried peaches, and enriched cereals and breads are also good sources.

Persons in high-risk populations require diet instruction with emphasis on including foods with high-iron content into the daily meals. Mothers of infants should be encouraged to breast feed (since the iron in breast milk is well absorbed) or to use formulas that have been fortified with iron (5). Iron-rich foods such as fortified infant cereals or a liquid-iron preparation may be prescribed by the physician according to the age and maturation of the infant. (Refer to Chapter 4 for a complete discussion on the nutritional needs of infants and children.)

Special attention should be given to the dietary intake of the adolescent because of the energy demands on the body resulting from growth and the blood loss associated with the onset of menses in teenage girls (6). Teenagers may tend to skip meals, restrict food intake because of concern about weight gain, and consume foods that are low in nutrients.

In addition to an adequate intake of iron in the diet of the pregnant woman, the physician will generally prescribe iron supplements to help the body meet the increased demand during this period of stress (7). Women with heavy menstrual flow may also require additional iron intake (dietary as well as supplemental).

Special attention should be given to encouraging adequate dietary iron intake for the elderly, since iron deficiency is common. Chronic disease states may lead to the deficiency, but frequently, inadequate intake is often the major cause.

Iron toxicity is possible, but it is generally not a problem, because of the way in which the body processes the iron. Although iron toxicity has been noted in individuals who consume excessive numbers of iron supplements, extremely large quantities of dietary iron would need to be ingested over a long period of time before toxic reactions occur, unless the individual has a genetic defect (hemochromatosis) in which the stores of iron are uncontrolled (8).

NURSING INTERVENTIONS FOR NUTRITIONAL DISORDERS

Work closely with the dietitian in planning diet instruction for those persons in the high-risk groups for iron-deficiency anemia (infants, adolescents, women of childbearing age, the elderly, and persons of low-socioeconomic status).

Potential alteration in nutrition; less than body requirements related to lack of interest in food secondary to sore, inflamed mouth.

- Be aware that the elderly may be more prone to developing iron-deficiency anemia because of the presence of other chronic diseases such as achlorhydria or blood loss resulting from undetected gastrointestinal lesions (9).

Knowledge deficit related to
- **nutritional requirements and food choices.**
- **hazards of decreased blood count and/or hemoglobin levels.**

- Instruct the patient to:
    eat sufficient iron-containing foods such as liver, red meats, fish, poultry, and legumes (10);

    eat meats and vegetables together to enhance absorption from the vegetable (nonheme iron source);

    drink citrus juices when taking iron supplements to enhance absorption, since the ascorbic acid helps to convert ferric salts to the ferrous, soluble form of iron salts;

    avoid the use of antacids within one hour of meals;

    refrain from drinking coffee and tea with meals since these beverages inhibit nonheme iron absorption from food (especially important for anemic individuals);

    refrain from self-medicating with iron supplements if they suspect anemia, since this habit may mask a serious condition such as chronic blood loss associated with cancer of the colon.
- Note that although iron supplements taken with citrus juice or on an empty stomach are better absorbed, patients may take the supplement with food if gastric irritation is a problem.

Continued

NURSING INTERVENTIONS *(continued)*

- Dilute liquid iron preparations and give through a straw to prevent staining of tooth enamel.
- Be aware that the ingestion of clay or starch (pica) by individuals in some cultures may predispose to iron-deficiency anemia by interfering with iron absorption.

Potential for injury; bleeding tendency secondary to an abnormal blood profile.

- Observe for alteration in the normal healing process. Healing may be delayed in those persons with severe anemia (iron less than 6 mg/100 ml).
- Monitor laboratory reports: hemoglobin, hematocrit, and iron levels in the blood; evidence of blood loss in gastrointestinal or genitourinary tracts.

Potential alteration in bowel elimination; constipation or diarrhea, secondary to gastric mucosal atrophy and/or drug-replacement therapy.

- Encourage the patient to increase fluid intake when taking iron supplements to prevent constipation.
- Remind the patient that stools will change color (black or dark green) while taking iron salts, since the gastrointestinal tract is the major route of excretion of iron.

Noncompliance related to diet and/or drug therapy.

- Oral iron preparations may be toxic in large quantities. All medications should be kept out of the reach of children to prevent accidental ingestion.

Vitamin-B$_{12}$ Deficiency (Including Pernicious Anemia)

Vitamin B$_{12}$ is an essential cofactor in the synthesis of DNA. If vitamin B$_{12}$ is deficient, an imbalance in the relationship of DNA, RNA, and protein synthesis becomes apparent and is manifested in tissues with rapidly reproducing cells such as bone marrow and gastric mucosal cells (11).

The liver is the primary storage site for vitamin B$_{12}$, which is also referred to as extrinsic factor. In order for vitamin B$_{12}$ to reach the liver, it undergoes a series of reactions. Vitamin B$_{12}$ is found in food sources of animal origin (meat, fish, poultry, eggs, and milk) only. None is contained in plant sources. When vitamin B$_{12}$ comes in contact with the intrinsic factor (protein secreted by the parietal cells of the stomach), a compound is formed that is transported to the mucosal cells of the distal ileum. This compound, which is insensitive to digestive enzymes, in the presence of calcium, can be absorbed

into the intestinal cell. After release from intrinsic factor, vitamin B$_{12}$ enters the bloodstream and is transported to the liver for storage. (See Chapter 2 for a full discussion of vitamin B$_{12}$.)

The anemia associated with vitamin-B$_{12}$ deficiency is referred to as a megaloblastic type of anemia. The red blood cells are larger in size than normal cells and have a characteristic oval shape. The cell membrane is under stress because the content of the cell is greater, leading to potential cellular destruction.

Deficiency of vitamin B$_{12}$ may not become apparent for several years (three to six) after the absorption of the vitamin ceases (11). This deficiency can occur at all ages. Vegans (individuals who consume no animal protein) can develop vitamin-B$_{12}$ deficiency. The majority of persons who manifest the deficiency, however, have an associated decrease or absence of intrinsic factor in the stomach. This condition is referred to as pernicious anemia.

Pernicious anemia usually affects adults past the age of 35. The cause is unknown; however, some theories cite hereditary tendencies, prolonged iron deficiency (which can predispose to gastric atrophy), or an autoimmune reaction within the gastric cells or against the intrinsic factor (12). In pernicious anemia, the nervous system as well as the red blood cells are affected.

Vitamin-B_{12} deficiency can also occur following gastrectomy (including partial) or in association with atrophy of the gastric mucosa. Patients who suffer from regional enteritis or following ileal resection (ileostomy) may also manifest signs of deficiency.

Symptoms of vitamin-B_{12} deficiency include those nonspecific symptoms associated with any form of anemia: pallor, anorexia, weight loss, and dyspnea. Specific signs and symptoms include smooth, sore tongue; paresthesias (tingling of the hands and feet and bowel and bladder disturbances); and altered mental states including hallucinations and depression.

The type of replacement therapy is dependent on the cause. If a nutritionally poor diet has been the etiology, the physician may prescribe oral vitamin-B_{12} supplements in addition to increasing animal products in the diet (13, 14).

Conditions like pernicious anemia, which involve impaired absorption of the vitamin, require more intensive replacement. Lifelong administration of vitamin B_{12} is required. Usually this involves monthly parenteral doses. Some physicians may prescribe daily oral replacement, especially for the elderly; however, the effectiveness of the

NURSING INTERVENTIONS
FOR NUTRITIONAL DISORDERS

Work closely with the patient and dietitian to plan a diet that contains adequate amounts of vitamin B_{12}.

Knowledge deficit related to
- **nutritional requirements and food choices.**
- **hazards of decreased blood count and/or hemoglobin levels.**
- **hereditary factors (pernicious anemia and sickle cell disease).**

- Instruct the patient with a deficiency resulting from inadequate absorption due to an alteration in the available intrinsic factor (pernicious anemia, following gastrectomy or associated with gastric atrophy) that lifelong replacement of vitamin B_{12} is required and eating a well-balanced diet is essential.
- Encourage vegans to request a prescription for a therapeutic level of the vitamin supplement, not OTC preparations.
- Instruct pregnant women who are vegans to inform the physician of their dietary preferences so that the vitamin-replacement therapy can prevent deficiency from developing in the fetus.
- Instruct patients following ileal resection (ileostomy) that lifelong vitamin-B_{12} supplements are required.

Activity intolerance related to inadequate oxygen supply secondary to a decreased number of red blood cells or inadequate hemoglobin concentration.

- Monitor laboratory results to note an increase in the mean corpuscular volume (MCV) and increase in the serum levels of vitamin B_{12}.

oral preparations has not been proven. Any patient receiving oral vitamin B_{12} should be closely monitored. Vitamin B_{12} is not toxic in large doses, and any excess is excreted by the kidneys.

Folic-Acid Deficiency

Like vitamin B_{12}, folic acid (folate) is a member of the B-complex family and is also a cofactor in DNA manufacture. Deficiency of this vitamin can lead to depressed synthesis and maturation not only of red blood cells, but also of white blood cells and platelets. Both folic-acid and vitamin-B_{12} anemias are referred to as megaloblastic because the red blood cells are larger and fewer in number than normal red blood cells. The cell membrane is also more fragile, which leads to a shorter life span.

Because of the close relationship between folic-acid deficiency and vitamin-B_{12} deficiency, a similar type of blood picture emerges, but the changes occur more rapidly, since unlike vitamin B_{12} there is virtually no conservation of folate. Both folic acid and vitamin B_{12} are essential during different phases of red blood cell maturation (15).

Folic acid is stored in the liver but in insufficient quantity. Folate is readily available and easily absorbed from green leafy vegetables and fresh fruits, fruit juices, liver, yeast, and nuts. (Refer to Chapter 2 for more information on folate.)

A deficiency of folic acid may be due to decreased dietary intake, malabsorption (including drug interactions), and increased requirement for the vitamin. Chronic alcoholics frequently suffer from this deficiency due to poor dietary intake as well as decreased folate metabolism caused by the action of alcohol. Elderly persons with unpredictable dietary intake patterns may also suffer from decreased folic-acid levels.

Patients suffering from malabsorption syndromes, such as sprue or regional enteritis, can experience a deficiency of a number of nutrients and micronutrients because the essential substances cannot be absorbed from the mucosa of the small intestine. (Refer to Chapter 7 for a discussion of malabsorption syndromes.) Drug therapy may also interfere with the absorption of folic acid. Patients who may be taking anticonvulsant drugs (such as phenytoin sodium (Dilantin) or phenobarbital), oral contraceptives, or antineoplastic drugs (such as methotrexate, an antimetabolite) used in the treatment of cancer may require folic-acid supplements.

An increased need for folate occurs in conditions in which rapid cellular growth occurs, such as during pregnancy. Patients who suffer from Hodgkin's disease or leukemia or other hemolytic diseases such as sickle-cell anemia also have an increased need for folic acid.

Signs and symptoms of folic-acid deficiency are similar to those associated with vitamin-B_{12} deficiency. The characteristic that distinguishes folic-acid deficiency from vitamin B_{12} deficiency is the lack of neurological symptoms.

Treatment of folic-acid deficiency is related to the cause. If the diet is inadequate, inclusion of foods that are high in folate should be emphasized. Fresh fruits and leafy green vegetables (such as spinach and broccoli), as well as liver, lean beef and veal, eggs, and wheat germ are good sources of folic acid.

Folic-acid supplements may be necessary for those persons who require more than diet modification. Pregnant women, persons on anticonvulsant drug therapy, or persons with any disease process that causes hemolysis (destruction) of blood cells may need oral vitamin supplements.

Replacement therapy with folic acid is never begun for a patient with megaloblastic anemia before blood tests reveal the cause of the anemia. Administration of folic acid may temporarily relieve some of the symptoms associated with a vitamin-B_{12} deficiency; however, the neurological manifestation will progressively worsen.

NURSING INTERVENTIONS FOR NUTRITIONAL DISORDERS

Work closely with the patient and dietitian to plan a diet that is nutritionally adequate and contains the necessary quantity of folic acid.

Knowledge deficit related to
- **nutritional requirements and food choices.**
- **hazards of decreased blood count and/or hemoglobin levels.**

- Inform persons who are preparing food that 50%–95% of folate may be destroyed by prolonged cooking (8).
- Instruct pregnant women to eat a nutritionally adequate diet rich in foods containing folic acid and to take supplements, if prescribed by the physician.
- Instruct mothers that an infant who is placed on goat's milk will require folic-acid supplements because of the low level of the vitamin in that milk (16).

Noncompliance related to diet and/or drug therapy.

- Monitor laboratory reports on those persons who are prone to developing folic-acid deficiency: chronic alcoholics, the elderly, pregnant women, persons on drug therapy (oral contraceptive, anticonvulsant, or antineoplastic drugs), and persons with hemolytic disorders (Hodgkin's, leukemia, or sickle-cell disease).
- Instruct persons who take oral contraceptive, anticonvulsant or antineoplastic drugs that folic-acid supplements may be required because of malabsorption of the vitamin.
- Inform patients that therapeutic levels of folic acid are available by prescription; only small amounts of folate are available in over-the-counter multivitamin preparations to prevent masking of symptoms associated with pernicious anemia.

HEMOLYTIC ANEMIAS

Hemolytic anemias are caused by a destruction of red blood cells from internal or external causes. Abnormalities may exist in the cell membrane (inherited or acquired), hemoglobin may be structurally abnormal due to low oxygen tension (sickle-cell disease), or physical trauma may damage the cells (prolonged exercise or extracorporeal circulation devices). This discussion is limited to sickle-cell disease (sickle-cell anemia).

Sickle-Cell Anemia

Sickle-cell disease is a genetic disorder in which an individual has two HbS hemoglobin genes in place of the normal HbA hemoglobin genes. Sickle-cell anemia is one of the most frequent forms of sickle disease, but it is only one of a number of diseases in this category.

Persons of varied ethnic backgrounds are particularly susceptible, especially those of Mediterranean, Caribbean, and Asian ancestry. Within the black population in the United States, sickle-cell disease occurs in approximately one in every 650 live births (11). It is also estimated that one in every 1000–1500 Hispanics is affected (17).

The sickling or abnormal, curved (crescent) shape of the red blood cells occurs due to a low oxygen tension. The hemoglobin within the cell forms crystalloid molecules that are less soluble and inhibit the exchange of oxygen. The red blood cells become rigid and inflexible, which causes an increase in the viscosity of the blood. The life-span of the altered cells is approximately 7–20 days, compared with the life span of normal cells of 120 days (18, 19).

During periods of sickle-cell crisis, circulation is slowed as the blood becomes more viscous, ultimately causing obstruction of arterioles, capillaries, and venules. Occlusion (obstruction) of the blood flow to the organs of the body and extremities causes edema and pain. Ulcerations on the extremities are common, and serious complications result as liver and kidney function are impaired.

Signs and symptoms associated with sickle-cell anemia are similar to other forms of anemia (see discussion earlier in this chapter), but symptoms of the "crises" also may be present. Persons may complain of severe pain associated with acute and chronic tissue damage. Gallstone formation is frequent because of the increased bile pigment that results from hemolysis. Potential for infection is greater, probably due to the decreased function of the spleen (repeated infarcts).

There is no cure for sickle-cell anemia at this time. Treatment protocols are based on prevention and management of the complications as they arise. Careful dietary management is essential for the patient with sickle-cell anemia.

The diet should be low in iron, since an excess of iron is usually present as a result of the increased by-products of red-blood-cell destruction. Foods containing vitamin C should be avoided with meals in order to decrease the amount of nonheme iron that may be absorbed from the foods (18, 20). An increase in the amount of folic acid is usually needed for red-blood-cell production. Even though an increase in the amount of zinc in the diet has been found to increase weight gain and the growing of body hair, zinc and copper utilization may be altered due to cellular destruction. Zinc replacement must be carefully monitored because these elements compete for the same binding sites on protein. An overabundance of one nutrient can produce a deficit of the other.

Fluid intake should be increased to about 2000–3000 ml, as tolerated, in order to decrease the viscosity of the blood in order to prevent stagnation in the microcirculation. The person should be instructed to avoid consuming alcohol, which could precipitate dehydration.

NURSING INTERVENTIONS FOR NUTRITIONAL DISORDERS

Work closely with the patient, physician, and dietitian to plan a diet, that will help correct the anemia without creating additional stress to the body.

Potential fluid-volume deficit related to decreased oral intake (sickle-cell disease).

- Monitor fluid intake and output and daily weight (during crisis).
- Instruct the patient to drink fluids liberally throughout the day (2000–3000 ml, or as prescribed) in order to prevent vascular occlusion.

Continued

NURSING INTERVENTIONS (continued)

- Encourage teachers to allow students with the diagnosis of sickle-cell anemia to consume additional fluids during school hours.

Potential alteration in tissue perfusion related to viscosity of blood and occlusion of blood flow (microcirculation) (sickle-cell disease).

- Instruct the patient to drink fluids liberally throughout the day (2000–3000 ml, or as prescribed) in order to prevent vascular occlusion.

Potential alteration in comfort; pain related to vascular occlusion.

- Administer analgesic medications as prescribed.

Knowledge deficit related to
- **nutritional requirements and food choices.**

- **hazards of decreased blood count and/or hemoglobin levels.**
- **hereditary factors (pernicious anemia and sickle-cell disease).**

- Instruct the patient to follow the diet prescription (especially for children and adolescents, since growth and maturation may be retarded due to a deficiency of nutrients).
- Advise the patient of the need for foods that contain vitamin C and to ingest these foods/fluids between meals to prevent the additional uptake of iron.
- Instruct the patient to avoid foods that are high in iron because of the increased supply and storage resulting from red-blood-cell destruction. (See Chapter 2 for iron sources.)
- Advise teachers of the importance of adequate fluid and food intake for the student during the school day.

BLOOD-LOSS ANEMIA

Acute Blood Loss

Acute blood loss can occur in those persons with a history of gastrointestinal disease, following traumatic accidents, or in conjunction with the use of prescription and non prescription drugs such as nonsteroidal anti-inflammatory agents and salicylates (aspirin).

Whatever the cause of the hemorrhage and following treatment (usually including blood transfusion), the fluid portion of the blood is replaced within 48–72 hours (21). The life of red blood cells is approximately 120 days, so that supportive therapy must be instituted to enable the body to replace the lost cells. Iron replacement is essential following hemorrhage. For every two milliliters of blood loss, approximately one milligram of iron is lost (20). Initially, dietary replacement alone is not suf-

ficient. Oral and/or parenteral administration of iron products may be prescribed.

Dietary management is important, however. The diet prescription will be determined by the cause of the blood loss. Ultimately, the diet will contain adequate kilocalories with liberal protein. Foods that are rich in vitamins B_{12}, C, and folic acid and the minerals zinc, iron, and copper are also included.

Chronic Blood Loss

The manifestations of anemia that result from chronic loss of blood are similar to those of iron-deficiency anemia. Chronic blood loss of two to four milliliters per day may lead to the development of iron-deficiency anemia (22).

Once the source of bleeding is identified, appropriate treatment can be instituted. Dietary management will be similar to that described under iron-deficiency anemia.

NURSING INTERVENTIONS FOR NUTRITIONAL DISORDERS

Work closely with the patient and dietitian to plan a diet that will enhance the body's iron supply.

Knowledge deficit related to
- **nutritional requirements and food choices.**
- **hazards of decreased blood count and/or hemoglobin levels.**

- Instruct patients that blood transfusions provide only temporary relief of anemia. Iron supplements and dietary management (long-term) are required to return iron levels to normal ranges.

- Instruct persons who are blood donors to eat foods that are high in iron to help replace losses.
- Plan teaching strategies for high-risk groups associated with potential chronic blood loss: women with heavy menstrual flow and the elderly.

(Refer to the section of this chapter dealing with iron deficiency anemia for additional suggestions.)

TOPIC OF INTEREST

It has been found that high doses of vitamin C through intake of supplements may affect the availability of vitamin B_{12} in food. It appears that megadoses of vitamin C destroy vitamin B_{12} and may convert some vitamin B_{12} into inactive forms (23). While taking megadoses of any vitamin or mineral is discouraged, it has been suggested that patients on large doses of vitamin C be checked regularly for vitamin-B_{12} deficiency.

SPOTLIGHT ON LEARNING

Pamela, a 26-year-old mother of two children, ages 5 and 3, has come to the clinic with complaints of fatigue and frequent colds. During the assessment, it is noted that Pamela's color is pale and her hair is dry and brittle. She also complains of some soreness of her mouth and tongue. She states that her menstrual periods are regular but the flow seems heavier than it was before her pregnancies.

The physician ordered blood studies, including plasma ferritin. The results indicated the following: hematocrit, 32%; hemoglobin, 10 g/dl; ferritin, 10 mg/dl. A diagnosis of iron-deficiency anemia was established, and Pamela was given ferrous-sulfate supplements by the physician. She was also encouraged to eat a nutritious diet and to get as much rest as possible. A nutrition consultation was arranged with the dietitian for the next visit, which is scheduled in four weeks.

Before Pamela leaves the clinic you are able to give her some preliminary information about her diet and iron supplements. The following questions should help you prepare for your discussion with Pamela.

1. What food sources should be included in Pamela's diet to provide additional iron intake?
2. What food combinations can help to enhance the absorption of iron from foods?
3. What additional information could you give Pamela about the diet of the children?
4. What instructions should be given to Pamela concerning the iron supplements with regard to increased absorption, possible gastric irritation, preventing constipation, and the appearance of the stool?

REVIEW QUESTIONS

1. Iron is important in the body because it:
   a. is essential for bones and teeth
   b. helps maintain gastric acidity
   c. helps regulate blood glucose
   d. is a constituent of hemoglobin

2. Which of the following food groups would be beneficial in increasing the hemoglobin levels in the body?
   a. sweet potatoes, peanut butter, cheese
   b. liver, green beans, strawberries
   c. eggs, skim milk, apple
   d. banana, oatmeal, grape juice

3. Iron-deficiency anemia is not frequently found in which of the following groups?
   a. young men
   b. adolescents
   c. pregnant women
   d. elderly men

4. Which of the following can interfere with nonheme-iron absorption?
   a. ascorbic acid
   b. well-done steak
   c. citrus juices
   d. EDTA

5. Physiological problems associated with decreased iron intake can predispose to which of the following?
   a. severe mental retardation
   b. red-blood-cell stasis in microcirculation
   c. decreased red-blood-cell count
   d. pernicious anemia

6. If a patient eats steamed spinach for dinner, which food should also be eaten to increase the absorption of iron?
   a. chicken
   b. whole-wheat bread
   c. white toast
   d. butter

7. Which of the following is not a good food source of iron?
   a. milk products
   b. enriched cereals and breads
   c. liver
   d. red meat

8. Which is the most common nutrient deficiency in children?
   a. folic acid
   b. vitamin B_{12}
   c. iron
   d. iodine

9. In order for the body to use the available vitamin B_{12} in foods, which of the following must be present in the stomach?
   a. intrinsic factor
   b. extrinsic factor
   c. an alkaline medium
   d. absence of ulceration

10. The patient with sickle-cell anemia generally will not need which alteration to the diet?
    a. increased fluids
    b. increased iron
    c. balanced nutrients
    d. midday snacks

ACTIVITIES

1. Select one of the meals you have eaten in the past three days, and identify the iron sources in your diet. Which foods provided heme iron and nonheme iron? Did you consume foods that would help in the absorption of iron? Which foods may have inhibited the absorption of iron?

2. Compare the iron requirements and stores for men and women. Why do men have less need for increased stores of iron?

3. Iron supplements (pharmacologic) may be required to treat iron deficiency in addition to nutritional enhancement of the diet for some patients. Identify the groups who are most at risk for developing iron-deficiency anemia. Why are these groups at risk?

4. Persons with sickle-cell anemia may need to reduce the amount of iron that is consumed in the diet. If iron is so important in the transportation of oxygen to the body cells, why is it prohibited in this form of anemia? Plan a simple breakfast that would be appropriate for this type of patient.

5. Prepare a diet assessment on a patient who has chronic blood loss. What adjustments to the former dietary pattern may be necessary to provide the required nutrients to assist the body in replacing red blood cells?

REFERENCES

1. Krause, M.V., and L.K. Mahan. *Food, nutrition and diet therapy: A textbook of nutritional care.* Philadelphia: W.B. Saunders, 1984.
2. Brittin, H.C., and C.E. Nossaman. Iron content of foods cooked in iron utensils. *Journal of the American Dietetic Association* 86 (1986):897–901.
3. Munoz, L.M., et al. Coffee consumption as a factor in iron-deficiency anemia among pregnant women and their infants in Costa Rica. *American Journal of Clinical Nutrition* 48 (1988):645–51.
4. Lopez, L.M., and J.P. Habicht. Food stamps and the iron status of the U.S. elderly poor. *Journal of the American Dietetic Association* 87 (1987):598–603.
5. Brady, M.S., et al. Specialized formulas and feeding for infants with malabsorption or formula intolerance. *Journal of the American Dietetic Association* 86 (1986):191–99.
6. Vigietti, G.C., and J.D. Skinner. Estimation of iron bioavailability in adolescents' meals and snacks. *Journal of the American Dietetic Association* 87 (1987):903–7.
7. Gorduek, V.R., et al. High dose carbonyl iron for iron deficiency anemia: A randomized double blind trial. *American Journal of Clinical Nutrition* 46 (1987):1029–34.

8. Robinson, C.H., et al. *Normal and therapeutic nutrition.* New York: Macmillan Publishing Company, 1986.

9. Carnevali, D.L., and M. Patrick. *Nursing management for the elderly,* 2d ed. Philadelphia: J.B. Lippincott Company, 1986.

10. Farley, M.A., et al. Adult dietary characteristics affecting iron intake: A comparison based on iron density. *Journal of the American Dietetic Association* 87 (1987):184–89.

11. Crapo, J.D., M.A. Hamilton, and S. Edgman. *Medicine and pediatrics in one book.* St. Louis: Hanley Belfus, Inc., The C.V. Mosby Company, 1988.

12. Thompson, J.M., et al. *Clinical nursing.* St. Louis: The C.V. Mosby Company, 1986.

13. Herbert, V. Recommended dietary intakes (RDI) of vitamin B_{12} in humans. *American Journal of Clinical Nutrition* 45 (1987):671–78.

14. Helman, A.D., and I. Darnton-Hill. Vitamin and iron stores in new vegetarians. *American Journal of Clinical Nutrition* 45 (1987):785–89.

15. Herbert, V. Recommended dietary intakes (RDI) of folates in humans. *American Journal of Clinical Nutrition* 45 (1987):661–70.

16. Committee on Nutrition, American Academy of Pediatrics. *Pediatric nutrition handbook.* Elk Grove Village: American Academy of Pediatrics, 1985.

17. *Public health information sheet, sickle-cell anemia: Genetic series.* March of Dimes, Birth Defect Foundation, 1983.

18. Gueldner, S.H., and S. Yu. Dysfunctions of erythrocytes. In *Adult nursing in hospital and community settings,* edited by L. Burrell. E. Norwalk: Appleton & Lange, 1990.

19. Rooks, Y., and B. Pack. A profile of sickle-cell disease. *Nursing Clinics of North America* 18 (1983):131–38.

20. Lewis, S.M., and I.C. Collier. *Medical-surgical nursing: Assessment and management of clinical problems.* New York: The McGraw-Hill Book Company, 1987.

21. Bullock, B.L., and P.P. Rosendahl. *Pathophysiology: Adaptations and alterations in function,* 2d ed. Glenview: Scott, Foresman and Company, 1988.

22. Krupp, M.A., M.J. Chatton, and L.M. Tierney. *Current medical diagnoses and treatment 1986.* Los Altos: Lange Medical Publications, 1986.

23. Herbert, V. Vitamin B_{12}. In *Nutrition reviews' present knowledge in nutrition,* 5th ed., edited by R.E. Olson, et al. Washington, D.C.: The Nutrition Foundation, Inc., 1984.

CHAPTER
11

NUTRITION AND THE PATIENT WITH RESPIRATORY DISORDERS

Objectives

After studying this chapter, you will be able to
- describe the metabolic consequences associated with chronic obstructive pulmonary disease and cystic fibrosis.
- explain the dietary management for patients with chronic obstructive pulmonary disease and cystic fibrosis.
- describe the rationale for the use of pancreatic-enzyme supplements for patients with cystic fibrosis.
- identify the nursing interventions for nutritional disorders associated with respiratory problems.

Overview

Diseases and conditions affecting the respiratory system can have an impact on nutrition in a variety of ways. When a person is suffering from an upper-respiratory condition that causes edema of the nasal passages, the sense of taste and smell may be temporarily affected. Generally, unless the condition involves an overwhelming infection or a severe case of the flu, the person is able to ingest appropriate nutrients to support the body during this period of stress, and no dire consequences result.

However, obstructive pulmonary conditions can lead to altered nutritional states, including malnutrition. The extent of the nutritional problems for the patient with severe pulmonary conditions is beginning to gain additional interest and emphasis by health-care professionals.

The focus of this chapter primarily is on the nutritional alterations related to chronic obstructive pulmonary diseases that are long-term and generally irreversible (emphysema, chronic bronchitis, and cystic fibrosis).

OBSTRUCTIVE PULMONARY DISEASES

Obstruction within the pulmonary system can occur in the air passages or in the lung tissue itself and can be acute or chronic. An example of an acute airway obstruction is asthma or acute bronchitis.

Chronic obstructive pulmonary (or lung) disease is frequently referred to by the acronyms, COPD or COLD. Chronic obstructive pulmonary disease is actually a group of diseases that have the common characteristic of obstruction to the airflow from the lungs (emphysema and chronic bronchitis). Some authors include asthma in this category.

A basic tissue defect and/or decrease in defense mechanisms within the lung tissues may precipitate the changes that occur in the bronchi or the parenchyma of the lung that lead to COPD (1). These nonspecific inflammatory processes that cause a chronic, productive cough (mucous expectorated), wheezing, and dyspnea may be precipitated by factors such as smoking, infection, or other inhaled irritant (1).

Many times, diagnosis is not made until the disease process is in the later stages; consequently, COPD has become the fifth leading cause of death in the United States. The mortality rate has tripled in the past 30 years (2).

Even though pulmonary emphysema and chronic bronchitis may share the common factor, damage that results from years of exposure to cigarette smoking, they are different disease processes.

Chronic bronchitis is characterized by excessive mucus production by the bronchial mucosa. This mucus can occlude the bronchi and predispose to a chronic productive cough and bronchospasm. Air becomes trapped behind the partial obstruction, which eventually leads to an increase in lung volume.

Pulmonary emphysema may coexist with chronic bronchitis, but emphysema differs in that the lung tissue that is distal to the terminal bronchioles becomes damaged. The alveolar destruction leads to airway collapse. Dyspnea is the predominant symptom because the gaseous exchange mechanism is upset. Carbon dioxide becomes trapped in the alveoli, and sufficient oxygen cannot enter. The patient develops hypoxia and can ultimately develop respiratory acidosis due to carbon dioxide retention. Further complications include cor pulmonale (right ventricular congestive heart failure) and edema to the liver and the extremities.

Treatment for COPD must be comprehensive. The patient and family must understand that this condition is chronic, long-term, and, many times, incapacitating. In addition to the nutritional concerns, the patient needs to understand the importance and role of medications (bronchodilators, antibiotics, corticosteroids, and expectorants) in helping to control symptoms. Bronchial hygiene, including natural (postural drainage) and mechanical means (intermittent positive pressure breathing) of clearing the airway must be understood. Supplemental oxygen therapy may be given to facilitate breathing. Exercises may be beneficial in order to learn to use accessory muscles (abdominal) to facilitate air exchange from the lungs.

Dietary management is frequently a complex matter for the patient with COPD. Poor nutritional status may develop because of a variety of factors. Dyspnea may interfere with the mechanical process of eating. During a meal, the distended stomach may restrict the movement of the diaphragm, or the flattened, restricted diaphragm may limit the expansion of the stomach. Gastric upset and anorexia may be related to medication intake (bronchodilators and/or steroids) or due to the increased production of sputum (3).

Caloric requirements are increased because of the energy required for breathing and because of the degree of tissue breakdown.

Malnutrition is common among COPD patients (4). The caloric needs of the patient increase as the disease process advances and becomes more severe, presumably due to the high energy cost of breathing (5). In addition to the caloric needs, adequate intake of vitamins A and C is essential in helping to prevent pulmonary infections and to help decrease the extent of tissue damage within the lungs (3).

The goals for nutritional support for the COPD patient are to maintain weight and lean body mass (if the patient is not overweight); assess energy requirements for the individual patient; and provide appropriate protein, carbohydrate, and fat to supply the metabolic needs (6).

The diet must be tailored to the individual needs of the patient. Most persons adapt to eating smaller quantities of food at more frequent intervals (five to six meals per day). Alteration in the consistency of the food (soft and/or liquid) and thorough chewing of the food may help to prevent respiratory distress because the softer food exerts less pressure on the diaphragm. Special dietary supplements, commercially prepared such as Pulmocare and Isocal HN or those prepared in the home may be beneficial to provide additional kilocalories without adding bulk. Avoidance of foods such as onions, peas, melons, and cabbage, which tend to produce gas following digestion, may also put less tension on the diaphragm.

Medication therapy may play a significant role in adversely affecting adequate nutrient intake. Bronchodilator drugs (xanthines, such as theophylline, and steroids, such as prednisone) can cause gastric upset. Caution the patient to check with the pharmacist to determine whether these drugs should be taken with milk or with food to reduce gastric irritation. Some sustained-release xanthine preparations may be too rapidly released in the presence of food and result in drug toxicity (7).

The type of diet can also affect the breakdown and absorption of xanthine preparations. Generally a diet that is low in carbohydrate and high in protein will increase the elimination (shorten the half-life) of the drug. Eating charbroiled foods can also speed the elimination of the drug from the body. Retention of the drug in the body is prolonged with a diet that is high in carbohydrate and low in protein.

Persons who take steroid preparations frequently excrete increased amounts of calcium. The low blood levels of calcium when combined with the inactivity that accompanies COPD can lead to osteoporosis. Increasing the calcium in the diet should be recommended. Food such as dairy products and green leafy vegetables low in oxalic acid should be included in the diet. Exercise can also help to increase bone mass.

It is imperative that the patient understand the importance of the role of diet in the treatment of chronic obstructive diseases of the lungs. Malnutrition can lead to alterations in lung tissue because of decreased defense mechanisms, thereby predisposing the person to infection. Respiratory muscle mass and strength may be reduced, and a person can develop a blunted respiratory response to hypoxemia, which ultimately leads to decreased ventilation (4, 6).

POSSIBLE NURSING DIAGNOSES

Potential alteration in nutrition; less than body requirements related to anorexia, dyspnea, and fatigue.

Knowledge deficit related to
- nutritional support and therapy.
- effects of drug therapy on food intake.

Potential for infection related to inadequate dietary intake.

Activity intolerance related to hypoxia, inability to carry out activities of daily living.

NURSING INTERVENTIONS
RELATED TO NUTRITIONAL DISORDERS

Work closely with the patient, dietitian, and physician to develop a dietary plan that will ensure optimum nutrition to meet the increased metabolic needs of the body.

Potential alteration in nutrition; less than body requirements related to anorexia, dyspnea, and fatigue.

- Encourage the patient to follow the diet prescribed by the physician. The diet is designed to meet the body's metabolic needs and to enhance the action of the medications.
- Teach the patient and family ways to incorporate additional kilocalories and protein into the diet (refer to Chapter 12).
- Perform bronchial hygiene treatments (postural drainage or intermittent positive pressure breathing (IPPB) treatment and exercise at least one hour before meals.
- Contact the social worker to arrange for Meals on Wheels for those persons who may need assistance in food preparation.

Knowledge deficit related to
- **nutritional support and therapy.**
- **effects of drug therapy on food intake.**

- Instruct the patient to
    eat smaller meals at more frequent intervals (five to six per day) to decrease the work load of the body;

    eat slowly and chew all foods well;

    use nasal oxygen during meals (if prescribed);

    use a liquid dietary supplement such as Pulmocare or Isocal HN rather than miss a meal;

    avoid gas-forming foods to reduce tension on the diaphragm.
- Encourage the patient to consume the necessary quantity of protein in the diet. Inadequate protein intake can decrease the colloid osmotic pressure within the lung and predispose to pulmonary edema.

Continued

NURSING INTERVENTIONS *(continued)*

- Monitor body weight. Weight gain may be indicative of fluid retention associated with steroid drug preparations or impending complications such as cor pulmonale.
- Monitor laboratory reports to note serum levels of xanthine drug preparations such as theophylline. Adverse reactions are likely to develop if the serum levels are above 20 mcg/ml (7).
- Encourage patients on xanthine drug preparations to:

  consult with the pharmacist before taking sustained-release drug preparations. The drugs may act more rapidly in a fasting state, making drug toxicity more likely;

  be consistent in the administration of drug preparations; take the medications with food or fasting, as prescribed, in order to receive the optimum action of the drug;

  notify the physician if signs of gastric irritation (burning, nausea, and/or vomiting) become apparent during drug therapy, since stress ulcers are common for COPD patients (see Chapter 7 for more details on gastric irritation);

  limit the use of coffee, tea, and chocolate, which contain methylxanthines. Blood levels in the body could increase;

  limit the intake of charbroiled foods because the drug can be eliminated more rapidly from the body;

  follow the diet prescription, since the breakdown and elimination of the drug from the body can be greatly affected. A diet that is high in protein and low in carbohydrate will speed the elimination of the drug from the body. Retention of the drug within the body can be prolonged with a diet that is high in carbohydrate and low in protein.

Potential for infection related to inadequate dietary intake.

- Instruct the patient to:

  eat foods that are rich in vitamins A and C to help maintain body defenses (refer to Chapter 2);

  drink liberal quantities of fluids (two to three quarts per day) in order to liquefy bronchial secretions (unless contraindicated by another medical condition such as heart failure).

Activity intolerance related to hypoxia; inability to carry out activities of daily living.

- Encourage the patient to:

  use foods that require minimal preparation (fresh fruits and vegetables and vegetables that require no peeling, such as baked potatoes, summer squash, broccoli, and cauliflower);

  use a blender or food processor to puree foods if necessary;

  prepare meals ahead of time; rest 30 minutes to one hour before eating;

  use a microwave oven for food preparation, if available.

- Contact the social worker to arrange for Meals on Wheels for those persons who may need assistance in food preparation.

Cystic Fibrosis

Cystic fibrosis is an inherited disease in which large quantities of viscous (thick, tenacious) mucus is secreted by the exocrine glands (external secreting) of the pancreas, bronchi, and small intestine. The sweat glands and saliva also excrete large amounts of sodium chloride. The liver and organs of the reproductive system may also be affected. This disease is the most common inherited, fatal disease of childhood and affects 1 in 1600–2000 children (2, 8, 9). Approximately 10 million persons in the United States are carriers of the recessive gene (10).

The abnormal, thick mucus can accumulate in the exocrine ducts of the target glands and predispose to a variety of problems. Structural deformities can occur that can lead to destruction of the tissue within that gland.

Chronic obstructive pulmonary disease can occur because of the blockage of the small bronchioles. Recurrent infections usually occur that ultimately lead to destruction of lung tissue, pulmonary hypertension, and eventually respiratory failure. Pancreatic insufficiency results from the blockage of the exocrine ducts of the pancreas. Fibrotic tissue replaces normal functioning pancreatic tissue and leads to steatorrhea (fatty stool) and ultimately malnutrition, since the enzymes necessary to aid in the digestion of, predominantly, fats, but also carbohydrates and protein are not broken down and absorbed from the small intestine. Cirrhosis of the liver is possible because the bile ducts become blocked. Obstruction of the ducts can predispose to the development of portal hypertension and esophageal varices (see chapter 7).

Because of the advances in recognition and treatment of cystic fibrosis, increasing numbers of children who have the disease are living until childbearing age. It has been found that most men afflicted with cystic fibrosis are infertile because the vas deferens is blocked before birth. Although women with cystic fibrosis have structurally normal reproductive systems, the abnormally thick cervical mucus makes it difficult for the sperm to fertilize the egg.

Even though there are no structural deformities in the sweat glands, there is an increased excretion of sodium chloride. The increased loss of electrolytes can lead to increased fluid losses, especially during periods of fever or hot weather. Diagnosis of cystic fibrosis is confirmed by the abnormal results of the sweat test, in which increased amounts of sodium and chloride are detected. Prenatal diagnosis and screening are still in the research stages.

The primary goal of treatment is to improve the quality and duration of life. Since malnutrition can have an impact not only on growth patterns, but also on resistance to infection and function of the lungs, it is essential that strong emphasis be placed on nutritional support for the patient. Treatment regimens are principally symptomatic and supportive. Preventive measures must be taken for all persons with cystic fibrosis. Daily postural drainage procedures to prevent stasis of mucus in the pulmonary tree is frequently required. Prompt identification and control of pulmonary infections are essential so that appropriate antibiotic therapy may be instituted as early as possible.

The energy needs of the child with cystic fibrosis are 130%–150% greater than the RDA for children of comparable age (8). Prior to diagnosis, the child with cystic fibrosis can consume extremely large quantities of food but manifest as much as a 50% deficit in energy due to kilocalories lost from malabsorption (11, 12). The increased appetite may not be consistent at all times. Anorexia may occur at times when infections are present, when the child is unusually fatigued, or when abdominal distention results from malabsorption of nutrients. Generally, cystic fibrosis patients have increased metabolic demands as well as nutrient losses due to malabsorption.

The diet for cystic fibrosis must be tailored to each child, but it is usually high in kilocalories and protein, with fat levels determined by individual tolerance. A digestant, pancrelipase, which is a pancreatic-enzyme replacement (Cotazym, Pancrease, or Viokase), is given with meals and snacks to aid in the digestion of fat, carbohydrate, and protein. Pancrelipase powder is given before meals or during meals, mixed with a fruit such as applesauce or cereal, to infants or small children who are not able to swallow the replacement in capsule form. The dosage of the drug is calculated for each individual patient in an attempt to ensure a maximum of one to two bowel movements a day.

Malnutrition can result from malabsorption and fecal loss of nutrients as well as from the stress of frequent episodes of pulmonary infections. Oral dietary supplements as well as nocturnal nasogastric feedings may be required to provide additional nutrient intake. It may be helpful for the child to eat several small meals (five to six per day) in order to prevent gastric distress and to possibly increase food intake. Some patients, especially those with advanced stages of the disease, may prefer gastrostomy or jejunostomy feeding rather than insertion of a nasogastric tube every night. Research is being conducted as to the advantages of the various methods of providing supplemental caloric intake. Currently, parenteral nutrition is also being used for some patients. The long-term

clinical benefits have not been thoroughly evaluated (13).

Because of fat malabsorption, water-soluble forms of the fat-soluble vitamins, vitamins A, D, E, and K, may be prescribed. In addition, a therapeutic multivitamin, as well as calcium and iron supplements, may also be prescribed. Micronutrient replacements are essential to help promote optimum growth. At times when salt replacement becomes necessary, such as during periods of fever or exercise, the physician may recommend the use of salt tablets rather than the oversalting of foods.

Infants under one year of age may have a formula such as Pregestimil, a protein hydrolysate formula that contains medium-chain triglycerides. Pregestimil may be prescribed if fats are not well tolerated. Pancreatic-enzyme supplements may not be required with this type of formula; however, if a standard formula preparation is used, it is necessary to administer pancreatic-enzyme supplements. Introduction of new foods to the diet should be gradual in order to determine the type of food best tolerated by the infant.

POSSIBLE NURSING DIAGNOSES

Potential alteration in nutrition, less than body requirements related to
- malabsorption and loss of fats and fat-soluble vitamins in the stool.
- anorexia secondary to labored breathing.
- vomiting secondary to chronic coughing.

Knowledge deficit related to
- nutritional support and therapy
- effects of drug therapy on food intake.

Alteration in elimination; diarrhea and/or constipation related to insufficient or excessive pancreatic enzyme enhancement.

Potential fluid-volume deficit related to increased concentration of sodium and chloride in the sweat.

NURSING INTERVENTIONS
RELATED TO NUTRITIONAL DISORDERS

Work closely with the patient, dietitian, and physician to help create a diet that will provide optimum nutrition and promote growth for the infant or child with cystic fibrosis.

Potential alteration in nutrition; less than body requirements related to
- **malabsorption and loss of fats and fat-soluble vitamins in the stool;**
- **anorexia secondary to labored breathing.**
- **vomiting secondary to chronic coughing.**

- Provide adequate intake; food requirements may be 130%–150% greater than the RDA for normal children (8).
- Monitor all food intake to determine which foods are best tolerated.
- Record body weight and height to determine whether the child is consistent with norms for age.
- Offer small quantities of food at more frequent intervals (five to six meals per day) in addition to supplements, if necessary.
- Offer food replacement if vomiting has occurred following severe coughing.
- Perform chest physical therapy and postural drainage at least 30 minutes to one hour prior to meals to prevent vomiting.
- Instruct parents in the procedure for nasogastric tube insertion, if appropriate.
- Teach parents methods to prevent complications associated with nocturnal nasogastric tube feedings; e.g., positioning of the child and checking for proper tube placement.
- Instruct parents in the procedure for administering feedings by means of a gastrostomy or jejunostomy tube.

Knowledge deficit related to
- **nutritional support and therapy.**
- **effects of drug therapy on food intake.**

- Instruct the family to:
    attempt to encourage the child to consume the necessary kilocalories and protein throughout the day;

    offer smaller quantities of food at more frequent intervals;

    introduce new food gradually, to determine the individual tolerance;

    avoid foods that cause diarrhea, noting that individual response is unique;

    encourage the child to consume adequate kilocalories during periods of stress, such as infection and fever;

    administer the vitamin and mineral supplements as prescribed;

    communicate with teachers so that they understand the importance of snacks between meals, snacks (such as ice cream and cookies) during school parties must be given with pancreatic-enzyme replacement;

    administer pancreatic enzymes as prescribed by the physician, since these are essential for the child to digest and use the nutrients; however, doses must be individualized;

    be aware that the activity of the enzyme will vary for each child, since the action of the enzyme is dependent on the pH of the intestine;

    administer pancrelipase 30 minutes to one hour prior to meals in order to aid

Continued

NURSING INTERVENTIONS *(continued)*

in digestion and absorption of nutrients (enzyme replacements are usually given concurrently with snacks);

sprinkle powdered or enteric coated forms of pancrelipase on fruit (applesauce) or cereal for infants who cannot swallow the capsule form of the drug. Enteric-coated preparations should never be crushed; spheres should be sprinkled on the food if necessary;

avoid sprinkling pancreatic enzyme on protein food, for it will begin immediate food breakdown and make food unpalatable;

avoid mixing pancrelipase in formula, not only because the taste will be altered, but also because it will be difficult to determine the exact dosage of the enzyme if the entire quantity of formula is not consumed;

keep a supply of pancrelipase in the school office or where designated, for easy access by the child.

Alteration in elimination; diarrhea and/or constipation related to insufficient or excessive pancreatic-enzyme replacement.

- Monitor all stools. Large, foul-smelling stools are indicative of fat malabsorption (steatorrhea); the dose of pancrelipase may need to be increased.

- Monitor the number of stools per day. One to two stools is optimum.
- Note that constipation may be relieved by decreasing the dose of pancrelipase.
- Inform teachers that the child may need to be excused to the bathroom more frequently than other children.

Fluid-volume deficit related to increased concentration of sodium and chloride in the sweat.

- Encourage adequate fluid intake as determined by the age of the child and any physiological alteration, such as fever, vomiting, diarrhea, and increased physical exertion.
- Avoid oversalting food as a means of sodium and chloride replacement. The child can develop a liking for heavily salted foods. This practice could predispose to problems as an adult if complications that involve edema formation occur.
- Keep salt tablets on hand when sodium and chloride may need to be replaced, such as during hot weather, during and after physical exercise, or during episodes of fever.

TOPIC OF INTEREST

A recent study involving cystic fibrosis patients examined whether nutrition counseling based on self-management skills could improve caloric intake (14). The age range of the patients who participated was 4 to 29 years, and they were studied over a four-year period. Rather than prescribing a specific diet and expecting compliance, the nutritionists encouraged the patients to actively participate in treatment. After teaching general nutrition guidelines, the patients were helped to set their own goals for increasing caloric intake in small, gradual steps. Results indicated that patients were able to increase body weight and maintain it over a four-year period. Allowing patients to shape and individualize their treatment seems to be much more successful than dictating dietary prescriptions, especially in the treatment of a chronic illness such as cystic fibrosis.

SPOTLIGHT ON LEARNING

Ms. Goldman, the mother of a child with cystic fibrosis, asks your advice in helping her plan a diet (including snacks for school) for her 10-year-old son. Jason weighs 46 lb (21 kg) and is 29 in. tall. Ideally, Jason should consume 120–150 kcal and 3–4 g of protein per kilogram of body weight (10).

Visit the library and consult food tables so that you may give Ms. Goldman some suggestions for foods that would help to provide the nutrients and kilocalories for Jason.

REVIEW QUESTIONS

1. Patients with COPD have high energy needs and are prone to malnutrition. Which of the following is not a reason for this?
   a. dyspnea
   b. frequent pulmonary infections
   c. distention of the stomach and flattening of the diaphragm
   d. exercises to strengthen the accessory muscles to facilitate breathing

2. Which of the following vitamins are essential for helping to maintain body defenses to fight infection?
   a. A and C
   b. B and K
   c. D and E
   d. C and K

3. Persons taking xanthine drug preparations should not follow which of the following dietary guidelines?
   a. limit the use of charbroiled foods
   b. increase the protein content of the diet
   c. be alert for signs of gastric irritation
   d. limit the use of coffee, tea, and chocolate

4. Which of the following activities may not be of benefit in helping the patient with COPD to consume more adequate nutrition at mealtime?
   a. eat small meals at frequent intervals
   b. use foods that require minimal preparation
   c. perform bronchial hygiene treatments 10–15 minutes before meals
   d. blend foods that may be difficult to chew

5. Food preparation can be a challenge for the COPD patient. Which of the following suggestions may not be appropriate?
   a. prepare meals immediately before eating to avoid extra trips to the kitchen
   b. use fresh fruits and vegetables
   c. blenderized foods may be easier to eat
   d. arrange for delivery of Meals on Wheels

6. Helping the family deal with the challenges associated with cystic fibrosis is of vital importance. Which of the following suggestions is not appropriate?
   a. eat small meals at frequent intervals
   b. offer food replacement after an episode of vomiting following a severe coughing spell
   c. eat three meals a day to facilitate pancreatic enzyme utilization
   d. introduce new foods gradually to determine the child's tolerance

7. Pancreatic-enzyme supplements are central to the absorption of the necessary nutrients from the foods that are eaten. Which of the following is not appropriate?
   a. mix pancrelipase in the formula to make it easier for the infant to swallow
   b. mix the pancrelipase on fruit or cereal
   c. give the enzyme 30 minutes to one hour before meals and with snacks
   d. sprinkle the enteric-coated spheres on nonprotein food for children who cannot swallow the capsules

8. Vitamin replacement is essential for the child with cystic fibrosis. Which of the following vitamins must be given in a water-soluble form to aid in absorption?
   a. vitamin B-complex
   b. vitamins A, B-complex and C
   c. niacin
   d. vitamins A, D, E, and K

9. Which of the following diets would be best for a child with cystic fibrosis?
   a. high kilocalorie, high protein, low fat
   b. moderate kilocalorie, low protein, low fat
   c. high kilocalorie, high protein, fat as tolerated
   d. moderate kilocalorie, high protein, fat as tolerated

10. Which of the following is not included in the goals for nutritional support of the COPD patient?
   a. maintain a desirable body weight
   b. assess the energy requirements of the body
   c. provide appropriate nutrients to supply metabolic need
   d. limit fluid intake

ACTIVITIES

1. Invite a pharmacist or dietitian to class to discuss the commercial supplements used in the treatment of COPD. The discussion should feature nutrient composition and rationale for the nutrients included. Arrange for a taste-testing if possible.

2. Review protein, fat, and carbohydrate digestion. Explain why individuals with cystic fibrosis have difficulty digesting these nutrients.

3. Mr. Brow has COPD and has been losing weight. The physician tells you that Mr. Brow is suffering from protein-kilocalorie malnutrition. What ideas can you discuss with Mr. Brow to increase the protein and caloric content of his diet?

REFERENCES

1. Petty, T.L. *Chronic obstructive pulmonary disease*, 2d ed. New York: Marcel Dekker, Inc., 1985.
2. Bullock, B.L., and P.O. Rosendahl. *Pathophysiology: adaptations and alterations in function*. 2d ed. Glenview: Scott, Foresman and Company, 1988.
3. McCauley, K., and T.E. Weaver. Cardiac and pulmonary diseases: Nursing implications. *Nursing Clinics of North America* 18(1983):81–96.
4. Fiaccadori, E., et al. Hypercapnic-hypoxemic obstructive pulmonary disease (COPD): Influence of severity of COPD on nutritional status. *American Journal of Clinical Nutrition* 48(1988):680–85.
5. Keim, N.L., et al. Dietary evaluation of patients with chronic obstructive pulmonary disease. *Journal of the American Dietetic Association* 86(1986):902–6.

6. Pingleton, S.K., and G.S. Harmon. Nutritional management in acute respiratory failure. *Journal of the American Medical Association* 257(1987):3094–99.

7. Olin, B.R. *Facts and comparisons. Loose-leaf drug information service.* St. Louis: J.B. Lippincott Company, 1989.

8. Gerson, W.T., P. Swan, and W.A. Walker. Nutrition support in cystic fibrosis. *Nutrition Reviews* 45(1987):353–60.

9. Crapo, J.D., M.A. Hamilton, and S. Edgman. *Medicine and pediatrics in one book.* St. Louis: Hanley Belfus, Inc., The C.V. Mosby Company, 1988.

10. Robinson, C.H., et al. *Normal and therapeutic nutrition.* New York: Macmillan Publishing Company, 1986.

11. Corey, M., et al. *Nutritional support.* Cystic Fibrosis Club Abstract 25–67, 1985.

12. Marcotte, J.E., et al. Effects of nutritional status on exercise performance in advanced cystic fibrosis. *Chest* 90(1987):375–79.

13. Mansell, A.L., et al. Short-terms pulmonary effects of total parenteral nutrition in children with cystic fibrosis. *Journal of Pediatrics* 104(1984):700–705.

14. Luder, E., and J.A. Gilbride. Teaching self-management skills to cystic fibrosis patients and its effect on their caloric intake. *Journal of the American Dietetic Association* 89(1989):359–64.

CHAPTER
12
NUTRITION AND THE PATIENT WITH CANCER

Objectives

After studying this chapter, you will be able to
- describe alterations in metabolism that occur in cancer.
- list the symptoms of cancer and the side effects of its treatment modalities that may have nutritional consequences.
- specify a nutrition plan that increases the protein and kilocalorie content of the diet.
- recognize the advantages and disadvantages of enteral and parenteral feedings.
- explain the dietary guidelines for reducing cancer risk.
- identify nursing interventions for nutritional disorders that may be associated with cancer.

Overview

The term cancer refers to a large group of diseases characterized by abnormal growth and extension of cells. Currently, cancer accounts for approximately 20% of all deaths in the United States each year, exceeded only by coronary heart disease (1). Most cancers have an external cause; that is, they are related to what we eat, drink, and smoke, and where we work or live rather than to genetic factors. In fact, as much as 80% of all cancers may be related to our environment (2).

The most common cancers for men in the United States are lung cancer and prostate cancer. Breast cancer is the most common cancer for women. Colorectal cancer ranks next in incidence for both men and women (3). The effects of cancer may exert a tremendous physical, emotional and financial toll on the patient. The metabolic changes that occur, the side effects of treatment, and often the depression accompanying the disease may create a negative impact on nutritional status. The financial burden may be overwhelming as a result of the possible loss of job and income and the high cost of medical care. Attempts to improve the nutritional status may or may not be successful, depending on the stage of the disease; therefore, goals for nutrition intervention vary with medical-treatment goals.

THE METABOLIC EFFECTS OF CANCER

The deterioration in nutritional status that occurs in cancer superficially resembles starvation; however, derangements in metabolism occur in cancer that are distinct from the mechanisms in starvation.

Metabolism in Starvation

The preferred fuel for cell metabolism is glucose. In the initial stage of a fast, the body calls on stored carbohydrate (glycogen) for energy. Glycogen is converted to glucose and used in the energy-yielding pathways of glycolysis and the Kreb's cycle in the body cells. Glycogen storage in the body is limited, however, and soon other tissues must try to fill the gap left by limited glucose. A compensatory mechanism in the liver called gluconeogenesis is stimulated. Gluconeogenesis is the production of glucose from noncarbohydrate sources. The muscle tissue breaks down protein to amino acids to supply the liver with a source for conversion to glucose. The adipose tissue also responds by catabolizing stored triglyceride into fatty acids. The use of fat for energy entails different metabolic pathways, requiring less oxygen, yielding more energy for cellular reactions, and sparing protein (muscle tissue). The fatty acids follow two pathways. Some are transported directly to peripheral tissues to be used for energy, and others are converted to ketones, which can also be used by many tissues for energy.

If this type of metabolic picture continued, death would occur quickly due to severe muscle wasting and dehydration. The body adapts to starvation, however, and shifts its use of body fuels. Basal metabolism slows, thus reducing energy needs. Gluconeogenesis continues but at a much lower rate so that less protein tissue is catabolized for body needs. Glucose continues to be used by only those cells that cannot use anything else as an energy source (red blood cells, white blood cells, nerve tissue). Even the brain's consumption of glucose declines. Tissues not entirely dependent on glucose shift to the use of fat, either as fatty acids or ketones, for the majority of their energy needs. Although the body can adapt to lack of food for a period of time, starvation ultimately leads to death. (Refer to Chapter 6 for a discussion of physiological stress.) A summary of body fuel use in starvation is pictured in Figures 12-1 and 12-2.

Metabolism in Cancer

In cancer, a failure of the normal homeostatic mechanisms occurs. Cancer patients do not appear to shift from the use of glucose to the use of fat stores for energy needs. Individuals in the advanced stages of cancer exhibit hyperglycemia associated with a marked resistance to insulin (4). It appears that an increase in glucose turnover occurs because the cancer patient is relying heavily on glycolysis for the majority of energy needs. The higher oxidation of glucose increases oxygen consumption in cancer patients, and these patients may exhibit weight loss.

Whole body protein metabolism increases, with a decreased synthesis and increased degradation of muscle tissue to provide the amino acids to the liver for gluconeogenesis (5). Also, the active, growing tumor is a nitrogen trap, stealing nitrogen-rich protein reserves from the host and flourishing despite the wasting occurring in the patient

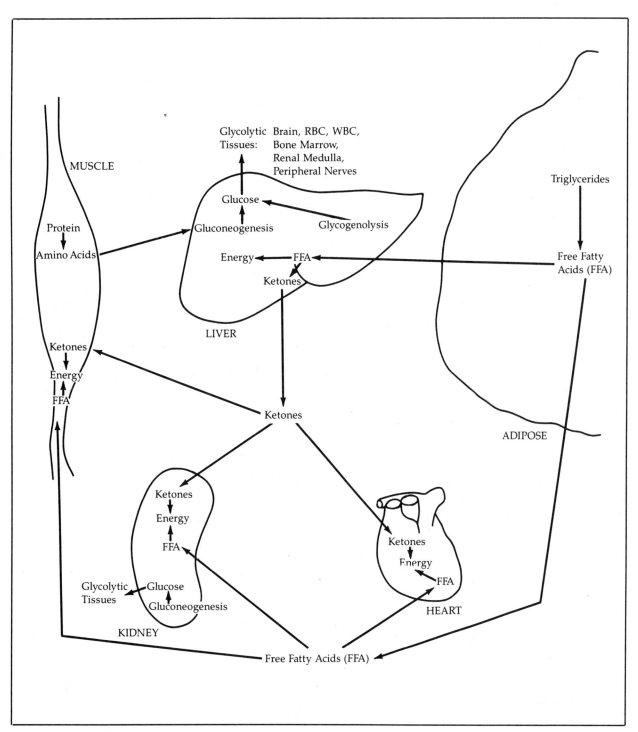

Figure 12-1. Initial stage of starvation.

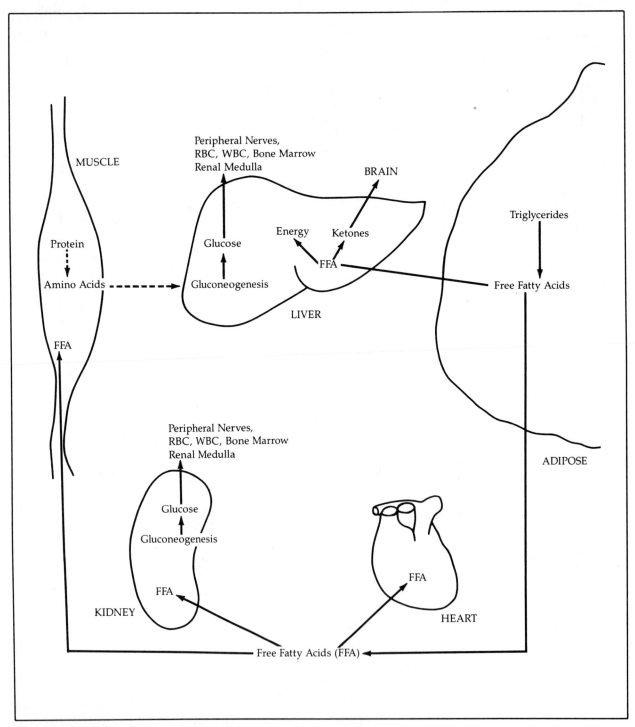

Figure 12-2. Adaptation to starvation.

(4, 6). The increased protein turnover results in higher protein needs of the patient.

Adipose tissue is also catabolized in the cancer patient. The depletion of body fat is a characteristic feature of extreme malnutrition associated with cancer. While an increase in free fatty acids occurs as a result of adipose-tissue catabolism, it does not appear that the fatty acids are used for energy. Thus, to the detriment of the host, glucose continues to be the preferred energy source.

Energy expenditure in individuals with cancer is affected by body size and cell metabolism, nutritional status, degree of starvation, antineoplastic therapy (chemotherapy or irradiation), tumor type, and duration of the disease (6). About half of cancer patients have an abnormal resting energy expenditure. Of these, some have increased caloric requirements, and others have lower than normal metabolic rates. As a result, generalizations about caloric needs are difficult to make, and ongoing nutritional assessment of the patient becomes critical.

ASSESSMENT OF THE PATIENT WITH CANCER

When cancer patients are initially admitted to the hospital or clinic, and throughout their treatment, assessments are made of their nutritional status. Extensive laboratory and clinical measures are completed, because the nutritional status of the individual affects the delivery of antineoplastic therapy. Biochemical parameters, such as pre-albumin, are measured and monitored. A posthydrational serum albumin of less than 3.5 g/dl could be indicative of malnutrition.

Clinical Assessment

Anthropometric measures are used to determine the body fat and lean mass of the individual. Included in the anthropometric assessment are weight and height measurements, triceps skinfold measures, and arm muscle and mid-upper-arm circumference measurements. The procedures for taking the anthropometric measures are discussed in detail in Chapter 15. A dietary assessment is completed to ascertain usual food patterns. A rough estimate of recent caloric and nutrient intake, as well as changes in intake, can be made through the use of dietary recalls and food frequency forms. Information on recent weight changes, food preferences, and food aversions can be obtained through a careful dietary history.

Malnutrition, a frequent complication in cancer, can be caused by a number of factors: metabolic effects of the cancer itself, a mechanical obstruction in the digestive tract, anorexia, mucositis, dysgeusia (taste distortion), nausea and vomiting, diarrhea resulting in malabsorption of nutrients, and food refusal (7). In addition to a serum albumin of less than 3.5 g/dl, two of the following criteria must be satisfied: a recent weight loss of more than 10% of body weight, weight for height less than the 10th percentile, mid-arm circumference less than the 10th percentile, and/or triceps skinfold thickness less than the 10th percentile (8). If malnutrition continues, cachexia can result. Cachexia is a condition of ill health characterized by severe weight loss, wasting of body tissues, and multiple vitamin deficiencies. Cachexia is difficult to halt or reverse once it appears.

MANAGEMENT OF THE PATIENT WITH CANCER

The medical management of patients with cancer includes surgery, chemotherapy, radiation, immunotherapy, or a combination of these treatments. Each of these modalities has side effects. Surgery creates a tremendous physiological stress for the body and affects nutritional needs.

Chemotherapeutic drugs can be administered by mouth, by injection into a muscle, or by infusion into a vein. Rapidly proliferating tissues are most susceptible to the effects of the drugs. Therefore, the drugs not only affect cancer cells, but other cells as well, such as the cells in the mucous linings of the gastrointestinal tract, the skin, hair, and bone marrow. Mouth sores (stomatitis), bleeding gums, nausea and vomiting, constipation, diarrhea, and development of food aversions are often side effects of chemotherapy.

Radiation therapy is administered from a source outside the body or via the insertion of radioactive implants into the body. The side effects of radiation are dependent on the part of the body exposed to radiation. Radiation of the head, neck, and chest can result in mouth soreness, decreased saliva production, and difficulties in swallowing. Taste alterations are also a side effect of radiation to the head and neck. Patients may experience sour, bitter, burning, or metallic tastes in foods, diminished taste sensitivity, or a complete loss of taste (9). Radiation to the abdomen or bowel frequently results in nausea, vomiting, and diarrhea.

Nutrition therapy has an adjunctive role in cancer treatment; that is, it is not part of the cure for cancer, but it often facilitates the full delivery of the primary treatment. Well-nourished individuals usually experience fewer treatment delays, fewer complications from infections, and an increased feeling of well-being (7, 10). The disease itself and the various cancer treatments make the maintenance of good nutritional status a difficult challenge.

Side Effects and Their Management

Stomatitis, Bleeding Gums. Good oral hygiene is required to remove food and bacteria from the mouth, to promote healing of any sores that develop, and to freshen the mouth before meals. Dentures may need to be removed while eating, if gums are irritated. Soft foods are easier to chew and swallow than high-fiber foods. Cold foods may be easier to tolerate than hot foods, which may irritate tender tissues. Citrus fruits and citrus-fruit juices may need to be avoided if they burn or sting the mouth.

Decreased Saliva Production. A decrease in saliva production and difficulties in swallowing can be counteracted through the use of gravies and sauces. Avoidance of high sugar foods is imperative to avoid tooth decay when saliva is decreased. However, for the patient who is terminally ill, it will be necessary to determine whether the increased caloric intake is more critical than preventing dental caries. Tart foods, such as lemonade, can help to stimulate saliva production if stomatitis is not present. Chewing sugar-free gum or sucking on sugarless hard candies can also be helpful. Frequent rinsing of the mouth may help to lubricate and soothe the mucosa.

Taste Alterations. The most common foods for which taste distortion occurs are meats, vegetables, and sweets, especially chocolate (9, 11, 12). If taste sensitivity is diminished, extra seasoning or marinating of food may help encourage intake. When patients are not eating, a discussion of the types of foods that might taste good and provision of these foods are often helpful.

Food Aversions. Food aversions can occur to previously enjoyed foods when they are consumed immediately prior to chemotherapy (7). Careful monitoring of intake prior to chemotherapy may help to provide suggestions to patients on what to eat. Also, it is best for the patient to avoid a favorite food immediately before chemotherapy treatment to decrease the risk of developing an aversion to that food.

Nausea and Vomiting. Nausea and vomiting may be a problem for some patients who are undergoing treatment with chemotherapy or irradiation. In order to avoid nausea and vomiting, the cancer patient may want to limit fluid intake at mealtime. Fluids may be taken between meals to avoid fullness in the stomach and pressure on the diaphragm. Small, frequent meals containing high-carbohydrate, low-fat foods, such as fruits, breads, saltines, noodles, rice, jams and jellies, and fruit ices, may be easier to tolerate than large meals served less frequently. (Refer to Chapter 7 for additional information and suggestions for controlling nausea and vomiting.) If nausea continues to be a problem despite the conservative measures, it may be necessary to obtain an order for an antiemetic drug such as promethazine (Phenergan) from the physician.

Constipation. Constipation, which may be precipitated by the drug therapy, the disease process itself, or the consumption of soft or liquid foods, can be counteracted by increasing fluid and fiber intake. (See Chapter 7 for a discussion of constipation.)

Diarrhea. The cancer patient may suffer from diarrhea due to an alteration in the ability to digest and eliminate foods. Diarrhea is treated by lowering the fiber content of the diet. In addition, the patient may have to avoid lactose-containing foods if radiation to the bowel caused a temporary lack of the enzyme lactase, which is needed to digest lactose (see Chapter 7). Lactose-containing foods include milk and milk products. Fermented milk products, such as cheese and yogurt, may or may not be tolerated, depending on the degree of lactose intolerance. Liquids should be encouraged to avoid dehydration. Potassium levels need to be monitored as well, since diarrhea can result in high potassium losses. Foods high in potassium, such as canned or fresh fruits (bananas) and cooked vegetables, can be offered. (Sources of potassium are listed in Chapter 9.) If the patient is unable to ingest adequate amounts of potassium-rich foods, a supplement may need to be prescribed by the physician. (A detailed discussion of diarrhea is included in Chapter 7.)

Weight Loss. Protein and kilocalorie needs may be increased as a result of the metabolic changes that occur with cancer. Cancer treatment can also cause increased needs. The side effects of chemotherapy can result in weight loss; therefore, maintenance of good nutritional status by increasing kilocalorie and protein intake before and between treatments is critical. The physical stress caused by radiation and surgery also increase kilocalorie and protein needs (see Chapter 6). One recommendation for weight maintenance is to provide 115%–130% of the kilocalories needed for resting energy expenditure. Kilocalories as high as 150% of resting expenditure may be required to increase weight (6).

Suggestions for increasing the kilocalorie and protein content of the diet include the following:

- Add cheese to sauces, casseroles, and vegetables, or use cheeses as a topping for sandwiches.
- Add nonfat dry milk to liquid milk for a high-protein drink.
- Use milk instead of water when making cooked cereals and hot cocoa.

- Offer nutritious snacks, such as cheese, peanut butter and crackers, milkshakes, commercial enteral supplements (such as Ensure or Enrich), yogurt, puddings, custards, and nuts, to increase intake.
- Use peanut butter on toast instead of butter to increase protein. The peanut butter in combination with the bread makes a complete protein.
- To increase intake without excessive volume, offer one of the numerous commercial liquid supplements that are available. These are high in kilocalories, protein, vitamins, and minerals.

Special Considerations

Surgery. A cancer patient going into surgery should have a good nutritional status. A high-protein, high-kilocalorie diet prior to surgery can help if the patient has experienced weight loss. Postoperatively, the first priority is for replacement of body fluids via intravenous therapy. When nourishment by mouth is permitted, a progression from clear liquids to full liquids to a soft diet, and finally, to a regular diet is usually followed. (See Chapter 7.)

Enteral Nutrition. Enteral nutrition is considered to be an aggressive nutritional therapy. When a patient is unable to eat or cannot consume adequate kilocalories, tube feedings are sometimes initiated. In enteral feedings, a tube is inserted through the nose to the stomach (nasogastric) or jejunum (nasojejunal), or through an opening directly into the pharynx (pharyngostomy), esophagus (esophagostomy), stomach (gastrostomy), or jejunum (jejunostomy) (8). The route of entry is often dictated by the problems patients have. No matter where the tube is inserted, the common factor for all enteral feedings is the use of the digestive tract.

Numerous enteral preparations (commercial products) are available from pharmaceutical manufacturers (see Appendix E), since few hospitals continue to make tube feeding mixtures. Commercial tube feedings provide carbohydrate, protein, fat, and 100% of the U.S. RDA for vitamins and minerals. Carbohydrate in the formulas is usually corn syrup, sugar, maltodextrin, hydrolyzed corn starch or a combination of these sources. Fat is in the form of corn or soy oil, or medium-chain triglycerides, and protein can be in the form of calcium and/or sodium caseinates, soy protein isolate or egg albumin in regular formulas. In elemental formulas, the protein is supplied via peptides and amino acids.

Before instituting a tube feeding, an assessment of benefits versus risks is essential. (See Table 12-1.) In addition to the complications listed in Table 12-1, a number of researchers have questioned the interaction between the composition of some of the enteral feedings and cancer treatment. Elemental enteral feedings were thought to provide advantages over other enteral formulas because of the readily usable nutrient sources. Unfortunately, it has been shown in experimental animals that elemental tube feedings increase the toxicity of chemotherapeutic drugs (13).

Total Parenteral Nutrition (TPN). Total parenteral nutrition, another aggressive nutrition therapy, is nutrition provided directly to the bloodstream and is used when feedings cannot be given through the gastrointestinal tract. The central catheter may be inserted into the superior vena cava by way of the internal jugular or subclavian veins. Many patients who are debilitated require numerous peripheral venous infusions so that a central line may be the most reliable for nutritional support. Peripheral parenteral nutrition (PPN) may be used for those persons who are less debilitated and may receive nutrients via other routes, including oral (8, 14). Originally, TPN was considered to be the answer to alleviating or preventing malnutrition, and improving the outcome of patients receiving curative surgery, radiation therapy, or chemotherapy, but it has not quite reached expectations.

In patients receiving chemotherapy, TPN may have a positive or negative effect or no effect on nutritional status and response to treatment. The general feeling is that TPN should not be administered on a routine basis to provide nutritional support for patients undergoing chemotherapy, in

order to reduce the side effects of the treatment or to minimize weight loss. Total parenteral nutrition is recommended only for patients who have lost a significant amount of weight and who cannot regain weight by normal use of the gastrointestinal tract (15). One advantage of TPN is that it can be tailored to the needs of the individual patient. Some positive benefits of TPN have been observed in cancer patients undergoing surgery and radiation therapy, but because the studies involved small numbers of patients, no generalizations are possible.

Complications of TPN can include infection, fluid and electrolyte imbalance, metabolic disturbances such as cholelithiasis, bone disorders such as osteomalacia (softening of the bones), or hypo- or hyperglycemia. Infection may be a problem due to phlebitis or the introduction of microorganisms at the insertion site, or through contamination of the hypertonic glucose solution that provides an ideal medium for microbial growth. Solutions should be stored in the refrigerator until they are used. The container should be dated with an indication of the time the infusion was begun. Solutions should not hang at room temperature for longer than 12 hours (14). Patients who undergo TPN are particularly prone to sepsis. Additional problems related to TPN include hemothorax (blood in the pleural cavity), pneumothorax (air in the pleural cavity), venous puncture and hemorrhage, thrombosis (blood clots), or fatal air embolism (14, 16, 17). Clearly, a careful assessment of risks versus benefits is required before instituting TPN.

Home Parenteral Nutrition (HPN). The use of HPN for the cancer patient is controversial. It is used only after dietary modification, enteral supplementation, and antidiarrheal agents prove unsuccessful (18). HPN is the use of total parenteral nutrition in the home setting. HPN carries similar risks to hospital TPN and requires extensive patient and family training. Home nursing supervision is essential for the patient on HPN.

The aggressive nutritional therapies described may or may not be useful adjuncts to the active treatment of cancer. Usefulness depends on assessment of the patient, the goals of treatment, and other nutritional therapies tried. While aggressive nutrition intervention may have a place in active cancer treatment, health professionals do not agree on its role in the treatment of terminal cancer patients.

Table 12-1. INDICATIONS FOR USE AND POSSIBLE COMPLICATIONS OF ENTERAL FEEDINGS

ENTRY	INDICATIONS FOR USE	POSSIBLE COMPLICATIONS
Nasogastric	Preferred route when needed for only short periods of time. Can be used to supplement oral feeding, providing increased nutrients. Useful when oral feeding is impossible due to ulceration, bleeding, presence of a tumor, or as a result of surgery, radiation or chemotherapy.	Subjective distress, rhinitis, sinusitis, mucosal injury, fluid overload, electrolyte imbalance, hyperglycemia, bloating, diarrhea, aspiration, nasopharyngeal stenosis when use is prolonged.
Nasojejunal	Used when gastric outputs are high.	See above.
Pharyngostomy/ Esophagostomy	Used when nasal route is contraindicated. Used when necessary for prolonged periods.	Soft tissue irritation, pulmonary aspiration, carotid artery erosion.
Gastrostomy	Used in advanced but stable cancer.	Gastric leakage, resulting in peritonitis.
Jejunostomy	Used in the absence of a stomach, or in the case of an obstruction.	Incomplete digestion, malabsorption, leakage, small-bowel fistulization, small-bowel obstruction, jejunal varices.

Sources:

M.M. Meguid, S. Eldar, and A. Wahba, "The Delivery of Nutritional Support. A Potpourri of New Devices and Methods," *Cancer* 55 (1985):279–89.

C. Arnold, "Nutrition Intervention in the Terminally Ill Cancer Patient." *Journal of the American Dietetic Association* 86 (1986):522–23.

B.E. Hearne, et al., "Enteral Nutrition Support in Head and Neck Cancer: Tube vs. Oral Feeding During Radiation Therapy," *Journal of the American Dietetic Association* 85 (1985):669–77.

Nutrition and the Terminally Ill
Cancer Patient

The definition of terminal varies, but a reasonable recent definition is a life expectancy of three months or less for a patient who is not receiving curative treatment (19). The goal of nutrition support for the terminal patient is to provide comfort. Dietary modifications (pureed foods, soft foods) should be made to accommodate the patient's capabilities. Commercial enteral supplements may also be prescribed. Patients should be encouraged to eat and/or drink whatever they can. If symptoms of the disease, such as pain, nausea, and/or depression, are adversely affecting intake, medications can be prescribed by the physician to control the symptoms. TPN or enteral feedings are to be considered only if such aggressive intervention helps maintain or improve the quality of life but not necessarily prolong the agony of dying (20).

POSSIBLE NURSING DIAGNOSES

Possible alterations in oral mucous membrane related to
- altered nutritional/fluid intake.
- treatment modalities: chemotherapy and radiation.
- inadequate oral hygiene.

Potential alteration in nutrition; less than body requirements related to
- nausea and vomiting.
- anorexia.
- disease process.
- treatment modalities.

Potential alteration in bowel elimination; diarrhea related to
- disease process.
- treatment modalities.

Potential fluid-volume deficit related to
- nausea and vomiting.
- diarrhea.

- inability to ingest fluids.
- lack of desire for fluids.

Potential alteration in bowel elimination; constipation related to
- dietary intake, lack of fiber, consistency of food.
- treatment modalities.
- disease process.

Potential alteration in skin integrity related to altered nutritional status.

Knowledge deficit related to
- disease process.
- treatment modalities and their relationship to nutritional status.

NURSING INTERVENTIONS FOR NUTRITIONAL DISORDERS

Work closely with the patient and family and the dietitian and physician to develop and implement a diet plan that will help to reverse the catabolic effects of cancer.

Possible alterations in oral mucous membrane related to
- **altered nutritional/fluid intake.**
- **treatment modalities: chemotherapy and radiation.**
- **inadequate oral hygiene.**

- Administer analgesic or antiemetic medication at least 30 minutes prior to mealtime, if prescribed.
- Advise patients to avoid extreme temperatures; offer cool or room-temperature foods and fluids if the oral cavity is sensitive.
- Be aware that patients who use viscous xylocaine to relieve pain in the mouth may refuse to continue the use of the medication because of its unpleasant taste.

Potential alteration in nutrition; less than body requirements related to
- **nausea and vomiting.**
- **anorexia.**
- **disease process.**
- **treatment modalities.**
- Encourage frequent oral hygiene.
- Make the mealtime enjoyable, visually as well as socially.
- Encourage fluid intake between meals to reduce gastric distention and prevent nausea and vomiting.
- Obtain an order for an alcoholic beverage, such as wine, to stimulate the appetite, if the patient desires and if it is not contraindicated by other treatment modalities.
- Encourage relatives and friends to bring favorite foods to entice the patient to eat.
- Understand that loss of taste may cause food rejection.
- Be aware that breakfast may be the best meal of the day.

Potential alteration in bowel elimination; diarrhea related to
- **disease process.**
- **treatment modalities.**

- Monitor fluid intake and output.
- Monitor laboratory reports; note alterations in electrolytes.
- Instruct the patient to:
    avoid fatty foods;

    drink fluids between meals;

    avoid high fiber foods.

Potential fluid-volume deficit related to
- **nausea and vomiting.**
- **diarrhea.**
- **inability to ingest fluids.**
- **lack of desire for fluids.**

- Monitor fluid intake and output.
- Offer a variety of fluids at frequent intervals.
- Remember that juices can be frozen into cubes or slush and may be more readily acceptable.

Potential alteration in bowel elimination; constipation related to
- **dietary intake, lack of fiber, consistency of food.**

Continued

NURSING INTERVENTIONS (continued)

- **treatment modalities.**
- **disease process.**

- Instruct the patient to:
  increase fluid intake;

  eat foods that are high in fiber content;

  add one to two tablespoons of bran to foods such as casseroles or cooked cereals;

  add grated, raw foods to the diet if chewing is difficult.

Potential alteration in skin integrity related to altered nutritional status.

- Monitor laboratory reports; note albumin levels to detect potential problems with skin breakdown.
- Encourage and increase protein intake in the diet.

Knowledge deficit related to
- **disease process.**
- **treatment modalities and their relationship to nutritional status.**

- Instruct persons regarding risk factors and measures that may be helpful in preventing the development of cancer.
- Instruct the patient to:
  eat a balanced diet to maintain strength and prevent infection;

  increase the amount of protein and kilocalories in the diet to offset the effects of the various treatment modalities: chemotherapy, radiation, and/or surgery;

  weigh himself two times per week and keep a record;

  eat smaller meals more frequently;

  avoid eating favorite foods before chemotherapy or irradiation, when prone to nausea; an aversion to those foods may develop;

  eat nutritious snacks and keep these close at hand at all times;

  avoid tart or citrus foods if stomatitis is present;

  avoid highly spiced foods if stomatitis is present;

  limit greasy or fried foods, which may stimulate nausea;

  allow other people to prepare the meals if the aroma of food stimulates nausea;

  choose soft or blended foods if swallowing is difficult;

  supplement diet as prescribed by the physician and determined by weight loss;

  rinse mouth before and after eating;

  chew sugarless gum or suck on sugarless hard candies to increase salivation;

  be aware that taste may be altered due to treatment modalities and/or the extent of the disease process;

  chew all foods well to extract flavors, and vary the intake of different food to enhance the perception of a variety of flavors.

TOPIC OF INTEREST

Research continues to determine ways to prevent cancer as well as identify risk factors that predispose to the development of cancer. In 1982, the Committee on Diet, Nutrition and Cancer of the National Research Council released a set of dietary guidelines for reducing the risk of cancer (1). The Committee indicated that the National Cancer Institute should review the guidelines on a regular basis (21).

The American Cancer Society has outlined the dietary and environmental factors that may be helpful in reducing the risk of cancer. (See Table 12-2 for a summary of these factors.)

Other work on factors that contribute to cancer risk indicates that while the mechanisms are unknown, obesity contributes to the development of breast and endometrial cancer in postmenopausal females and colon and prostate cancer in

Table 12-2. FACTORS FOR REDUCED CANCER RISK

PROTECTIVE FACTORS
Eat more cruciferous vegetables.[1]
Eat more high-fiber foods.
Eat foods rich in Vitamins A and C.
Prevent obesity by increasing exercise and lowering caloric intake.
RISK FACTORS
Limit fat consumption.
Minimize salt-cured, smoked, nitrite-cured foods.[2]
Stop smoking.
Moderate alcohol intake.
Limit expsoure to the sun's rays.
Limit exposure to x-rays, estrogens, harmful chemicals.

(Adapted with permission from "Taking Control. 10 Steps to a Healthier Life and Reduced Cancer Risk," The American Cancer Society, 1985.)

[1]Cruciferous vegetables are named for their cross-shaped blossoms. They include cauliflower, cabbage, brussels sprouts, broccoli, turnips, rutabagas.

[2]In some parts of the world (China, Japan, Iceland), salt-cured and smoked foods increase cancer of the esophagus and stomach.

males (22). Some researchers have gone so far as to claim that the key to the relationship between obesity and cancer is not the fat in the diet, suggested by interim guideline number one, but the balance among energy consumption, retention, and expenditure (23). Supporting this theory are the studies that show a decreased cancer risk associated with physical exercise (24), and a prospective study showing no substantial reduction in the incidence of breast cancer when fat was moderately restricted (25). Finally, though only demonstrated so far in rats and mice, omega-3 fatty acids seem to exert an anticarcinogenic effect through disturbance of prostaglandin synthesis (26). These types of studies will need to be examined carefully when the dietary guidance for reducing cancer risk is reviewed.

Cancer development is a result of environmental and genetic factors. Alterations in life-style can help reduce the risk of developing cancer. Early detection is of prime importance and is under an individual's control. Cancer treatment has progressed considerably, and the cure rate is increasing. Nutritional support is critical to ensure the full benefits of treatment and to combat side effects.

SPOTLIGHT ON LEARNING

A terminally ill cancer patient under your care is thinking of trying a macrobiotic diet to cure her cancer. She asks what your view is.

Macrobiotic diets emphasize grains and beans, and sometimes include fruit and salads. Animal and dairy products are eliminated. The diets are typically high in volume and low in kilocalories, thus making it highly unlikely that the diet will meet the nutritional needs of the patient with cancer.

Questionable dietary therapies for cancer are often used when patients are unhappy with their treatment and feel as though they lack control in their treatment. Often, the problem can be traced to lack of communication with their care takers. Many times (especially in the case of terminally ill patients), family members exert pressure to try an alternative therapy in the hopes that the cancer will be cured.

1. What is your view of macrobiotic diets and why?
2. What types of things can you do to help the patient feel more in control?
3. How can you improve the communication between the patient and the hospital staff?

REVIEW QUESTIONS

1. From which of the following do most body tissues satisfy their energy needs once they adapt to starvation?
   a. amino acids
   b. fat
   c. glycogen
   d. glucose

2. Cancer causes a failure of the normal homeostatic mechanisms, and the preferential fuel source becomes which of the following?
   a. amino acids
   b. fatty acids
   c. ketones
   d. glucose

3. Which of the following is not included in the criteria for malnutrition?
   a. serum albumin less than 3.5 g/dl
   b. recent weight loss of greater than 10% of body weight
   c. triceps skinfold thickness less than the 10th percentile
   d. nausea and vomiting

4. Which is not a side effect of cancer treatment?
   a. mouth sores
   b. diarrhea
   c. constipation
   d. increased appetite

5. Which of the following will not help in managing nausea?
   a. avoiding liquids at meals
   b. eating high-carbohydrate, low-fat foods
   c. extra seasoning of food
   d. eating salty foods, avoiding overly sweet foods

6. Which of the following is not a food included on a clear liquid diet?
   a. apple juice
   b. gingerale
   c. gelatin
   d. vegetable juice

7. Which of the following would not increase protein and kilocalorie intake?
   a. using jellies and jams instead of butter on toast
   b. mixing nonfat dry milk into liquid milk
   c. using milk instead of water in cooked cereals
   d. offering a commercial liquid supplement

8. Enteral nutrition involves use of which of the following?
   a. the digestive tract
   b. the subclavian vein
   c. the jugular vein
   d. the deep brachial vein

9. What is the goal of nutrition support for terminally ill cancer patients?
   a. to rebuild body tissues
   b. to provide comfort
   c. to cure the cancer
   d. to counteract the effects of curative treatment

10. Which of the following does the American Cancer Society recommend for reducing cancer risk?
    a. decrease total consumption of fiber-containing foods
    b. increase kilocalorie consumption to build immunity
    c. increase use of supplements providing vitamins A and C
    d. use alcohol in moderation

ACTIVITIES

1. Review the dietary guidelines for reducing cancer risk. List the types of changes that would be required in your diet to follow the guidelines. Decide on one change and try to incorporate it for at least a week. Describe the obstacles faced and the success encountered in changing your diet.

2. Change the following menu to increase the kilocalorie, protein, and fiber content.

Breakfast
Fruit juice
Toast with butter and jelly
Coffee
Milk

Lunch
Chicken broth
Roast-beef sandwich
Cherry-flavored gelatin with canned fruit
Milk

Dinner
Baked chicken breast
Carrots
Baked potato with butter
Ice cream
Tea

3. Contact a representative from a pharmaceutical company or a local dietitian to explain the different types of supplemental and enteral feedings available. Arrange a tasting session and rate the feedings on taste appeal.

4. Go to a local supermarket and list the high-fiber products you can find. If possible, have a tasting session of some of the products.

5. Interview a nurse involved in the treatment of terminally ill cancer patients to discuss the approach to care used at his or her facility. If a number of facilities are in the vicinity, compare approaches.

REFERENCES

1. Committee on Diet, Nutrition and Cancer, Assembly of Life Sciences, National Research Council. *Diet, nutrition and cancer.* Washington, D.C.: National Academy Press, 1982.
2. U.S. Department of Health and Human Services, Public Health Service, National Institutes of Health. *Diet, nutrition and cancer prevention: A guide to food choices.* NIH Publication No. 85-2711, 1984.
3. American Cancer Society. *Cancer Facts and Figures—1987.* New York: American Cancer Society, 1987.
4. Heber, D., et al. Malnutrition and cancer: Mechanisms and therapy. Part 1. *Nutrition International* 2 (1986):184–87.
5. Dickerson, J.W.T. Nutrition in the cancer patient: A review. *Journal of the Royal Society of Medicine* 77 (1984):309–15.
6. Dempsy, D.T., and J.L. Mullen. Macronutrient requirements in the malnourished cancer patient: How much of what and why? *Cancer* 55 (1985):290–94.
7. Sherry, M.E.G., S.N. Aker, and C.L. Cheney. Nutrition assessment and management of the pediatric cancer patient. *Topics in Clinical Nutrition* 2 (1987):38–48.
8. Meguid, M.M., S. Eldar, and A. Wahba. The delivery of nutritional support. A potpourri of new devices and methods. *Cancer* 55 (1985):279–89.
9. Mattes, R.D. Effects of health disorders and poor nutritional status on gustatory function. *Journal of Sensory Studies* 1 (1986).275–90.
10. Carter, P., et al. Energy and nutrient intake of children with cancer. *Journal of the American Dietetic Association* 82 (1983):610–15.
11. Markley, E.J., D.A. Mattes-Kulig, and R.I. Henkin. A classification of dysgeusia. *Journal of the American Dietetic Association* 83 (1983):578–80.
12. U.S. Department of Health and Human Services, Public Health Service, National Institutes of Health. *Eating hints: Recipes and tips for better nutrition during cancer treatment.* NIH Publication No. 83-2079, 1983.
13. ———. Interaction of elemental diets and chemotherapeutic agents. *Nutrition Reviews* 46 (1988):24–25.
14. Robinson, C.H., et al. *Normal and therapeutic nutrition.* New York: Macmillan Publishing Company, 1986.

15. Darbinian, J.A., and A.M. Coulston. Parenteral nutrition in cancer therapy: A useful adjunct? *Journal of the American Dietetic Association* 82 (1983):493–500.

16. Klein, G.L., and D. Rivera. Adverse metabolic consequences of total parenteral nutrition. *Cancer* 55 (1985):305–8.

17. Shils, M.E., and V.R. Young, eds. *Modern nutrition in health and disease.* 7th ed. Philadelphia: Lea and Febiger, 1988.

18. Marein, C., et al. Home parental nutrition. *Nutrition in Clinical Practice* 1 (1986):179–92.

19. Arnold, C. Nutrition intervention in the terminally ill cancer patient. *Journal of the American Dietetic Association* 86 (1986):522–23.

20. Wade, E.V., and R. Jain. Nutritional support: Enhancing the quality of life of the terminally ill patient with cancer. *Journal of the American Dietetic Association* 84 (1984):1044–45.

21. Cleveland, L.E., and A.B. Pfeffer. Planning diets to meet the National Research Council's guidelines for reducing cancer risk. *Journal of the American Dietetic Association* 87 (1987):162–68.

22. Simopoulos, A.P. Obesity and carcinogenesis: Historical perspective. *American Journal of Clinical Nutrition* 45 (1987):271–76.

23. Pariza, M.W. Dietary fat, kilocalorie restriction, ad libitum feeding and cancer risk. *Nutrition Reviews* 45 (1987):1–7.

24. Frisch, R.E., et al. Lower lifetime occurrence of breast cancer and cancers of the reproductive system among former college athletes. *American Journal of Clinical Nutrition* 45 (1987):328–35.

25. Willett, W.C., et al. Dietary fat and the risk of breast cancer. *New England Journal of Medicine* 316 (1987):22–28.

26. Karmali, R.A., J. Marsh, and C. Fuchs. Effect of omega-3 fatty acids on growth of a rat mammary tumor. *Journal of the National Cancer Institute* 73 (1984):457–61.

CHAPTER
13

NUTRITION AND THE PATIENT WITH DIABETES MELLITUS

Objectives

After studying this chapter, you will be able to
- classify the major types of diabetes mellitus.
- describe the consequences of insufficient and total lack of insulin.
- identify the altered metabolic pattern that occurs in a patient with diabetes.
- explain the nutritional assessment of a patient with diabetes.
- discuss the importance of the role of diet in the treatment of diabetes.
- describe the effects of exercise on dietary requirements and insulin utilization.
- discuss the various dietary patterns required according to the type of insulin that is prescribed.
- discuss the effects of oral hypoglycemic agents on the dietary pattern.
- identify the nursing interventions for nutritional disorders associated with diabetes mellitus.

Overview

Diabetes mellitus is a complex, chronic syndrome characterized by altered metabolism of carbohydrate, protein, and fat. The classic sign, hyperglycemia, is due to either a deficient secretion of insulin by the beta cells of the pancreas or a nonutilization of insulin by the cells of the body. Diabetes is estimated to affect approximately 11 million people in the United States (1). Total rates increase with age, and approximately one-half million new cases are diagnosed each year.

CLASSIFICATION OF DIABETES MELLITUS

The National Institutes of Health, in 1979, outlined a classification system for diabetes that is based on a therapeutic rather than a pathophysiological classification. This new classification system, which has also been endorsed by the American Diabetes Association, categorizes diabetes mellitus as follows (2):

- Type I, insulin-dependent diabetes mellitus (IDDM)
- Type II, noninsulin-dependent diabetes mellitus (NIDDM)
- Diabetes mellitus associated with other conditions
- Impaired glucose tolerance (IGT)
- Gestational diabetes mellitus

Type I and Type II diabetes mellitus are different disorders but share a common factor, alteration in or utilization of endogenous insulin.

Insulin-dependent diabetes mellitus, which is an irreversible disease, seems to occur in younger persons (under age 40). The insulin deficiency is due to pancreatic beta-cell destruction that may be immunologically mediated and may also be related to an infectious or toxic environmental agent in a person who is genetically sensitive (3). Persons with IDDM are prone to ketosis (accumulation of waste products of fat breakdown due to inadequate carbohydrate metabolism). Since the beta cells do not produce insulin, insulin must be provided.

Approximately 90% of the cases of diabetes in the United States are classified as NIDDM (4). Noninsulin-dependent diabetes mellitus occurs most frequently in adults over the age of 40, and individuals who have this disease are resistant to ketosis. Genetic predisposition plus environmental factors such as the urban life-style, including lack of exercise, appear to be responsible for the development of NIDDM. The degree, duration, and distribution of excess body fat is a significant environmental factor. In the United States, more than 80% of NIDDM patients have excess body fat (5).

Strong evidence indicates that individuals who are 20%–30% overweight are at an increased risk for developing NIDDM, and that risk rises with increasing weight. Upper body (android) obesity seems to have a stronger association with NIDDM than lower body (gynoid) obesity (5).

Diabetes mellitus that may be associated with other disease conditions and syndromes is directly related to the primary condition, such as pancreatic or hormonal disorders, or drug or chemical toxicity. The fourth category, impaired glucose tolerance, includes persons who manifest an abnormal glucose level somewhere between the normal and the diabetic plasma glucose level. It is not known whether these cases will progress to overt diabetes. The nurse must be aware of the importance of counseling persons with IGT to have repeat blood glucose screenings and seek medical attention when symptoms become apparent.

Gestational diabetes mellitus is glucose intolerance that occurs during pregnancy. Special care must be taken with these patients due to the increased risk of perinatal mortality and complications during pregnancy.

OVERVIEW OF INSULIN ACTION IN NORMAL METABOLISM

Insulin is a hormone that is synthesized in and secreted from the beta cells in the islets of Langerhans. Release of insulin is a constant process; i.e., there is a basal level of circulating insulin always maintained in order to control levels of glucose in the bloodstream. The normal range of blood glucose is 70–120 mg/dl. An increase in insulin secretion occurs when food is eaten, because the digestion of food provides the availability of substrate (glucose, fatty acids, and amino acids) needed for cell metabolism and tissue synthesis. As shown in Figure 13-1, insulin is essential in some tissues for the uptake and use of glucose for energy. An anabolic (building) hormone, insulin promotes lipogenesis, proteogenesis, and glycogenesis. Insulin also inhibits the catabolic hor-

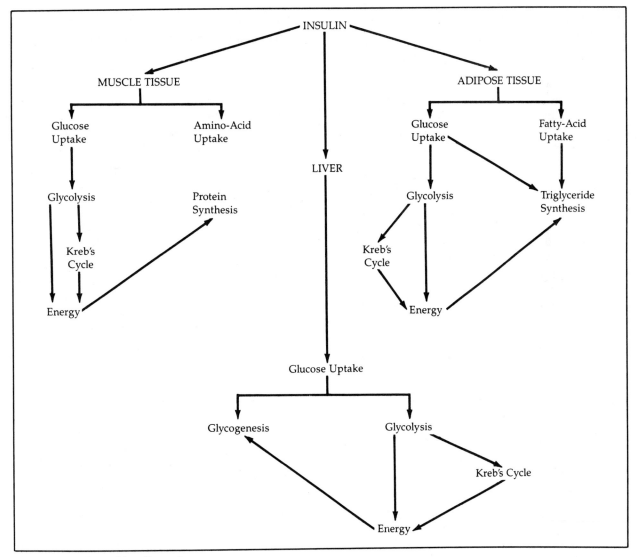

Figure 13-1. Normal insulin action.

mones (glucagon, epinephrine, cortisol, and growth hormone) and therefore prevents the breakdown of muscle tissue, adipose tissue, and glycogen. Insulin-dependent tissues, or those that require insulin for the metabolism of glucose, are the skeletal muscle and adipose tissue. The red blood cells, the brain, and the liver are dependent on an adequate glucose supply but are not directly dependent on insulin for glucose transport. The metabolic disturbances that occur in diabetes are a result of the effect of insulin deficiency on the major insulin-dependent tissues: skeletal muscle and adipose tissue.

DISTURBANCES IN GLUCOSE METABOLISM: HYPERGLYCEMIA

With a deficiency or lack of insulin, the transport of glucose from the bloodstream and into the cells of insulin-dependent tissues is impaired. Glucose circulates in the blood but cannot enter the cells to be used for energy. Therefore, these tissues react as though no glucose is available, despite increased blood glucose levels. Without insulin to inhibit breakdown of muscle and adipose tissue, catabolism occurs (Figure 13-2).

The cellular need for glucose continues, since glucose is the preferential source of energy. Com-

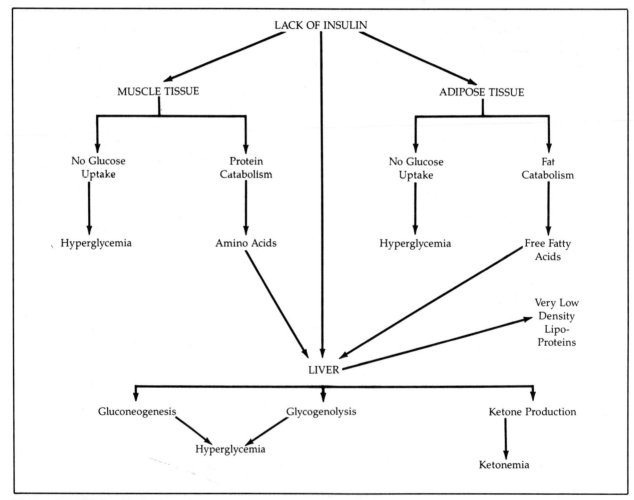

Figure 13-2. Effect of lack of insulin.

pensatory mechanisms (gluconeogenesis and glycogenolysis) triggered in the liver attempt to meet the need for cellular glucose. Gluconeogenesis is the formation of glucose from noncarbohydrate sources, e.g., amino acids derived from muscle catabolism and glycerol from fat metabolism. Glycogenolysis is the breakdown of glycogen into glucose. Because glycogen storage in the body is limited, gluconeogenesis is the major source of glucose production. The infusion of glucose into the bloodstream combined with the failure of cellular uptake of glucose due to a lack of insulin, results in elevated serum glucose or hyperglycemia.

Glucose that remains in the bloodstream produces an osmotic effect on both interstitial and intracellular fluids. The resulting fluid shifts give rise to the classic symptoms polyuria (increased urination) and polydipsia (increased thirst). Polyphagia (increased appetite) associated with weight loss occurs as a result of the breakdown of muscle and adipose tissue for energy.

With continued gluconeogenesis, muscle wasting results. In the adipose tissue, enhanced lipolysis occurs from the absence of insulin and the need for an energy source other than glucose. Fatty-acid levels rise in the blood and are picked up by the liver and peripheral tissues to be oxidized or synthesized into lipids. The increased amount of free fatty acids entering the liver has two main effects. Some of the free fatty acids are converted into triglycerides, which are released into the blood as VLDL. The liver also oxidizes large quantities of free fatty acids for energy, and an excessive formation of ketone bodies results. When hepatic production of ketone bodies exceeds the capacity of the peripheral tissues to use them as an energy substrate, ketonemia (elevated ketones in the blood) follows. (See Figure 13-3.)

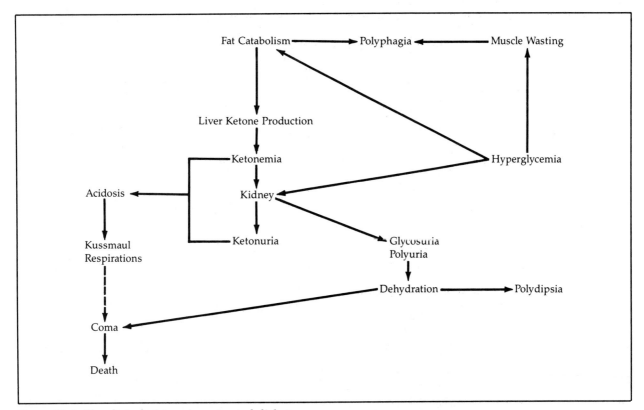

Figure 13-3. The clinical picture in untreated diabetes.

In Type II diabetes, obesity is commonly part of the clinical picture. The state of obesity itself results in metabolic alterations that contribute to the development of NIDDM in susceptible individuals. These include an increased insulin secretion, a decreased insulin sensitivity (or increased insulin resistance), and an increase in serum triglycerides and free-fatty-acid turnover (4). During the development of obesity, insulin production and secretion increases to accommodate the increased number of kilocalories ingested. The increased secretion of insulin can exhaust the pancreas (6). Even with higher circulating levels of insulin, hyperglycemia continues because the cells become insulin resistant. The insulin receptors are degraded faster than they are synthesized resulting in fewer insulin receptors on the cell surface to which the hormone can bind and exert its action. Therefore, glucose cannot enter the cells and remains circulating in the blood at high levels.

Laboratory Assessment

Elevated blood glucose (hyperglycemia) is a characteristic finding in diabetes. In Table 13-1, the normal values for plasma glucose and the criteria for classifying adults and children as having diabetes or IGT are listed.

Glucose monitoring is essential for determining the levels of circulating glucose. Fasting blood sugar, postprandial (two hours following meals) blood sugars, and glucose-tolerance tests are routinely performed.

Because the level of blood glucose is higher than normal, more glucose is present in the kidney tubular filtrate. The glucose exceeds the amount that can be reabsorbed from the kidney tubule and is excreted in the urine. Urinalysis may help to note the presence of glucose and ketone bodies in the urine. Urine testing for glucose on a routine basis has largely been replaced by the use of capillary-glucose monitoring. Routine measurement of ketone bodies in the urine is a valuable tool in detecting possible diabetic ketoacidosis (DKA) in individuals with Type I diabetes.

Self-glucose monitoring involves the measurement of capillary blood glucose levels. This method does not require the presence of a laboratory to give the report of the blood test. Portable, battery-operated scanners, such as Glucometer (Ames Company) and Glucoscan (Lifescan, Inc.), can measure the blood glucose levels when capillary blood is applied to a glucose oxidase paper strip such as Dextrostix or Visidex.

Glycosylated hemoglobin (hemoglobin A_{1C}) is a new diagnostic tool that reflects the concentration of glucose in the red blood cells during their life span (approximately 120 days). Hemoglobin A_{1C} is formed during periods of hyperglycemia, when the glucose molecules attach themselves to hemoglobin. This is a valuable detection tool in the diagnosis of diabetes mellitus.

Complications of Diabetes

Both acute and chronic complications of diabetes may present problems for the patient. Acute complications, such as DKA are usually associated with IDDM. Ketone bodies, acid substances that result from fat metabolism when there is insufficient glucose for the cell, increase in the blood stream. As the metabolic acidosis occurs, the body attempts to compensate and rid itself of the excess acid by increasing the rate and depth of respirations (Kussmaul breathing). Excess carbon dioxide and ketones are exhaled from the lungs; these ketone bodies give the breath a sweet, fruit-like odor. The compensation is temporary, however. Immediate treatment including insulin, intravenous fluid, and electrolyte replacement and support of vital signs is essential, or death will result.

Hypertonic, hyperosmolar, nonketotic coma occurs in NIDDM patients and results from severe hyperglycemia (blood glucose may exceed 800 mg/dl) and dehydration. The excess glucose exerts an osmotic action to pull fluids from the intracellular and interstitial spaces. Unless sufficient insulin, fluids, and electrolytes are administered, death may result from hyperglycemic shock.

Hypoglycemia (insulin reaction) may be classified as an acute complication, and may result from too large a dose of insulin or oral hypoglycemic agent, causing a significant drop in blood glucose. (Hypoglycemic reaction is discussed later in this section.) Chronic complications may involve the blood vessels (macro and micro), nerves (periph-eral and autonomic), skin and mucous membrane, and frequent infections.

Diabetes mellitus is a major risk factor for coronary artery disease and peripheral vascular disease. Additionally, it is a leading cause of amputa-

Table 13-1. BLOOD GLUCOSE VALUES IN THE NORMAL AND DIABETIC STATE

NORMAL PLASMA GLUCOSE VALUES*
- Fasting plasma glucose $\leq$ 115 mg/dl
- 2-hour plasma glucose < 140 mg/dl
- Oral-glucose-tolerance test** of plasma glucose values between zero time and 2 hours < 200 mg/dl

DIABETES MELLITUS, NONPREGNANT ADULTS
- Unequivocal elevation of plasma glucose; i.e., $\geq$ 200 mg/dl and classic symptoms of diabetes
- Fasting plasma glucose $\geq$ 140 mg/dl on two occasions.
- Fasting plasma glucose < 140 mg/dl and 2-hour plasma glucose $\geq$ 200 mg/dl with one intervening value $\geq$ 200 mg/dl following a 75 g glucose load

DIABETES MELLITUS, CHILDREN
- Classic symptoms of diabetes with random plasma glucose $\geq$ 200 mg/dl
- Fasting plasma glucose < 140 mg/dl and 2-hour and one intervening value $\geq$ 200 mg/dl following a glucose load

GESTATIONAL DIABETES
Two or more of the following plasma glucose concentrations met or exceeded using a 100 g glucose load:
- Fasting plasma glucose 150 mg/dl
- 1-hour plasma glucose 190 mg/dl
- 2-hour plasma glucose 165 mg/dl
- 3-hour plasma glucose 145 mg/dl

IMPAIRED GLUCOSE TOLERANCE
- Fasting plasma glucose < 140 mg/dl
- 2-hour plasma glucose $\geq$140 mg/dl and < 200 mg/dl with one intervening value $\geq$ 200 mg/dl following a 75 g glucose load.

(From "Office Guide to Diagnosis and Classification of Diabetes Mellitus and Other Categories of Glucose Intolerance," *Diabetes Care*, 4, no. 2 (1981):335.) Copyright 1981 by the American Diabetes Association, Inc. Reprinted with permission.

*Serum and plasma glucose values are 10%–15% higher than blood glucose measurements because blood glucose measurements include insulin-independent red blood cells, which metabolize glucose and have the effect of reducing the values.

**In the past, the standard glucose load used in an oral-glucose-tolerance test was 100 g, which takes 5 hours to leave the stomach. Because the test is normally 2 hours and 75 g of glucose leaves the stomach at the same rate yielding the same results as a larger load, the smaller glucose load was been chosen to be the standard.

tion, blindness, and renal failure in the United States. Inadequate glycemic control is believed to be the common mechanism causing functional alterations in the peripheral and autonomic nerves, retina, and kidney tissues (7).

Disturbances in nerve tissue, or neuropathy, characteristically affect the legs. Pain and numbness are frequent complaints. Autonomic nerve damage can also result in incontinence, impotence, and nausea and vomiting. The diabetes-induced pathological changes in the retina, retinopathy, are one of the leading causes of blindness in the United States.

The incidence of nephropathy, or kidney disease, appears to be rising in individuals with diabetes, primarily because they are living longer and are experiencing the complications of years of altered carbohydrate metabolism. In the United States today, diabetes is the leading cause of end-stage renal disease. (The characteristics of renal disease and its treatment are discussed in detail in Chapter 8.)

MANAGEMENT OF DIABETES MELLITUS

Medication

Individuals with Type I diabetes require the use of insulin. In Type II diabetes, oral hypoglycemic drugs that stimulate the pancreatic beta cell to release insulin are sometimes prescribed.

Insulin. Much has been learned about insulin since its discovery in 1921. Three types of insulin are commonly used to treat diabetes: beef insulin, pork insulin, and human insulin. Beef insulin is slightly more antigenic (stimulates the formation of antibodies) than pork insulin due to differences in the amino acids which comprise the polypeptide chains. Human insulin is not obtained from humans, but it can be made by altering the amino-acid pattern of pork insulin to make it identical to the amino-acid pattern of human insulin. Because of the projected increase in the number of persons who will be needing to take insulin, researchers feared insufficient quantities of insulin from animal origin would be available in the future. A synthetic human insulin produced from recombinant DNA technology was developed. Human insulin is the least allergenic (capable of producing an allergic response) of all the insulins. Most individuals with diabetes use animal insulin. However, all newly diagnosed diabetic individuals as well as those not well controlled on animal insulin are started on human insulin.

The standard strength of insulin today is U100, which refers to units of insulin per milliliter of solution. Other available strengths are U40 for children and adults who may require smaller doses and U500 for severe cases of insulin resistance (8). Insulin may be administered by subcutaneous or intravenous routes. Only regular insulin may be administered intravenously.

Insulin is classified according to the speed with which it is released and absorbed by the body. Three categories exist: rapid-acting, intermediate-acting, and long-acting insulin (Table 13-2). To maintain near normal blood-glucose concentrations, injections of a combination of rapid-acting and either intermediate or long-acting insulin is often prescribed. The nurse must help the patient assess the relationship between dietary intake and the action of the insulin.

Insulin pumps, or continuous subcutaneous insulin infusion (CSII) with external pumps, are used by some individuals with Type I diabetes with the goal of achieving near-normal glycemic control. The use of the pump is expensive and requires active involvement of the patient in glucose monitoring and decision making related to the treatment regimen. Only rapid-acting insulin is used with the insulin pump, since it must be infused on a continuous basis. Capper et al. (9) reported that the main advantage of the pump cited by patients was increased mealtime flexibility; however, less adherence to dietary recommendations was observed in CSII versus conventional (insulin injection) therapy. A potential problem with pump therapy is the lack of any type of insulin depot in the body at any one time. With pump failure, metabolic decompensation would be rapid (10).

Table 13-2. INSULIN FORMULATIONS

TYPE OF INSULIN	ONSET (hours)	PEAK (hours)	DURATION (hours)
Rapid Acting			
Regular	½–1	2½–5	6–8
Semilente	1–1½	5–10	12–16
Intermediate Acting			
NPH	1–1½	4–12	24
Lente	1–2½	7–15	24
Long Acting			
Protamine Zinc	4–8	14–24	36
Ultralente	4–8	10–30	>36

Source: Insulin preparations, *Drug Facts and Comparisons*, 1988 ed., p. 375. Used with permission from *Drug Facts and Comparisons*. 1988 ed., St. Louis: Facts and Comparisons, a division of the J.B. Lippincott Company.

Oral Agents. Oral hypoglycemic or antidiabetic agents are sometimes prescribed for individuals with Type II diabetes when diet and exercise alone do not control blood glucose levels. The oral medications are sulfonylureas, which stimulate the beta cells to secrete more insulin. Sulfonylureas can be used only when some beta-cell function is present in the pancreas and are, therefore, unsuitable for individuals with IDDM. Currently, controversy surrounds the oral agents, and issues concerning safety, value, and criteria for choosing the best candidates have not been resolved. Questions have arisen regarding the effect of the oral agents on increasing the risk of developing coronary heart disease. Second-generation oral hypoglycemic agents have been developed. These drugs can be taken in smaller doses and generally have fewer side effects. Bonheim (11) has delineated the following criteria for choosing NIDD candidates for whom oral agents are suitable:

- They are near (not below) ideal body weight;
- They have no allergy to sulfonylureas or sulfa drugs;
- They have no evidence of kidney or liver disease; and
- They are not pregnant.

When oral agents are prescribed, the patients must be carefully monitored in the same manner as those patients who are controlled with insulin.

Diet Therapy

The goals for the nutritional management of diabetes mellitus, as enumerated by the American Diabetes Association (12), are to:

- Restore normal blood glucose and maintain optimal lipid levels;
- Maintain normal growth in children and adolescents and maintain a reasonable weight in adolescents and adults;
- Provide adequate nutrition to support pregnancy and lactation;
- Maintain consistency in the timing of meals and snacks to prevent widely varying levels of blood glucose;
- Determine a meal plan for an individual based on his or her life-style;
- Manage weight for obese persons with NIDDM; and
- Improve health via optimal nutrition.

An appropriate meal plan is considered to be an essential part of the treatment of both Type I and

Type II diabetes. While the same dietary principles are followed in both IDDM and NIDDM, the emphasis differs. Day-to-day consistency in intake is crucial in maintaining near normal glycemia on an insulin regimen. The timing of eating and the number of meals and snacks are determined by an assessment of the individuals' needs influenced by life-style variables, physicial activity, type of insulin used, and extent of blood glucose control (12). Three regular meals, a bedtime snack, and one or more snacks between meals is currently recommended.

Tight glycemic control through aggressive treatment carries with it the risk of an insulin reaction, which is a severe hypoglycemic episode. An insulin reaction or hypoglycemia occurs when more insulin is circulating in the body than is needed at the time. This can result from an increased dose of exogenous insulin or oral hypoglycemic agent, a decreased intake of food, or stress. Symptoms of an insulin reaction include blurred vision, headache, tremors, sweating, faintness, and loss of consciousness. Swift treatment through administration of readily available carbohydrate, such as orange juice or candy (if conscious) or intravenous glucose (if unconscious) is required. Once the symptoms have subsided, the patient should eat a more complex carbohydrate such as bread or cereal to prevent recurrence. Untreated, an insulin reaction can result in coma, brain damage, and death.

In Type II diabetes, kilocalorie restriction is emphasized in overweight individuals as a means to decrease blood glucose. Evidence supports that such restriction reduces hyperglycemia even before a desirable body weight is achieved. It appears that the reduction in kilocalorie intake provides the early benefits of better glycemic control.

The recommendations for the meal plan for diabetes have recently been updated by the American Diabetes Association (12). It is important to note that the recommendations (Table 13-3) are guidelines that need to be tailored according to each individual's life-style.

Kilocalories. The kilocalorie level in diabetes management is determined by body weight, age, gender, and activity level of the individual. As mentioned earlier, the majority of NIDDM individuals are overweight, making caloric restriction necessary. Moderate caloric restriction (500–1000 kcal less than daily requirements) is preferred because the goal is to promote permanent behavior changes in dietary intake. Severe caloric restrictions do not result in permanent behavior change and are only used for limited periods under very close medical supervision.

Carbohydrate. Current dietary recommendations for the prevention and management of most chronic diseases encourage an increase in carbohydrate intake, with an emphasis on complex versus simple carbohydrate, and diabetes is no exception. The percentage recommended for diabetes management is flexible, and must be individualized according to blood glucose levels, lipid levels, and eating patterns (12). Evidence indicates that a higher carbohydrate intake causes no significant changes in glycemic control when compared with a lower carbohydrate intake (13).

Dietary Fiber. Foods should be selected that are good sources of dietary fiber. In particular, soluble dietary fiber, such as that contained in legumes, oats, oat bran, barley, and high-pectin fruits is recommended for inclusion in the meal plan, since improved glucose tolerance has been reported using this type of fiber (14). Insoluble dietary fiber, found in wheat bran and bran-containing products such as breads and cereals, is important for the maintenance of normal bowel function and can delay glucose absorption. Though no maximum intake has been defined, the American Diabetes Association has set the limit at 50 g daily. Fiber supplements are not recommended because they often produce nausea, flatulence, feelings of fullness and abdominal discomfort in some individuals (14). Food sources of dietary fiber are listed in Chapter 7.

Sucrose. In patients with NIDDM who are lean and showing no evidence of hyperlipidemia due to carbohydrate sensitivity, a small amount of sucrose as part of a mixed meal can be included. Five percent of the carbohydrate kilocalories is the limit that has been set (5). For example, approximately three teaspoons of sugar is equal to 5% of the

Table 13-3. DIETARY RECOMMENDATIONS FOR INDIVIDUALS WITH DIABETES

VARIABLE	RECOMMENDATION
Kilocalories	Ingest enough to achieve and maintain desirable body weight
Carbohydrate	55%–60% of kilocalories
Dietary fiber	40 g; low kilocalorie diets should contain 25 g 1000 kcal
Sucrose	Depends on metabolic control and body weight
Protein	Similar to the RDA of 0.8 g protein per kilogram body weight
Fat	Less than 30% of total kilocalories, replace saturated fat with unsaturated fat
Cholesterol	Less than 300 mg per day
Sodium	1000 mg/1000 kcal, not to exceed 3000 mg daily
Vitamins/minerals	Under normal circumstances, no supplementation is needed
Alternative sweeteners	Acceptable
Alcohol	Caution

Source: American Diabetes Association, "Nutritional Recommendations and Principles for Individuals with Diabetes Mellitus: 1986," *Diabetes Care* 10(1987):126–32.

carbohydrate kilocalories in a meal plan containing 1800 kcal, with 60% of the total kilocalories from carbohydrate:

1800 kcal times .60 = 1080 carbohydrate kcal
1080 kcal times .05 = 54 sucrose kcal
54 kcal ÷ 16 kcal per teaspoon sugar = 3⅜ teaspoons sugar.

The decision to include sucrose is highly individual.

Protein. RDA for protein is similar in diabetic and nondiabetic individuals. If complications involving the kidney occur, a reduction in protein is necessary (See Chapter 8 for specific dietary recommendations in renal disorders.)

Fat and Cholesterol. Because diabetes is a major risk factor for cardiovascular disease, the recommendations for fat and cholesterol intake are similar to the American Heart Association's Dietary Guidelines for Healthy American Adults: fat should be reduced to less than 30% of total kilocalories, and cholesterol intake should not exceed 300 mg per day. If diabetic individuals continue to demonstrate elevated LDL levels despite following the fat and cholesterol recommendations, further reductions are necessary.

Sodium. Because of the increased risk of vascular disease for diabetic individuals, the American Diabetes Association guidelines for sodium intake are similar to the American Heart Association recommendations, a maximum intake of 3000 mg per day. (Methods for reducing dietary sodium are listed in Chapter 9.)

Vitamins and Minerals. Supplementation, under normal circumstances, is not necessary in diabetes. Exceptions occur when a very low kilo-calorie diet is followed. The majority of diabetic individuals have no evidence of micronutrient deficiency (15).

Alternate Sweeteners. Sweeteners may be classified as noncaloric and caloric. Noncaloric sweeteners are not metabolized by the body, and therefore do not affect blood glucose. Saccharin and acesulfame potassium are examples of noncaloric or alternate sweeteners. Fructose, sorbitol, and mannitol are examples of caloric sweeteners that must be accounted for in the total daily kilocalorie intake. Fructose, sorbitol, and mannitol have approximately the same caloric value as sucrose and other carbohydrates—four kilocalories per gram. Fructose does not require insulin for its initial digestion; however, it can be transformed to glucose in the liver. Once glucose is formed, insulin is necessary for its metabolism. Sorbitol and mannitol, known as sugar alcohols, are absorbed more slowly than other carbohydrates. Large doses can have a laxative effect.

Aspartame is a combination of the two amino acids, phenylalanine and aspartic acid. Although it contains the same number of kilocalories, aspartame is approximately 200 times sweeter than sucrose. Therefore, only small amounts are needed to sweeten foods, and using aspartame does not add substantial kilocalories to foods. Aspartame is considered to be safe for use by individuals with diabetes mellitus (16).

Alcohol. Alcohol cannot be converted to glucose or aminio acids. It can be used only for heat production; it cannot be converted to fat and stored for muscular activity. It does not require insulin for metabolism but actually potentiates the effect of insulin. In diabetic individuals, alcohol prolongs the effect of insulin injections, making hypoglycemia a possible dangerous side effect. Alcohol can be included in the meal plan when diabetes is well controlled. The following guidelines have been established by the International Diabetes Center in Minneapolis for the use of alcohol in the meal plan of individuals with diabetes (17):

- Diabetes must be well controlled. Alcohol use is contraindicated in individuals with

elevated triglycerides, gastritis, pancreatitis, or renal or cardiovascular disease.
- Moderation is essential. Moderation is defined as less than 6% of total daily kilocalories from alcohol on no more than one or two occasions weekly.
- When taken, alcohol should be limited to two equivalents. One equivalent of alcohol equals 1.5 oz of distilled beverages, 4 oz of dry wine, 3 oz of dry sherry, or 12 oz of beer (preferably light).
- Alcohol should not be taken on an empty stomach. Alcohol intake should be limited to shortly before, during, or right after a meal.
- In NIDDM, the kilocalories from alcohol should be calculated into the meal plan as fat exchanges. For a person whose IDDM is well controlled, the occasional use of alcohol can be considered an "extra."
- Drinks high in sugar content, such as liqueurs and mixed drinks, should be avoided. In addition to the alcohol content, the carbohydrate content of beer and sweet wines needs to be taken into consideration.
- Meals and snacks must be eaten on time to avoid the possibility of hypoglycemia.
- Visible identification should be worn; e.g., Medic-Alert tag or bracelet.
- Individuals on oral medications for diabetes need to recognize the possibility of an interaction between the sulfonylureas and alcohol.

Dietetic Foods. Many consumers erroneously believe that "dietetic" foods are foods specially formulated for individuals with diabetes and as such contain no kilocalories. Dietetic foods are not necessarily calorie-free foods. According to the Food and Drug Administration, foods may be labelled as "dietetic" when they are low calorie or reduced in kilocalories (18). Dietetic foods must therefore be counted as part of the daily meal plan. Because dietetic foods are specialty products, consumers usually must pay a premium price for them. Use of dietetic foods is not required when following a diabetic diet.

Exercise

It is well validated that exercise decreases the need for insulin. Exercise is an adjunct in the treatment of diabetes and is encouraged in NIDDM and in controlled IDDM. Besides cardiovascular benefits and better weight control, exercise can result in increased insulin sensitivity and improved glucose tolerance (19). Prior to embarking on an exercise program, individuals older than 30 years of age who have had diabetes for 10 years or more should seek physician approval (12).

Alterations in insulin dose and/or food intake are necessary when individuals with IDDM exercise, because glucose uptake by the exercising muscle is enhanced, thus decreasing insulin need. To avoid low blood sugar (hypoglycemia), supplemental carbohydrate snacks are recommended before, during, or after exercise for individuals with IDDM or NIDDM controlled through oral medications. Guidelines for carbohydrate supplementation are outlined in Table 13-4.

Individuals with IDDM may also need to adjust insulin dose and timing in activities longer than two hours. Because of the extreme variations among individuals, adjustments to the insulin dose should be based on the particular individual's previous experience. Individuals with NIDDM controlled by diet alone do not need extra food before or during exercise. In fact, regular exercise will aid in the expenditure of kilocalories and promote weight loss when combined with kilocalorie restriction.

Table 13-4. GUIDELINES FOR CARBOHYDRATE SUPPLEMENTATION DURING EXERCISE

EXERCISE INTENSITY	DURATION	BLOOD GLUCOSE PRIOR TO ACTIVITY	CARBOHYDRATE RECOMMENDED BEFORE ACTIVITY
Very low level	—	>100 mg/dl	None
Moderate	—	100–180 mg/dl	10–15 g: 1 piece of fruit, 4 oz fruit juice, or 6 saltine-type crackers
Moderate	1 hour	>180 but <300 mg/dl	None
Strenuous	1–2 hours	<100 mg/dl	50 g: whole sandwich plus 1 glass of milk
Strenuous	1–2 hours	100–180 mg/dl	25–50 g: half sandwich plus 1 fruit or 1 glass of milk
Strenuous	1–2 hours	>180 mg/dl	10–15 g: 1 piece of fruit, 4 oz fruit juice, or 6 saltine-type crackers

Source: M.J. Franz, "Exercise and the Management of Diabetes Mellitus," *Journal of the American Dietetic Association* 87(1987):872–80.

Cautions. Individuals with poorly controlled IDDM, that is, those exhibiting marked hyperglycemia and ketoacidosis, will experience an intensification of the diabetic state as a result of exercise. The initiation of exercise should therefore be delayed until adequate glucose control is achieved (19).

Neuropathy, retinopathy, and nephropathy may worsen as a result of strenuous exercise (19). Foot damage is a possible complication in individuals with neuropathy. Additionally, damage can occur in any body part that has sustained pathological nerve changes. Blood-pressure increases during exercise may place added stress on eye vessels already weakened by retinopathy. The protein losses in the urine following exercise may or may not be harmful in individuals with kidney complications. More research is needed to assess the effect of exercise on renal physiology in diabetic nephropathy.

Illness

Any type of illness is a stress to the body and, therefore, alters insulin requirements. Fever and severe infection stimulate the hormones released during stress and increase blood glucose. As a result, the need for insulin increases. Even when the individual with IDDM does not feel well enough to eat, exogenous insulin must continue to be administered. Carbohydrate liquids should be consumed every hour. A record should be kept of the type and amount of the liquid consumed. If vomiting occurs, broth or bouillon should be included to replace electrolytes. Liquids or semiliquids should not be taken for more than 36 hours without contacting the physician.

Surgery

Requirements for insulin increase during surgery, since it, too, represents a major stress on the body. Additional insulin is required postoperatively and is reduced to preoperative levels as recovery takes place. Initially, carbohydrate in the form of glucose is supplied intravenously. Once the patient is reintroduced to food, the normal progression from clear-liquid to full-liquid to soft and, finally, to a regular diabetic diet is followed. Only the carbohydrate content of the clear-liquid diet is calculated. Once a full-liquid diet can be tolerated, calculations for protein and fat in addition to carbohydrate are completed.

Patients who take oral hypoglycemic drugs are placed on insulin prior to and during surgery. When the patient is able to tolerate oral foods, the insulin may be discontinued and the oral hypoglycemic drug resumed, as prescribed.

Patient Education

When diabetic patients are discharged from the hospital, they assume responsibility for their own care. They must know how to control their blood glucose and be able to check on the adequacy of their efforts.

Measurements of Blood Glucose Control. The goal in therapy for diabetes is to achieve near normal glucose control, on the assumption that complications of diabetes may be averted with tight glycemic control. The patient should learn to perform self-monitoring of blood glucose (SMBG), which is used by over 1 million patients (20). Accurate records of blood glucose levels help in the management of diabetes.

The Meal Plan. The principles of dietary management specified earlier are usually taught to the patient using the exchange-system concept. The food-exchange system first came into being in 1950 to overcome problems often occurring when individuals tried to follow a diet to help control diabetes (21). Previous diets for diabetes were plagued by problems such as lack of variety, inflexibility, difficulty in understanding and teaching, and nutritional inadequacy. These problems worked against following the dietary principles on a long-term basis, which is essential to good glycemic control.

The exchange lists used to develop meal plans for individuals with diabetes are different food groups that have similar protein, fat, carbohydrate, and kilocalorie contents. There are six exchange lists:

1. Starch and bread exchange
2. Meat exchange
3. Vegetable exchange

4. Fruit exchange
5. Milk exchange
6. Fat exchange

Each list contains a variety of foods in varying amounts so that one exchange from a particular list provides approximately the same amount of protein, fat, carbohydrate, and kilocalories. For example, one starch and bread exchange provides 3 g of protein, a trace of fat, 15 g of carbohydrate, and 80 kcal. Items included as one bread exchange are one slice of bread, ½ cup cooked cereal, or ½ cup of mashed potatoes. One fruit exchange contains 0 g of protein, 0 g of fat, 15 g of carbohydrate, and 60 kcal. Examples of one fruit exchange are one apple, one peach, or ½ of a grapefruit. It is important to note that bacon and chitterlings are considered to be fat exchanges, not meat exchanges. The patient must become familiar with foods on the various lists to make appropriate substitutions.

Based on an individual's life-style, a daily meal plan is developed with a specific number of exchanges from each list. A detailed booklet containing the lists, *Exchange Lists for Meal Planning*, may be purchased from the American Dietetic Association. Helpful features in the booklet include a symbol for high-fiber foods (foods containing three or more grams of fiber per serving); a symbol for high-sodium foods (foods containing more than 400 mg of sodium per serving); management tips; and a list of combination foods that fit into more than one exchange list, such as soup, casseroles, and pizza.

Because some individuals may not be able to fully comprehend the exchange lists, a simplified tool is available. Called "Healthy Food Choices," it contains specific recommendations, such as "Eat less fat" and "Eat less sugar." The booklet opens into a poster with six groups of foods in categories by kilocalories. The reading level of "Healthy Food Choices" is sixth or seventh grade (21).

No matter what type of educational tool is chosen, one thing is certain: The use of preprinted diets is strongly discouraged (12). Preprinted diets are not individualized and therefore do not take into account all of the variables that affect dietary behavior. A realistic, individualized meal plan developed with plenty of patient involvement is more successful in terms of permanent behavior change (22).

POSSIBLE NURSING DIAGNOSES

Potential alteration in nutrition; less than body requirements related to insufficient nutrient intake or utilization to meet the demands for growth and activity.

Potential alteration in nutrition; greater than body requirements related to excess intake and/or lack of exercise (Type II).

Knowledge deficit pertaining to the disease process and the relationship of
- nutrition (meal planning).
- weight control.
- exercise.
- interrelationship of drug therapy and diet and energy needs during periods of stress (illness, infection, fever).
- signs and symptoms of hypo or hyperglycemia.
- signs and symptoms of complications.
- pregnancy.

Potential noncompliance related to the complex nature of the disease and treatment regimen.

Potential ineffective coping (individual and family) related to self-care.

Potential fluid-volume deficit related to inadequate disease control (hyperglycemia).

NURSING INTERVENTIONS
FOR NUTRITIONAL DISORDERS

Work closely with the patient, physician and dietitian to develop a meal plan that will meet the energy needs of the patient.

Potential alteration in nutrition; less than body requirements related to insufficient nutrient intake or utilization to meet the demands for growth and activity.

- Caution the patient about the importance of early detection of the signs of hypoglycemia. Carry simple carbohydrate substances (Lifesavers candy for example) and consume as needed to prevent a severe reaction.
- Caution the patient that hypoglycemia may occur during exercise because the insulin requirements are lowered. Carbohydrate should be consumed prior to exercise and should be readily available during and after exercise.
- Instruct the patient to call the physician if illness persists for more than 36 hours or if oral fluids cannot be retained.

Potential alteration in nutrition; greater than body requirements related to excess intake and/or lack of exercise (Type II).

- Stress the importance of establishing goals for kilocalorie reduction and increased physical activity (if appropriate) for the patient with NIDDM.
- Instruct the patient in the importance of eating complex carbohydrate foods rather than foods that are high in refined sugar.

Knowledge deficit pertaining to the disease process and the relationship of
- **nutrition (meal planning).**
- **weight control.**

- **exercise.**
- **interrelationship of drug therapy and diet and energy needs during periods of stress (illness, infection, fever).**
- **signs and symptoms of hypo- or hyperglycemia.**
- **signs and symptoms of complications.**
- **pregnancy.**

- Stress the importance of consistency in meal composition and appropriate timing of meals to coincide with insulin action. Three meals plus a bedtime snack and one or two snacks between meals are recommended.
- Instruct the patient in the proper use of caloric and noncaloric sweeteners.
- Help the patient evaluate dietetic foods that are available on the grocery shelves. Instruct the patient that special dietetic foods that are expensive are not necessary to follow the diabetic diet. For example, dietetic fruits do not need to be purchased. Fruits packed in unsweetened fruit juices are considered to be acceptable fruit exchanges. Exchange lists devised by the American Diabetes Association and the American Dietetic Association will help to provide variety in the diet.
- Instruct the patient who prefers an occasional alcoholic beverage that this source of carbohydrate can be planned into the diet. Alcohol intake should be limited to shortly before, during, or right after a meal.

Continued

NURSING INTERVENTIONS (*continued*)

Potential noncompliance related to the complex nature of the disease and treatment regimen.

- Assess the patient's usual eating habits and life-style.
- Attempt to ascertain the level of understanding and assess the importance the patient attaches to changing behaviors.

Potential ineffective coping (individual and family) related to self-care.

- Encourage the patient to schedule follow-up appointments with a dietitian on a regular basis. The American Diabetes Association Task Force on Nutrition and Exchange Lists recommends that all adults with diabetes be seen by a nutritionist every six months to one year (5).

Potential fluid-volume deficit related to inadequate disease control (hyperglycemia).

- Encourage the patient to schedule regular medical follow-up visits in order to prevent or delay serious complications associated with diabetes mellitus.

TOPIC OF INTEREST

The Glycemic Index

In recent years, work has been done measuring blood glucose responses which occur when various foods are eaten (23, 24). The glycemic index is an attempt to classify individual foods according to the extent to which they increase blood glucose levels rather than by similarities in their carbohydrate content (21). The flattest glycemic response has been observed for foods in the legume class, while the highest glycemic response occurred when root vegetables and grains were eaten (25).

The glycemic effect of food is greatly influenced by food form; rate of ingestion, digestion, and absorption; method of cooking; and the presence of other components such as fiber, fat, and protein. While the American Diabetes Association stated that glycemic indexing may be used in a simplified form as part of the exchange system, the organization has not condoned its widespread use until further work is completed (12).

Clinical Trials

Because of the increasing life span of the population, there will undoubtedly be more evidence of complications ("opathies" such as retinopathy, neuropathy, nephropathy) associated with IDDM and NIDDM. It has always been assumed that tighter glycemic control results in fewer complications; however, little data have been collected to substantiate this viewpoint. In fact, many of these complications occur despite good control and management on the part of the patient. A large collaborative seven-year clinical trial has been initiated to study the relationship between blood glucose control and vascular complications in IDDM. The study should provide new insights into the treatment of diabetes mellitus.

SPOTLIGHT ON LEARNING

Following is a listing of the kilocalorie, protein, fat, and carbohydrate content for the different food exchanges.

EXCHANGE LIST	CARBOHYDRATE	PROTEIN	FAT	KCALS
		Grams		
Starch/Bread	15	3	trace	80
Meat				
Lean		7	3	55
Medium fat	—	7	5	75
High fat	—	7	8	100
Vegetable	5	2	—	25
Fruit	15	—	—	60
Milk				
Skim	12	8	trace	90
Low fat	12	8	5	120
Whole	12	8	8	150
Fat	—	—	5	45

The exchange lists are the basis of a meal-planning system designed by a committee of the American Diabetes Association and the American Dietetic Association. While designed primarily for people with diabetes and others who must follow special diets, the exchange lists are based on principles of good nutrition that apply to everyone. ©1986 American Diabetes Association, Inc., American Dietetic Association.

Apply the preceding lists to the case of a male patient who is 27 years old and weighs 154 lbs (70 kg). He is a computer programmer, swims regularly, and plays occasional tennis. He was diagnosed as having Type I diabetes at age 13. His usual dietary intake is as follows:

Breakfast	*Exchanges*
1 cup cereal	2 starch
1 cup whole milk	1 whole milk
2 slices white toast	2 starch
2 tsp margarine	2 fat
½ cup orange juice	1 fruit
Coffee	

Lunch

Sandwich:	
2 slices white bread	2 starch
1 tbs mayonnaise	3 fat
3 oz roast beef	3 medium-fat meat
1 peach	1 fruit
Diet soda	

Dinner

3 oz fish baked with	3 lean meat
1 tsp margarine	1 fat
½ cup carrots	1 vegetable
1 baked potato with	1 starch
2 tbs sour cream	1 fat
Tea	

Snack

1 cup ice cream	2 starch, 4 fat
2 small gingersnap cookies	1 starch, 1 fat

TOTAL EXCHANGES	CARBOHYDRATE	PROTEIN	FAT	KCALS
	Grams			
10 starch	150	30	trace	800
1 whole milk	12	8	8	150
12 fat	—	—	60	540
2 fruit	30	—	—	120
3 medium-fat meat	—	21	15	225
3 lean meat	—	21	9	165
1 vegetable	5	2	—	25
Totals	197	82	92	2025

Percent of Total Kilocalorie Intake

- Carbohydrate: 197 carbohydrate times 4 kcal per gram = 788 kcal; 788 kilocalories ÷ 2025 kcal = 38%
- Protein: 82 g protein times 4 kcal per gram = 328 kilocalories; 328 kcal ÷ 2025 kcal = 16%
- Fat: 92 fat times 9 kcal per gram = 828 kcal; 828 kcal ÷ 2025 kcal = 41%.

Comparison of Ideal and Actual Intake

	CARBOHYDRATE	FAT	PROTEIN	KCALS
Ideal	55%–60%	Less than 30%	10%*	2300**
Actual	38%	41%	16%	2025

*Ideal protein needs are calculated as follows: 70 kg body weight times 0.8 g protein per kilogram = 56 g. Percentage of protein calculation: 56 g protein times 4 kcal per gram = 224 kcal; 224 kcal ÷ 2300 = 9.7% or 10%.

**Based on moderate activity

1. What changes are needed in this person's meal plan?
2. What changes should be made in food selection to increase kilocalories and carbohydrate (including dietary fiber) and decrease fat and protein?

REVIEW QUESTIONS

1. What is Type I diabetes?
   a. insulin dependent diabetes
   b. insulin independent diabetes
   c. noninsulin dependent diabetes
   d. gestational diabetes

2. Which of the following is not caused by lack of insulin?
   a. increased protein catabolism
   b. increased fat catabolism
   c. increased glycogenolysis
   d. decreased gluconeogenesis

3. How is a slice of bacon characterized for purposes of the exchange lists?
   a. one fat exchange
   b. one meat exchange
   c. one meat and one fat exchange
   d. two meat exchanges

4. In selecting another fruit instead of half of a banana, which is the best choice?
   a. 6 oz grape juice
   b. 8 oz orange juice
   c. small apple
   d. 2 cups cantaloupe

5. Which of the following is not a goal of the nutritional management of diabetes mellitus?
   a. restore normal blood glucose and maintenance of optimal lipid levels
   b. prescribe appropriate insulin to accommodate the meal plan
   c. maintain consistency in the timing of meals and snacks to prevent widely varying levels of blood glucose
   d. manage weight for obese persons with NIDDM

6. In Type II diabetes, what is the most important dietary consideration?
   a. kilocalorie restriction
   b. consistency in intake from day to day
   c. number of meals and snacks
   d. avoidance of an insulin reaction

7. What are the current carbohydrate- and fat-intake recommendations for individuals with diabetes?
   a. carbohydrate, 35%–40% of kilocalories; fat, less than 30% of kilocalories
   b. carbohydrate, 70%–75% of kilocalories; fat; less than 10% of kilocalories
   c. carbohydrate, 55%–60% of kilocalories, fat, less than 40% of kilocalories
   d. carbohydrate, 55%–60% of kilocalories; fat; less than 30% of kilocalories

8. How much carbohydrate should be taken prior to exercise of moderate intensity when blood glucose falls in the range of 100–180 mg/dl?
   a. 10–15 g
   b. 25–50 g
   c. 50 g or more
   d. 5 g

9. How may illness and surgery affect blood glucose level?
   a. decrease
   b. no change
   c. increase
   d. not an important factor

10. Which of the following is not a characteristic of the exchange lists for meal planning?
    a. they provide variety and flexibility in the meal plan
    b. they allow for individualization of the diet
    c. they categorize foods that have similar protein, fat, and carbohydrate content
    d. they are preprinted and standardized diets

ACTIVITIES

1. Record food intake and time of eating for one day. What changes would you have to make (if any) if you found that you were insulin dependent?
2. Recall your food intake from the previous day. Using the booklet *Exchange Lists for Meal Planning,* classify the foods you ate into the appropriate exchanges.
3. Using *Exchange Lists for Meal Planning,* devise a meal plan for yourself that conforms to the following: 1800 kcal, 60% of kcal from carbohydrate, 25% of kcal from fat, and 15% of kcal from protein

   - Carbohydrate calculation: .60 times 1800 kcal = 1080 kcal ÷ 4 kcal per gram carbohydrate = 270 g of carbohydrate daily.
   - Fat calculation: .25 times 1800 kcal = 450 kcal ÷ 9 kcal per gram fat = 50 g of fat daily.
   - Protein calculation: .15 times 1800 kcal = 270 kcal ÷ 4 kcal per gram protein = 68 g of protein daily.

REFERENCES

1. U.S. Department of Health and Human Services, Public Health Service. The Surgeon General's report on nutrition and health. Summary and recommendations. 1988. DHHS (PHS) Publication No. 88-50211.
2. Office guide to diagnosis and classification of diabetes mellitus and other categories of glucose intolerance. *Diabetes Care* 4(1981):335.
3. MacDonald, M.J., L. Liston, and I. Carlson. Seasonality in glycosylated hemoglobin in normal subjects. Does seasonal incidence in insulin-dependent diabetes suggest specific etiology? *Diabetes* 36(1987):265–68.
4. Katzeff, H.L. Noninsulin dependent diabetes mellitus: Nutrition and lifestyle. *Current Concepts and Perspectives in Nutrition* 5(1986):1–8.
5. Wheeler, M.L., L. Delahanty, and J. Wylie-Rosett. Diet and exercise in noninsulin-dependent diabetes mellitus: Implications for dietitians from the NIH consensus development conference. *Journal of the American Dietetic Association* 87(1987):480–85.
6. ———. Diabetes mellitus in an obese woman. *Nutrition Reviews* 45(1987):51–54.
7. Winegrad, A.I. Does a common mechanism induce the diverse complications of diabetes? *Diabetes* 36(1987):396–406.
8. Karam, J.H. Insulins 1983: Overview and outlook. *Clinical Diabetes* 1(1983):1 and 3–10. .
9. Capper, A.F., S.W. Headen, and R.M. Bergenstal. Dietary practices with persons with diabetes during insulin pump therapy. *Journal of the American Dietetic Association* 85(1985):445–49.
10. Kaye, R. Research and practice in the treatment of insulin-dependent diabetes: A survey of 53 diabetologists. *Pediatrics* 74(1984):1079–85.
11. Bonheim, R. The second generation. *Diabetes Forecast* (March/April 1983): 29–31.
12. American Diabetes Association. Nutritional recommendations and principles for individuals with diabetes mellitus: 1986. *Diabetes Care* 10(1987):126–32.
13. Hollenbeck, C.B., et al. The effects of subject-selected, high carbohydrate, low fat diets on glycemic control in insulin dependent diabetes mellitus. *American Journal of Clinical Nutrition* 41(1985):293–98.
14. Anderson, J.W., et al. Dietary fiber and diabetes: A comprehensive review and practical application. *Journal of the American Dietetic Association* 87(1987):1189–97.
15. Mooradian, A.D., and J.E. Morley. Micronutrient status in diabetes mellitus. *American Journal of Clinical Nutrition* 45(1987):877–95.
16. Nehrling, J.K., et al. Aspartame use by persons with diabetes. *Diabetes Care* 8, no. 5. (1985):415–17.
17. Franz, M.J. Diabetes mellitus: Considerations in the development of guidelines for the occasional use of alcohol. *Journal of the American Dietetic Association* 83(1983):147–55.
18. Food and Drug Administration, HHS. 21 CFR. Chapter 1, 105.66 (e), 1985.

19. Franz, M.J. Exercise and the management of diabetes mellitus. *Journal of the American Dietetic Association* 87(1987):872–80.

20. American Diabetes Association, Centers for Disease Control, Food and Drug Administration, and National Institute of Diabetes and Digestive and Kidney Diseases. Consensus statement on self-monitoring of blood glucose. *Diabetes Care* 10(1987):95–99.

21. Franz, M.J., et al. Exchange lists: Revised 1986. *Journal of the American Dietetic Association* 87(1987):28–34.

22. Hauenstein, D.J., M.R. Schiller, and R.S. Hurley. Motivational techniques of dietitians counseling individuals with Type II diabetes. *Journal of the American Dietetic Association* 87(1987):37–42.

23. Jenkins, D.J.A., et al. Glycemic index of foods: A physiological basis for carbohydrate exchange. *American Journal of Clinical Nutrition* 34(1981):362–66.

24. Jenkins, D.J.A. The glycaemic response to carbohydrate foods. *The Lancet* 2, no. 8399 (August 18, 1984):388–91.

25. Beebe, C.A. Self blood glucose monitoring: An adjunct to dietary and insulin management of the patient with diabetes. *Journal of the American Dietetic Association* 87(1987):61–65.

CHAPTER
14

NUTRITION AND THE PATIENT WITH SELECTED METABOLIC DISORDERS

Objectives

After studying this chapter, the student will be able to

- describe the metabolic consequences of hyperfunction and hypofunction of the thyroid, adrenal and parathyroid glands, arthritis, gout, and osteoporosis.
- explain the dietary management for patients with hyperfunction and hypofunction of the thyroid, adrenal and parathyroid glands, arthritis, gout, and osteoporosis.
- differentiate between the dietary approaches for a patient with hyperfunction versus hypofunction of the thyroid, adrenal and parathyroid glands.
- identify nursing interventions for nutritional disorders associated with selected metabolic disorders.

Overview

A variety of metabolic disorders are covered in this chapter. The nutritional alterations required for persons with endocrine gland dysfunctions (pancreas—hyperinsulinism, adrenal, thyroid and parathyroid) are included. In addition, nutritional implications related to osteoporosis, arthritis, and gout are addressed. (Refer to Chapter 13 for a discussion of diabetes mellitus.)

HYPOGLYCEMIA (HYPERINSULINISM)

Hypoglycemia (blood glucose below 50 mg/dl) occurs when there is too much serum insulin present for the available glucose in the bloodstream. This condition may also be referred to as hyperinsulinism. The cause of hypoglycemia may be organic, functional, reactive, induced, or idiopathic.

Organic causes of hypoglycemia may be due to tumors or hyperplasia of the islet cells of the pancreas, may be associated with liver diseases such as cirrhosis, or in combination with other endocrine disorders such as adrenocortical insufficiency or hypothyroidism. Functional hypoglycemia may be associated with an oversecretion of insulin following simple carbohydrate ingestion. This type of hypoglycemia may also occur following gastric surgery (dumping syndrome), when large quantities of simple carbohydrate enter the small intestine more rapidly than usual.

Following periods of stress or anxiety, reactive hypoglycemia that closely mimics reactions observed in diabetic patients, may occur. Reactive hypoglycemia should be medically diagnosed if at all possible (1). Hypoglycemia can be induced, especially in the adult diabetic patient who takes exogenous doses of insulin and abuses alcohol (2). Idiopathic hypoglycemia is particularly difficult to diagnose, since there is frequently no known cause.

Signs and symptoms of hypoglycemic reactions are manifested by two major response patterns: those related to the increased secretion of epinephrine by the sympathetic nervous system and those related to a deficient supply of glucose to the brain (the brain stores no glucose). Manifestations of a hypoglycemic reaction vary among individuals.

The reaction that occurs in response to increased epinephrine may include tachycardia, palpitations, pallor, increased perspiration, hunger, irritability, and tremors. These reactions usually occur more rapidly in response to hypoglycemia. If the hypoglycemia continues, the neurological responses to decreased glucose supply to the brain may become apparent. These signs and symptoms may include headache, lack of concentration, loss of memory, confusion, convulsions, and ultimately coma. The strange behavior that may accompany hypoglycemia may mimic intoxication from alcohol.

In order to accurately diagnose hypoglycemia, it is imperative to determine the level of the blood glucose while the patient is manifesting the symptoms. Relief of symptoms by ingestion of carbohydrate is also a diagnostic criterion (3).

Prevention is the preferred treatment for hypoglycemia. Emphasis on nutritional aspects of control must be understood by the patient. Dietary modifications are required, and the diet prescription is individualized based on the patient's history of reactions after ingestion of various carbohydrate foods. In general, however, the diet is moderate in protein, carbohydrate, and fat. Carbohydrates that are rapidly absorbed should be included in mixed meals rather than eaten alone, and the individual may fare better on five to six meals per day.

The mixed diet provides for a more gradual release of glucose into the bloodstream so as not to precipitate a hypoglycemic reaction. Complex carbohydrates may be substituted for simple carbohydrates (sugars) to help moderate the available glucose levels in the bloodstream, depending on the patient's reaction to these foods. Alcoholic-beverage intake is usually restricted, because alcohol inhibits gluconeogenesis (formation of glucose from noncarbohydrate food sources).

In emergency situations, however, the treatment would be similar to that for a hypoglycemic reaction following insulin injections or associated with antidiabetic agents such as Micronase. Ten to 15 g of quick-acting carbohydrate, such as four ounces soda pop or orange juice, several pieces of hard candy, or two teaspoons of jelly, must be administered. If the symptoms have not subsided within 10 minutes, the treatment can be repeated. Once the symptoms have subsided, the patient should be encouraged to consume a meal or snack containing protein and complex carbohydrate, such as cottage cheese and crackers or ½ meat sandwich (4). If the symptoms persist, the patient should notify the physician.

POSSIBLE NURSING DIAGNOSES

Potential alteration in nutrition; more than body requirements related to excess carbohydrate intake or availability.

Potential alteration in nutrition; less than body requirements related to insufficient balance of nutrient intake.

Knowledge deficit related to the disease process and the relationship of
- nutrition (meal planning).
- signs and symptoms of hypoglycemia.

Potential noncompliance related to the nature of the disease process and treatment regimen.

Potential ineffective coping related to self-care.

Potential sleep disturbance pattern related to need for food during the night-time hours.

NURSING INTERVENTIONS
FOR NUTRITIONAL DISORDERS

Work closely with the patient, dietitian, and physician to plan a diet that will help achieve relatively stable levels of glucose in the blood-stream.

Potential alteration in nutrition; more than body requirements related to excess carbohydrate intake or availability.

- Instruct the patient to:
    eat a well-balanced mixed diet that is moderate in protein, carbohydrate, and fat. It may be helpful to eat five to six small meals per day;

    limit the consumption of caffeine-containing substances, such as coffee, tea, colas, and chocolate, since caffeine can increase the blood glucose levels;

avoid the use of carbohydrate foods that produce symptoms of low blood glucose;

use the exchange lists (see Chapter 13) when calculating food intake.

Potential alteration in nutrition; less than body requirements related to insufficient balance of nutrient intake.

- Instruct the patient to:
    consume a mixed diet as prescribed to allow for a more gradual release of glucose into the bloodstream;

    eat six smaller meals per day to provide for a more constant supply of glucose.

Continued

NURSING INTERVENTIONS (continued)

Some patients may require a snack at 3 am;

restrict intake of alcoholic beverages since alcohol inhibits gluconeogenesis;

use complex carbohydrates in place of simple carbohydrates if symptoms occur after ingestion of the latter.

Knowledge deficit related to the disease process and the relationship of
- **nutrition (meal planning).**
- **signs and symptoms of hypoglycemia.**

- Instruct the patient about the relationship of food intake to glucose availability in the bloodstream and secretion of insulin by the pancreas.
- Teach the patient the signs and symptoms of a hypoglycemic reaction (sympathetic or central-nervous-system-related reactions).
- Teach the patient measures that may be used to treat a hypoglycemic reaction.

Potential noncompliance related to the nature of the disease process and treatment.

- Encourage the patient to follow the diet prescription as outlined to prevent episodes of hypoglycemia related to the type of foods ingested as well as the time intervals between meals and snacks.

Potential ineffective coping related to self-care.

- Provide information on the relationship of the disease process to nutritional intake in order to enhance feelings of control.

Potential sleep disturbance pattern related to need for food during the night-time hours.

- Stress the importance of taking food during the night in order to prevent early morning hypoglycemia.
- Suggest that the patient take naps during the day or go to bed at an earlier hour to provide for necessary sleep if night-time feedings are required.

THYROID DISORDERS

The thyroid gland, which lies below the larynx, consists of two lobes connected by an isthmus. The gland secretes the thyroid hormones thyroxin (T_4) and triiodothyronine (T_3), which are responsible for the metabolic rate of the body and for growth and development. Calcitonin, which is important for bone and calcium metabolism, is also secreted. Another function of the gland is to store iodine.

Hyperthyroidism

Hyperthyroidism occurs when the thyroid gland secretes an excessive amount of thyroid hormone. This, in turn, causes an increase in the metabolic rate and activity of the body. Additional caloric support is necessary to help the body meet the increased energy demands. It is felt that hyperthyroidism may be an autoimmune disorder, with a genetic predisposition, and is generally more common in women.

Excess thyroid hormone predisposes to a variety of disorders, including Graves disease (toxic diffuse goiter), thyroiditis, and thyrotoxicosis. Manifestations of the condition may be seen in many systems throughout the body.

Symptoms of hyperthyroidism may be seen in the weight loss, nervousness, and exophthalmus (prominent, bulging eyes) presented by the patient. Weakness is often a frequent complaint, despite the increased appetite, because of the catabolic effects of the increased hormone secretion on the protein tissues of the body. All the systems of the body will be affected by the increased thyroid hormone levels in the body. Increases in urinary output may be noted as well as tachycardia. The stress created on the heart can predispose to cardiac complications such as heart failure.

Treatment protocols are aimed at reducing the secretion of the thyroid hormones. These may involve surgical removal of the gland or a portion of the gland; a chemotherapeutic approach with the use of antithyroid drugs such as propylthiouracil or tapazole; and radioactive iodine to suppress the thyroid hormone secretion. Iodine (in the form of potassium iodide) is frequently used to stimulate the thyroid gland to store increased amounts of the

hormones. In the course of treatment, as thyroid hormones are suppressed, hypothyroidism may be precipitated. The discussion of hypothyroidism follows in this section.

Dietary management includes a high-kilocalorie (4000-5000 kcal), high-protein (100-125 g) diet until normal nutrition can be achieved (3). The diet may need to be supplemented with vitamins, especially A, B-complex, and C and minerals such as calcium. If, in the course of treatment, the thyroid is completely removed or destroyed, iodine replacement will also be required. The patient should be encouraged to eat foods at frequent intervals to relieve the hunger and prevent negative nitrogen balance from occurring. Liberal quantities of milk and milk products should be consumed.

POSSIBLE NURSING DIAGNOSES

Potential alteration in nutrition; less than body requirements secondary to increased metabolic demands of the body.

Potential fluid-volume deficit secondary to increased metabolic activity of the body.

Alteration in elimination; diarrhea related to increased peristaltic activity of the intestine secondary to increased metabolic activity.

Knowledge deficit related to
- increased caloric needs of the body secondary to increased metabolic activity.
- effects of drug therapy on food intake.

NURSING INTERVENTIONS FOR NUTRITIONAL DISORDERS

Work closely with the patients, dietitian, and physician in planning a diet that will help to meet the increased energy needs of the body.

Potential alteration in nutrition; less than body requirements secondary to increased metabolic demands of the body.

- Instruct the patient in the role of the diet in helping to prevent catabolic losses, especially of protein tissue, due to increased thyroid hormone secretion.
- Encourage the patient to snack throughout the day. Carbohydrate intake may be liberal. Continued

NURSING INTERVENTIONS (continued)

- Encourage the patient to consume greater quantities of milk and milk products to offset the losses of calcium salts.
- Advise the patient to limit the use of caffeine-containing substances (coffee, tea, colas, chocolate) as well as alcohol and tobacco.
- Encourage the patient to relax and eat in a pleasant, non-stimulating environment.

Potential fluid-volume deficit secondary to increased metabolic activity of the body.

- Encourage liberal fluid intake, 2000-3000 ml (unless contraindicated) to offset losses through increased perspiration and urination.
- Use decaffeinated beverages if desired to help increase fluid intake.
- Monitor intake and output if requested by the physician, but especially during times of illness involving fever or during prolonged exposure to the heat.

Alteration in elimination; diarrhea related to increased peristaltic activity of the intestine secondary to increased metabolic activity.

- Limit the use of caffeine-containing substances to prevent increased stimulation of peristalsis.
- Limit the use of high-fiber foods to prevent increased peristalsis.

- Avoid or limit the use of highly seasoned foods that may increase peristaltic activity, depending on individual sensitivity.

Knowledge deficit related to
- **increased caloric needs of the body secondary to increased metabolic activity.**
- **effects of drug therapy on food intake.**

- Instruct the patient in the role of the diet in helping to prevent catabolic losses, especially of protein tissues, due to increased thyroid hormone secretion.
- Involve the patient in planning the dietary regimen; hopefully this will encourage compliance.
- Instruct the patient that once the thyroid hormone secretions are controlled, dietary intake must be curtailed in order to prevent obesity.
- Instruct the patient to:
    dilute potassium iodide solution in water, juice (grape is particularly good), or milk to disguise the strong salty taste;

    sip the solution through a straw to prevent staining of the tooth enamel;

    take after meals to prevent gastric irritation.

- Instruct the patient to question the physician about using iodized salt and eating foods that are rich in iodine, such as shellfish while on drug therapy.

Hypothyroidism

Hypothyroidism results from a deficiency of thyroid hormones, which can lead to a general slowing of body processes precipitated by a decreased metabolic rate. Causative factors may include hypothalamic or pituitary disorders, thyroid hormone deficiency, and thyroid destruction that results from treatment of hyperthyroidism (surgical removal or use of radioactive iodine), or high intake of goitrogens (foods that inhibit the utilization of iodine by the thyroid gland, such as cabbage, rutabaga, turnips, mustard greens, horseradish, soybeans, and peanuts).

Hypothyroidism that occurs in infants or young children is referred to as cretinism. If untreated, cretinism can result in brain damage and mental retardation. Despite treatment, it has been found that prolonged juvenile hypothyroidism can result in permanent height deficit (5). Since iodized salt and food that contains iodine (seafood) are more readily available, this condition is not as prevalent in the United States. However, in several counties in the coal-rich areas of Kentucky, there is a high prevalence rate among 12- and 13-year-olds, despite adequate iodine intake. Researchers feel that there may be some environmental causes in addition to genetic causes (6). In third world countries, hypothyroidism continues to be a problem because of the deficient dietary intake of iodine.

Myxedema is the term used to describe an adult form of hypothyroidism. Women are affected more frequently, and the condition may occur following treatment for hyperthyroidism.

The clinical picture is characterized by a lower metabolic rate. The patient may gain weight, be mentally sluggish, become easily fatigued, manifest intolerance to cold, and be prone to constipation as a result of decreased gastrointestinal motility. Puffiness of the eyelids, face, and hands are usually noted due to edema caused by retention of hyaluronic acid (mucoprotein that binds the fluids in the skin) (7). Serum cholesterol and triglycerides may be elevated as a result of the decreased synthesis of fats.

Treatment for hypothyroidism involves lifelong hormone replacement and dietary management. Since the metabolic rate of the body is reduced, the kilocalories are generally limited, especially for those persons who are overweight. The diet should be well balanced, high in protein and fiber, low in carbohydrate and saturated fats, with adequate iodine intake. Fluid intake should be liberal (minimum of 2000 ml, unless contraindicated) in order to help prevent constipation and renal complications.

POSSIBLE NURSING DIAGNOSES

Potential alteration in nutrition; more than body requirements secondary to decreased metabolic demands of the body.

Alteration in elimination; constipation related to decreased gastrointestinal motility secondary to decreased metabolic activity and fluid retention in the tissues.

Knowledge deficit related to the decreased caloric needs of the body secondary to decreased metabolic activity.

Potential alteration in thought processes secondary to slowing of mental acuity and impaired memory.

NURSING INTERVENTIONS
FOR NUTRITIONAL DISORDERS

Work closely with the patient, dietitian, and physician to plan a diet that will meet the energy needs of the patient without causing weight gain.

Potential alteration in nutrition; more than body requirements secondary to decreased metabolic demands of the body.

- Instruct the patient regarding the importance of eating a well-balanced diet that will supply the needed energy. The diet should be high in protein and fiber, low in carbohydrate and saturated fat, with adequate iodine intake.
- Encourage the patient to eat five to six smaller meals per day to help prevent fatigue.
- Advise the patient to monitor weight. If weight gain is evident, caloric intake must be modified.
- Encourage the patient to use iodized salt.
- Advise the patient to limit the intake of goitrogenic foods such as those in the cabbage family.

Alteration in elimination; constipation related to decreased gastrointestinal motility secondary to decreased metabolic activity and fluid retention in the tissues.

- Encourage the patient to consume a high-fiber diet, including naturally laxative foods, such as bran, squash, and prunes, which will help stimulate peristalsis (refer to Chapter 7).

- Advise the patient to drink a minimum of 2000 ml per day (unless contraindicated) in order to prevent constipation.

Knowledge deficit related to the decreased caloric needs of the body secondary to decreased metabolic acitivity.

- Instruct the patient regarding the importance of eating a well-balanced diet that will supply the needed energy. The diet should be high in protein and fiber, low in carbohydrate and saturated fat, with adequate iodine intake.
- Encourage the patient to eat five to six smaller meals per day to help prevent fatigue.
- Advise the patient to monitor weight. If weight gain is evident, caloric intake must be modified.

Potential alteration in thought processes secondary to slowing of mental processes and impaired memory.

- Explain all instructions slowly and carefully, repeat as necessary. Validate all information given to the patient.
- Keep teaching sessions brief so as not to tire the patient.
- Provide written instructions regarding dietary information for easy reference.
- Instruct a family member as well as the patient, if at all possible.

ADRENAL DISORDERS

The adrenal glands are small but vital organs of the endocrine system. The glands are located in the retroperitoneal area (outside the peritoneum) and rest on the upper portion of each kidney. The cortex (outer portion) and the medulla (central portion) possess distinct physiological functions.

The medulla is responsible for secreting epinephrine and norepinephrine and helps to regulate the sympathetic nervous system. The cortical portion of the adrenal gland secretes glucocorticoids (cortisol), mineralocorticoids (aldosterone), and androgens (male sex hormones).

The hormones that are produced by the cortex are important in that they are involved in carbohydrate, protein, and fat metabolism. In addition, they help to determine how effectively the body can deal with stress situations such as infection and trauma.

The discussion in this section deals with alterations related to an excess secretion of cortical hormones (physiological or from exogenous forms such as steroid drugs), usually referred to as Cushing's syndrome, and deficiency of hormones, referred to as Addison's disease.

Cushing's Syndrome

Excess endogenous and exogenous (steroid drugs) forms of cortisol can precipitate Cushing's syndrome. Metabolism of carbohydrate, protein, and fat are affected. Increased carbohydrate metabolism produces a state of hyperglycemia that precipitates "steroid diabetes" (8). The hyperglycemia also results from a breakdown of protein so that the patient will manifest muscle wasting in the extremities as well as muscle weakness. The cause of the characteristic fat deposits, truncal obesity, and "buffalo hump" (fat pad across the shoulders) is unknown.

The characteristic "moon fact" that is due to extracellular fluid retention is the result of the sodium retaining effects of cortisol. The patient may also be predisposed to hypertension. Demineralization of the bone (loss of calcium), which can predispose to osteoporosis, may also be traced to the excess cortisol. Glucocorticoids interfere with vitamin D metabolism and upset calcium utilization by the body (9).

Dietary management is important for the patient with Cushing's syndrome or a patient who is being treated with corticosteroid drugs. The diet should be high in protein (at least one gram per kilogram per day) (10), low in carbohydrate (minimal quantities of simple carbohydrates), and low in cholesterol and sodium. Liberal amounts of potassium should be provided through incorporating meats, broths, fruits, and vegetables (including juices) into the diet as prescribed. Frequent, smaller meals (six to eight per day) may be beneficial, because hydrochloric acid secretion is increased when cortisol levels in the body are high. (Refer to Chapter 7 for a discussion of peptic ulcer management.) Foods containing calcium and vitamin D (such as milk), as well as oral supplements of these substances, may be prescribed for patients as corticosteroid therapy.

Ascorbic acid (vitamin C) is normally abundant in adrenal tissues. Corticosteroid therapy can deplete the stores of this vitamin in the tissues, and supplements may be prescribed.

POSSIBLE NURSING DIAGNOSES

Potential alteration in nutrition; less than body requirements related to disturbances in carbohydrate, protein, and fat metabolism.

Potential alteration in fluid volume; excess, related to increased amounts of sodium secondary to increased secretion of cortisol.

Potential for injury; pathological fractures (osteoporosis) related to altered calcium metabolism.

Knowledge deficit related to dietary management.

NURSING INTERVENTIONS FOR NUTRITIONAL DISORDERS

Work closely with the patient, dietitian, and physician to plan a diet that will complement the treatment regimen.

Potential alteration in nutrition; less than body requirements related to disturbances in carbohydrate, protein, and fat metabolism.

- Instruct the patient regarding the importance of adhering to the high-protein, low-carbohydrate, low-fat, low-cholesterol, and low-sodium diet in order to prevent the catabolic reactions and the complications associated with increased quantities of cortisol in the body.
- Advise the patient to avoid the use of concentrated sugars, because protein breakdown increases the available glucose and patients are frequently insensitive to insulin.
- Encourage the patient to consume liberal quantities of potassium-rich food (unless contraindicated), because of the loss of potassium associated with cortisol excess.
- Encourage the patient to eat several smaller meals per day (6-8) to reduce the risk of developing a peptic ulcer due to increased secretion of hydrochloric acid.

Potential alteration in fluid volume; excess related to increased amounts of sodium secondary to increased secretion of cortisol.

- Advise the patient to monitor body weight because of the extracellular fluid retention due to increased serum sodium. Notify the physician of weight gain over five pounds in one week.

- Caution the patient to adhere to the low-sodium diet to prevent further increases in serum sodium.
- Monitor blood pressure, since increases in blood pressure may indicate fluid retention.

Potential for injury; pathological fractures (osteoporosis) related to altered calcium metabolism.

- Instruct the patient to eat food rich in calcium and to take the prescribed supplements of calcium and vitamin D. Vitamin D is essential in calcium metabolism.

Knowledge deficit related to dietary management.

- Instruct the patient regarding the importance of adhering to the high-protein, low-carbohydrate, low-fat, low-cholesterol, and low-sodium diet in order to prevent the catabolic reactions and the complications associated with increased quantities of cortisol in the body.
- Instruct the patient to eat foods that are rich in vitamin C (see Chapter 2) in order to aid the body in the process of tissue healing and repair. A vitamin supplement may be prescribed.

Adrenal Insufficiency (Addison's disease)

Decreased production of glucocorticoids and mineralocorticoids can lead to Addison's disease, a complex metabolic disorder. Mineralocorticoid (aldosterone) deficiency results in decreased sodium absorption and can lead to excessive losses of sodium, chloride, and water through the urine, feces, and skin. Consequently, extracellular fluids are lost, acidosis develops, and serum potassium levels rise. If the process is not reversed, blood volume will be lost and cardiac output will decrease.

Deficiency of cortisol makes it almost impossible for the body to synthesize sufficient quantities of glucose, and severe hypoglycemia results. Weight loss, muscle wasting, anorexia, and fatigue are apparent, because the body attempts to use protein and fat for the needed glucose.

Treatment centers around lifelong hormone replacement. Dietary management is essential in conjunction with hormonal therapy. The diet should be designed to prevent hypoglycemic reactions (see discussion of hypoglycemia in this chapter). In order to maintain a more stable blood-sugar level, it is important for the patient to eat at least six meals and a late bedtime snack. All feedings should contain a mixture of protein, carbohydrate, and fat for more gradual glucose release. No meals should be skipped, and the person should carry a snack, such as fruit and nuts or cheese and crackers, at all times.

Large quantities of fluids should be consumed to maintain extracellular and intravascular fluid volume to prevent dehydration. Salt tablets may be prescribed in addition to eating highly salted foods. Special attention must be focused on potential fluid losses during periods of hot weather or during illness involving fever, vomiting, or diarrhea. Aldosterone may be necessary for some patient to maintain electrolyte balance.

Oral corticosteroid preparations should be taken with food, milk, or antacids to prevent gastric irritation by the drug. Patients on long-term drug therapy can develop Cushing's-like symptoms. (Refer to the discussion of Cushing's syndrome in this chapter.)

Supplements of vitamins B-complex and C may be needed to support the increased metabolic activity. Potassium supplements may also be required for some patients. Hyperkalemia or hypokalemia occurs in some patients; therefore, it is important to monitor blood chemistries and give increased amounts of potassium only when prescribed. (Food sources of potassium are detailed in Chapter 9.)

POSSIBLE NURSING DIAGNOSES

Potential alteration in nutrition; less than body requirements related to anorexia, nausea, and increased nutrient metabolism.

Potential fluid-volume deficit related to excessive losses of sodium and water secondary to polyuria, increased perspiration, and diarrhea.

Potential alteration in bowel elimination; diarrhea related to increased excretion of sodium and water.

Knowledge deficit related to
- dietary management.
- effects of drug therapy on food intake.

NURSING INTERVENTIONS FOR NUTRITIONAL DISORDERS

Work closely with the patient, dietitian, and physician to plan a diet that will complement the treatment regimen.

Potential alteration in nutrition; less than body requirements related to anorexia, nausea, and increased nutrient metabolism.

- Instruct the patient to:
  eat a diet that is similar to that described for the patient with hypoglycemia;

  carry a snack containing carbohydrate, protein, and fat at all times;

  eat six smaller meals and a large bedtime snack to provide for a more equal distribution of glucose throughout the day to prevent hypoglycemic reactions;

  eat all meals—do not skip a meal.

Potential fluid-volume deficit related to excessive losses of sodium and water secondary to polyuria, increased perspiration, and diarrhea.

- Instruct the patient to:
  drink large quantities of fluids (2000-3000 ml per day) to prevent dehydration;

  monitor intake and output, especially during periods of hot weather or during illness involving fever, vomiting, or diarrhea;

  eat highly salted foods and take salt tablets as prescribed to replace sodium and chloride losses.

- Assess tissue turgor to note signs of dehydration.
- Monitor blood pressure to note signs of dehydration.

- Monitor laboratory reports; note serum sodium and potassium levels to determine electrolyte balance.

Potential alteration in bowel elimination; diarrhea related to increased excretion of sodium and water.

- Instruct the patient to:
  monitor fluid losses resulting from diarrhea;

  replace fluids liberally (2000-3000 ml)—fluid output should equal fluid intake.

Knowledge deficit related to
- **dietary management.**
- **effects of drug therapy on food intake.**

Instruct the patient to:
eat a diet that is similar to that described for the patient with hypoglycemia;

eat all meals—do not skip a meal;

carry a snack at all times;

eat highly salted food and take salt substitutes as prescribed;

take vitamin supplements as prescribed because of increased metabolic activity;

take corticosteroid preparation with food, milk, or an antacid to prevent gastric irritation;

monitor weight pattern—weight loss may be indicative of inadequate control and weight gain may be indicative of fluid retention related to corticosteroid drug therapy.

PARATHYROID DISORDERS

The parathyroid glands are responsible for the calcium regulation throughout the body. Calcium is necessary for bone formation, maintaining contractility of cardiac and skeletal muscles, transmitting nerve impulses, and coagulation of blood.

Hypercalcemia

Hyperactivity of the parathyroid glands may be related to a number of disorders. Chronic elevation of the serum calcium level may be associated with chronic renal disease, pregnancy, hyperthyroidism, genetic mutations, and bone disorders including carcinoma (11). Vitamin D intoxication and increased consumption of antacids and milk associated with peptic-ulcer treatment may predispose to milk-alkali syndrome (see Chapter 7) and lead to increased blood levels of calcium (10).

Symptoms and clinical manifestations of hypercalcemia are related to the effect of the increased action of the parathyroid hormone on the bone, kidney, and gastrointestinal tissues (8). Bone resorption occurs that can lead to osteoporosis and pathological fractures (see discussion in this chapter). Increased serum calcium levels can predispose to renal calculi formation (see Chapter 8) and to decreased gastrointestinal motility. Bradycardia (slow pulse rate) may be apparent as conduction mechanisms in the heart are disturbed.

Treatment involves determining the underlying cause and providing the appropriate therapy. Dietary management includes a number of prophylactic measures to prevent complications associated with increased levels of serum calcium. Phosphates may be given in an oral or intravenous form to stimulate calcium deposit in the bony tissues. Liberal fluid intake is required (2000-3000 ml per day) in addition to an acid-ash diet, to help prevent the formation of calcium-base renal stones (see Chapter 8).

POSSIBLE NURSING DIAGNOSES

Potential fluid-volume deficit related to the need for forcing fluids to prevent renal calculi formation.

Potential alteration in elimination; constipation related to decreased gastrointestinal motility.

Knowledge deficit related to the dietary restrictions needed to prevent renal calculi and constipation.

NURSING INTERVENTIONS FOR NUTRITIONAL DISORDERS

Work closely with the patient, dietitian, and physician to plan the dietary interventions that may be important in the treatment of hypercalcemia.

Potential fluid-volume deficit related to the need for forcing fluids to prevent renal calculi formation.

Continued

NURSING INTERVENTIONS *(continued)*

- Instruct the patient to:

  drink at least 2000-3000 ml fluid per day;

  monitor intake and output;

  note signs of hematuria, which may be indicative of renal calculi formation.

Potential alteration in elimination: constipation related to decreased gastrointestinal motility.

- Instruct the patient to:

  drink at least 2000-3000 ml fluid per day;

  increase fiber-rich foods in the diet.

(Refer to Chapter 7 for additional suggested interventions to prevent constipation.)

Knowledge deficit related to the dietary restrictions needed to prevent renal calculi and constipation.

- Instruct the patient in the importance of consistent, liberal fluid intake and increasing the amount of fiber in the diet.
- Instruct the patient in the importance of following the acid-ash diet, if prescribed.

Hypocalcemia

Low serum levels of calcium may occur because of an inadequate amount of parathyroid hormone. The most frequent cause of hypocalcemia is the inadvertent removal of or damage to the parathyroid glands during thyroid surgery (12).

Symptoms of hypocalcemia include those related to neuromuscular dysfunction; muscle twitching and cramps as well as convulsions may occur, and the advanced stages are referred to as tetany. Bone-related problems can also develop due to defective bone formation, and this may lead to osteomalacia in adults and rickets in children.

Dental abnormalities may also be attributed to decreased levels of serum calcium.

Treatment involves replacement of parathyroid hormone as well as dietary emphasis on a high calcium diet with supplements of vitamin D to help in the absorption and storage of calcium in the body. Patients who suffer from lactose intolerance may require calcium supplements if no milk products, which are excellent sources of calcium, are not well tolerated. Some milk products such as cheese and yogurt may be better tolerated by these individuals than fluid milk.

POSSIBLE NURSING DIAGNOSES

Alteration in nutrition: less than body requirements related to low serum calcium levels secondary to inadequate parathyroid hormone.

Knowledge deficit related to:
- dietary management;
- effect of drug therapy on food intake.

NURSING INTERVENTIONS FOR NUTRITIONAL DISORDERS

Work closely with the patient, dietitian, and physician to plan a diet that will help to meet the calcium demands of the body.

Alteration in nutrition; less than body requirements related to low serum-calcium levels secondary to inadequate parathyroid hormone.

- Instruct the patient to:
  eat a diet that is high in calcium (see Chapter 2 for a discussion of calcium sources);

  have high-calcium snacks readily available;

  eat foods containing vitamin D to enhance the absorption of calcium in the intestine and to promote storage in the bones.

Knowledge deficit related to
- **dietary management.**
- **effect of drug therapy on food intake.**

- Instruct the patient to avoid taking calcium supplements with whole-grain cereals, breads, fresh fruits, and vegetables to allow for optimum absorption (13).
- Advise the patient to refrain from taking milk or antacids with calcium supplements to prevent milk-alkali syndrome.
- Monitor laboratory reports to note serum calcium levels.

JOINT AND BONE DISORDERS

Rheumatic diseases, which include arthritis and gout (gouty arthritis), are among a number of acute and chronic disorders that affect the joints, skin, and connective tissues of the body. This discussion focuses on nutritional alterations related to arthritis (rheumatoid, osteoarthritis, and gout) and osteoporosis. Osteoporosis can evolve from a number of metabolic disturbances in the body and frequently occurs concurrently with arthritis due to a lack of exercise.

Arthritis

Arthritis (inflammation of the joints) is a common disorder. Osteoarthritis, the most common form of arthritis, is usually limited to finger joints and weight-bearing joints (hips, knees, and spine) (14). This form of arthritis is frequently considered to be degenerative and associated with normal wear and tear on joints or following injury to a joint (Figure 14-1).

Rheumatoid arthritis is a systemic and puzzling form of arthritis. In addition to joint involvement, damage may occur to the skin, muscles, lungs, blood vessels, and nerves. (See in Figure 14-2.) The cause of rheumatoid arthritis is unknown; however, there may be a genetic link to the disease. Researchers have discovered a genetic marker (tissue type) in persons with rheumatoid arthritis. Some persons who possess that tissue type do develop rheumatoid arthritis in the future (15).

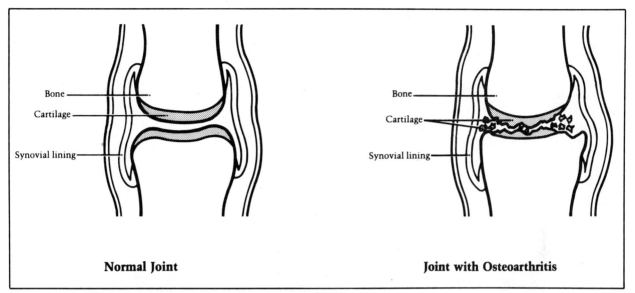

Figure 14-1. A normal joint versus a joint with osteoarthritis.
(From "Osteoarthritis," No. 4040 (Atlanta: Arthritis Foundation, 1986), reprinted with permission.)

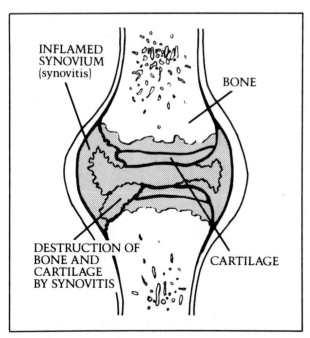

Figure 14-2. Destruction caused by rheumatoid arthritis. (From "Rheumatoid Arthritis," No. 4020 (Atlanta: Arthritis Foundation, 1985), reprinted with permission.)

Treatment protocols involve a combination of rest, exercise, and joint protection; control of pain and inflammation through the use of drugs; and surgical intervention for replacement of severely damaged, unstable joints. Much interest and controversy have centered around the dietary management of arthritis. At this time, there is no indication that special diets or supplements are of value, either in determining causative factors or cures for arthritis (16).

Nutritional recommendations for patients with arthritis include instructions to the patient to maintain ideal body weight; eat a balanced diet that includes a variety of nutrients and that is low in simple carbohydrates (sugars), fat, cholesterol, and sodium; consume only moderate amounts of alcohol; and include foods that will help to maintain the integrity of the immune system (16, 17, 18). Because arthritis patients take a number of drugs that can irritate the gastrointestinal tract (aspirin and nonsteroidal antiinflammatory agents) the patient is advised to take these drugs with food or at mealtime to reduce the potential side effects (nausea, vomiting, heartburn, or indigestion). Patients who take corticosteroid drugs may be prone to retain sodium and manifest edema and weight gain (refer to the discussion of corticosteroid drugs in this chapter).

Some of the slower acting antiarthritic drugs can also predispose a patient to a number of problems that may have an impact on nutritional status. Penicillamine may produce stomatitis (inflamma-tion of the mouth) and loss of taste; cytotoxic drugs can also lead to stomatitis.

Many patients with rheumatoid arthritis may have a problem with the mandibular (jaw) joints, which makes chewing difficult. The consistency of foods may need to be altered, and soft or blended foods may need to be substituted to enable the person to consume adequate nutrients.

POSSIBLE NURSING DIAGNOSES

Potential knowledge deficit related to the
- need to consume a balanced diet, low in simple carbohydrate, fat, and cholesterol, and low in sodium;
- need to maintain an ideal body weight to prevent stress on the affected joints;
- effect of drug therapy on food intake;
- need to adhere to a low kilocalorie diet to prevent stress on the affected joints (if overweight);
- myths associated with dietary management or unproven dietary cures.

NURSING INTERVENTIONS FOR NUTRITIONAL DISORDERS

Work closely with the patient, dietitian, and physician to plan a diet that will enhance the therapeutic regimen.

Potential knowledge deficit related to the
- **need to consume a balanced diet, low in simple carbohydrate, fat, and cholesterol, and low in sodium.**
- **need to maintain an ideal body weight to prevent stress on the affected joints.**
- **effect of drug therapy on food intake.**
- **need to adhere to a low kilocalorie diet to prevent stress on the affected joints (if overweight).**
- **myths associated with dietary management or unproven dietary cures.**

- Instruct the patient to:
  eat a balanced diet;

  maintain ideal body weight to prevent stress on the joints;

Continued

NURSING INTERVENTIONS *(continued)*

follow the diet prescription for lower intake of simple carbohydrate, fat, and cholesterol, if indicated:

restrict sodium intake, as prescribed, if taking corticosteroid drugs to prevent fluid retention;

avoid consuming caffeine-containing products (coffee, tea, chocolate, or colas) or alcoholic beverages before bedtime to enhance the quality of sleep (19);

take aspirin or nonsteroidal antiinflammatory drugs with food or at mealtime to prevent gastric irritation.

- Discuss the importance of modifying the consistency of the food (blend or use liquid supplements) if chewing food becomes difficult.

- Arrange for a physical or occupational therapy consultation to secure self-help feeding devices, if involvement of the joints of the hands makes it impossible for the patient to hold conventional feeding utensils.
- Arrange for a consultation with the dietitian and/or physical or occupational therapist for suggestions regarding ease of food preparation (peeling, slicing, sitting versus standing, etc.).
- Stress the importance of consulting with the physician before altering the diet in response to supposed dietary cures or supplements. For example, taking vitamin-D supplements can lead to vitamin intoxication, and eliminating foods such as those in the nightshade family (potatoes, tomatoes, and green peppers) deprives the body of vitamin C, which is important in the healing of tissues.

Gout

The family of rheumatic diseases includes gout, the only form of arthritis that can be controlled. Gout is a disease in which the purine (protein) metabolism of the body is altered and the by-product, uric acid, is increased in the bloodstream (hyperuricemia). When uric acid is excreted by the kidney, crystals form; these crystals may then be deposited in the tissues of the body. When the needlelike crystals are deposited in the joints, inflammation occurs; this deposit in the joint is referred to as a tophus (see Figure 14-3). The great toe (bunion) joint is one of the most frequently involved; however, any of the joints of the body may be affected (20).

Attacks of gout may occur suddenly (within hours), as compared with other forms of arthritis

that are slow and insidious in onset. In between attacks, the patient may have no signs or symptoms of joint inflammation. Repeated attacks may lead to joint destruction.

The treatment regimen, which includes drug therapy and emphasis on dietary management, will not cure gout but may help to control the disease process and allow the patient to remain in remission for long periods. Drug therapy has become increasingly important, because drugs like probenecid block the reabsorption of uric acid in the kidney tubules and allopurinol, reducing the production of uric acid in the body.

Dietary management (low-purine diet) may be used as an adjunct to help reduce the exogenous (dietary) sources of purines. The diet usually contains liberal amounts of carbohydrate (100 g per

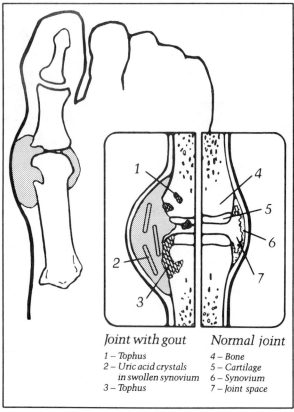

Joint with gout
1 – Tophus
2 – Uric acid crystals
    in swollen synovium
3 – Tophus

Normal joint
4 – Bone
5 – Cartilage
6 – Synovium
7 – Joint space

Figure 14-3. Comparison of a joint with gout and a normal joint.
(From "Gout," No. 4180 (Atlanta: Arthritis Foundation, 1982), reprinted with permission.)

day) and is low in fat and moderate in protein (10). Foods that are high in purine content, such as organ meats, meat extracts (broth, gravy, consomme), and shellfish (shrimp) are omitted. Protein intake is essential but should be restricted. Sources such as skim milk, cheese, and eggs are recommended. Meat intake should be limited (10).

Even though it has been found that alcohol does not precipitate an acute attack of gout, alcoholic-beverage intake should be maintained at a minimal to moderate level. Alcohol does increase uric acid production (10).

Fluid intake should be increased to a minimum of 2000–3000 ml per day. The dilute urine will help in the excretion of uric acid and prevent the settling of uric acid crystals within the urinary tract (uric acid calculi).

Maintaining ideal body weight can help to reduce the stress to the joints. Obese patients are instructed to follow a weight-reduction diet.

POSSIBLE NURSING DIAGNOSES

Potential knowledge deficit related to
- dietary management; low purine diet and/or weight-reduction diet to prevent stress on joints.
- effect of drug therapy on food intake.
- reducing or restricting alcohol intake to prevent formation of uric acid.

Potential fluid-volume deficit related to urinary calculi formation secondary to hyperuricemia.

NURSING INTERVENTIONS FOR NUTRITIONAL DISORDERS

Work closely with the patient, dietitian, and physician to plan a diet that will enhance the therapeutic regimen.

Potential knowledge deficit related to
- **dietary management, low-purine diet and weight-reduction diet to prevent stress on joints.**
- **effect of drug therapy on food intake.**
- **reducing or restricting alcohol intake to prevent formation of uric acid.**

- Instruct the patient to:

  follow the purine-restricted diet as prescribed to reduce uric-acid levels in the body;

  avoid fasting, because ketoacids formed by oxidation of fats encourage the body to retain urates;

  restrict alcohol intake as prescribed to prevent additional formation of uric acid;

  take medications with food or at mealtime to prevent gastric irritation.

Potential fluid-volume deficit related to urinary calculi formation secondary to hyperuricemia.

- Caution the patient to drink at least 2000–3000 ml of fluid per day to maintain a dilute urine in order to prevent the formation of uric acid calculi in the urinary tract.

Osteoporosis

When the rate of bone resorption exceeds the rate of bone formation, osteoporosis develops. Demineralization causes the bone to become porous and lose strength. The major clinical problem that can result is fractures, especially among the elderly (21).

Osteoporosis affects women more often than men. It is estimated that possibly half of all women in the United States over the age of 45 suffer from osteoporosis (22). A person who is thin with a small body build is also at risk. Steroid drugs, as well as aluminum-based antacids, may also predispose to osteoporosis by interfering with calcium metabolism. Prolonged immobilization, due to illness or lack of exercise can lead to bone demineralization.

It is obvious that many factors are involved in the development of osteoporosis. Researchers have not identified one single agent as the cause, but a number of factors seem to be involved. The decrease of hormone levels after menopause (estrogen in women and androgens in men) can lead to increased bone loss, but there may also be defects within the bone cells that influence the abnormal cellular activity (9, 21).

Treatment protocols involve prevention as a primary goal. In order to prevent osteoporosis in later life, it is beneficial to consume adequate amounts of calcium throughout life. Dietary management is an important aspect of the treatment. It has been suggested that calcium intake should be increased to 1500 mg, especially in postmenopausal women (21). The use of liberal quantities of milk and dairy products in the diet is essential; for example, an eight-ounce glass of milk contains approximately 300 mg of calcium (22). Calcium supplements may be required for some patients.

Vitamin D is essential for the utilization of calcium. Many of the elderly may be housebound and unable to receive the vitamin through the beneficial rays of the sun. Food sources of vitamin D are limited; therefore, supplements may be prescribed. Because vitamin D is a fat-soluble vitamin, careful monitoring of supplementation is required to avoid problems with toxicity (see Chapter 2).

Researchers found that persons who live in regions where the fluoride levels of the water are high have less incidence of osteoporosis, since fluoride seems to strengthen bone structure. Research is continuing in this area, because treatment costs could be minimal to add fluoride to a water system.

Caffeine, tobacco, and alcohol all have negative effects on calcium metabolism. The patient should be advised to limit the use of coffee, tea, colas, and chocolate. Alcoholic beverage intake should be limited to two drinks per day (21, 22).

High-fiber diets may bind calcium and decrease its absorption (10, 13). The patient should be advised to refrain from drinking milk and taking dietary supplements at mealtime, in order to obtain maximum absorption.

POSSIBLE NURSING DIAGNOSES

Potential alteration in nutrition; less than body requirements of calcium related to decreased dietary intake of calcium and vitamin D.

Potential for injury; fractures related to porous bone.

Knowledge deficit related to
- nutritional therapy.
- effect of drug therapy on food intake.

NURSING INTERVENTIONS FOR NUTRITIONAL DISORDERS

Work closely with the patient, dietitian, and physician to plan a diet that will enhance calcium metabolism in the body.

Potential alteration in nutrition; less than body requirements of calcium related to decreased dietary intake of calcium and vitamin D.

- Instruct the patient to:
  eat a balanced diet with sufficient kilocalories to maintain ideal body weight;

  include milk and dairy products in the diet to increase calcium intake.

Continued

NURSING INTERVENTIONS *(continued)*

Potential for injury; fractures related to porous bone.

- Instruct the patient to increase dietary calcium intake.
- Encourage the patient to exercise utilizing gravity (walk or swim) a minimum of three times per week to increase bone density.

Knowledge deficit related to
- **nutritional therapy.**
- **effect of drug therapy on food intake.**

- Instruct the patient to:
  eat a balanced diet with sufficient kilocalories to maintain ideal body weight;

  include milk and dairy products in the diet to increase calcium intake;

  take vitamin-D supplement as prescribed or get the vitamin through sunshine, in order to enhance calcium absorption;

  avoid the intake of large amounts of caffeine and alcohol, because these substances interfere with calcium metabolism;

  limit alcoholic beverage intake to two drinks per day.

- Caution patients who may be taking steroid preparations that these drugs may predispose to bone demineralization.
- Advise patients not to take aluminum-based antacids without physician knowledge. Aluminum can lead to altered calcium metabolism and bone demineralization.
- Instruct the patient to avoid taking a calcium supplement with whole-grain cereals, breads, fresh fruits, and vegetables to allow for optimum absorption (13).
- Encourage patients to drink liberal quantities of fluid, at least 2000 ml per day, to prevent formation of renal calculi.

TOPIC OF INTEREST

A supplement commonly used to increase calcium intake in postmenopausal women is calcium carbonate. For calcium to be absorbed, it must be in a soluble state. Gastric acid increases the solubility of calcium complexes. Although, generally, calcium supplements should be taken in the fasting state to enhance absorption, there is a major exception. Acid output by the stomach decreases with age, particularly after age 60, and the incidence of achlorhydria increases with age. As a result, absorption of calcium carbonate is decreased. It has been shown, contrary to usual recommendations, that in achlorhydric individuals, the calcium-carbonate supplement is better absorbed when taken with meals rather than in the fasting state (23).

SPOTLIGHT ON LEARNING

Adele Simpson is a 68-year old woman who was admitted with a fractured right femur. She fell at home, while she was making dinner. The fracture was pinned, and she has been in the orthopedic unit for the past two days.

Adele is undergoing an intensive rehabilitation program including physical therapy. The dietitian has completed a nutrition assessment. You note that the assessment indicates that Adele eats very few dairy products. She states, "I never liked to drink milk." The history and physical examination indicate that the fracture was probably the result of osteoporosis.

During the bath this morning, Adele asks you several questions about her condition. She wants to know how she could break her hip at her age. The doctor mentioned that her bones were "brittle" and she would have to work on increasing the strength of the bones. She tells you, "I'm too old to start improving the condition of my bones now!"

1. How can you respond to Adele's questions and comments?
2. What response can you make to Adele as to why it may have been possible for her to break her hip?
3. Identify measures that Adele might use to increase the strength of her bones. How might dietary modifications be of benefit to her? What foods should be included in her diet?
4. Adele stated that she does not like to drink milk. Share some ideas with her as to how she might increase the calcium content of her diet.
5. What is the relationship between vitamin D and calcium intake?

REVIEW QUESTIONS

1. Clara Smith, age 48, has been recently diagnosed as having a thyroid deficiency (simple goiter). Which of the following nutrients will most likely be deficient?
   a. calcium
   b. sodium
   c. iodine
   d. potassium

2. Ingestion of large amounts of which of the following foods may decrease thyroxine production in the body?
   a. melon
   b. corn
   c. milk
   d. cabbage

3. Mr. Peters will be taking prednisone for treatment of Addison's disease. Diet instruction regarding this drug should not include which of the following?
   a. administer with food or milk
   b. restrict salt intake
   c. encourage intake of food high in potassium
   d. notify the physician if gastrointestinal upset occurs

4. Ms. Jenner's parathyroid glands were inadvertently removed during thyroid surgery. Which of the following nutrients will most likely be deficient?
   a. calcium
   b. sodium
   c. iodine
   d. potassium

5. Which of the following is usually not used to treat osteoporosis?
   a. increased calcium intake
   b. increased fluid intake (two to three liters per day)
   c. regular exercise
   d. increased rest periods

6. An arthritic patient who is taking large doses of aspirin for relief of pain needs to increase the amount of vitamin C in the diet. Which of the following foods is not a good source of vitamin C?
   a. corn on the cob
   b. broccoli
   c. green peppers
   d. potatoes

7. Persons with gout are frequently asked to reduce the intake of purine-rich foods. Which of the following sources of protein should not be omitted?
   a. cheese
   b. liver
   c. sardines
   d. shrimp

8. Which of the following dietary guidelines should not be followed by persons suffering from hypoglycemia (hyperinsulinism)?
   a. eat six smaller meals per day
   b. consume a high-simple-carbohydrate, low-protein diet
   c. restrict intake of alcoholic beverages
   d. use complex carbohydrate in place of simple carbohydrate foods

9. Which of the following dietary guidelines is not included for a patient with hypothyroidism?
   a. use iodized salt
   b. eat five to six smaller meals per day to prevent fatigue
   c. include foods such as cabbage, peanuts and turnips to increase fiber
   d. monitor weight gain

10. Which of the following menu selections would indicate that the patient understood diet therapy principles related to treatment of osteoporosis?
   a. fried chicken, cole slaw, fresh apple, coffee
   b. broiled chicken, broccoli, pineapple and cottage-cheese salad, skim milk
   c. braised liver and onions, baby carrots, tossed salad, diet cola
   d. spareribs with sauerkraut, mashed potatoes, carrot-raisin salad, iced tea

ACTIVITIES

1. A 20-year-old college student has recently been diagnosed as hypoglycemic due to hyperinsulinism. He asks you to help him plan his diet, which should include 100 g (or less) of carbohydrate. Use the exchange list in Chapter 13 to assist you.

2. Endemic goiter has been virtually eliminated in the United States. Identify factors that have contributed to this. List foods that are good sources of iodine. Identify foods that can inhibit the use of iodine by the thyroid gland.

3. Describe the dietary modifications that will be required by the patient who will be taking corticosteroid drugs for the long-term management of arthritis symptoms.

4. Explain the nutritional implications of prolonged immobility associated with an extensive neuromuscular injury involving paralysis of the lower extremities.

5. Compare the dietary modifications that may be required for a young, thin person who suffers from rheumatoid arthritis and an elderly, obese person who has osteoarthritis of the spine.

REFERENCES

1. Fishbain, D.A., and D. Rotundo. Frequency of hypoglycemic delirium in a psychiatric emergency service. *Psychodynamics* 29 (1988):346–48.
2. Hershman, J.M. *Endocrine pathophysiology: A patient-centered approach.* 2d ed. Philadelphia: Lea & Febiger, 1982.
3. Robinson, C.H., et al. *Normal and therapeutic nutrition.* New York: Macmillan Publishing Company, 1986.
4. Lewis, S.M., and I.C. Collier. *Medical-surgical nursing: Assessment and management of clinical problems.* New York: The McGraw-Hill Book Company, 1987.
5. Riokees, S.A., H.H. Bode, and J.D. Crawford. Long-term growth in juvenile acquired hypothyroidism: The failure to achieve normal adult stature. *New England Journal of Medicine* 318 (1988):599–602.

6. Ziporyn, T. For many, endemic goiter remains a baffling problem. *Journal of the American Medical Association* 253 (1985):1846–47.

7. Bullock, B.L., and P.P. Rosendahl. *Pathophysiology: adaptations and alterations in function*, 2d ed. Glenview, IL: Scott, Foresman and Company, 1988.

8. Thompson, J.M., et al. *Clinical nursing*. St. Louis: The C.V. Mosby Company, 1986.

9. Raisz, L.G. Local and systemic factors in the pathogenesis of osteoporosis. *New England Journal of Medicine* 318 (1988):818–28.

10. Krause, M.V., and L.K. Mahan. *Food, nutrition and diet therapy: A textbook of nutritional care*. Philadelphia: W.B. Saunders Company, 1984.

11. Marx, S.J. Genetic defects in primary hyperparathyroidism. *New England Journal of Medicine* 318 (1988):699–701.

12. Brasier, A.R., and S.R. Nussbaum. Hungry bone syndrome:Clinical and biochemical predictions of its occurrence after parathyroid surgery. *American Journal of Medicine* 84 (1988):654–60.

13. Baer, C.L., and B.R. Williams. *Clinical pharmacology and nursing*. Springhouse: Springhouse Publishing Company, 1988.

14. Kushner, I., ed. *Understanding arthritis*. New York: Charles Scribner's Sons, 1984.

15. Pinals, R.S., and N.J. Zvaifler. *Arthritis medical information series: Rheumatoid arthritis*. 2d ed. Atlanta: Arthritis Foundation, 1987.

16. Panush, R., and R. Kimberly. *Arthritis diet guidelines and research*. Atlanta: Arthritis Foundation, 1987.

17. Kowsari, B., et al. Assessment of the diet of patients with rheumatoid arthritis and osteoarthritis. *Journal of the American Dietetic Association* 82 (1983):657–59.

18. Kremer, J.M., et al. Effects of manipulation of dietary fatty acids on clinical manifestations of rheumatoid arthritis. *Lancet* 1 (1985):184–87.

19. "News afp." Many factors affect quality of life for arthritis patients. *American Family Physician* 38 (1988):273–77.

20. Healey, L.A., and S.L. Wallace. *Arthritis medical information series: Gout*. Atlanta: Arthritis Foundation, 1986.

21. Fish, H.R., and R.F. Dons. Primary osteoporosis. *American Family Physician* 31 (1985):216–23.

22. Carpenter, J.R., and J.R.P. Tesser. *Arthritis medical information series: Osteoporosis*. Atlanta: Arthritis Foundation, 1987.

23. Recker, R.R. Calcium absorption and achlorhydria. *New England Journal of Medicine* 313 (1985):70–73.

CHAPTER

15

NUTRITION AND THE PATIENT WITH EATING DISORDERS

Objectives

After studying this chapter, you will be able to
- identify the determinants of energy balance.
- define obesity, anorexia nervosa, and bulimia.
- describe the major intervention methods for the treatment of obesity.
- list the criteria for diagnosis of anorexia nervosa and bulimia.
- identify dietary interventions for obesity, anorexia nervosa, and bulimia.
- identify nursing interventions for nutritional disorders associated with obesity, anorexia nervosa, and bulimia.

Overview

We live in a society preoccupied with our eating patterns. Diet books often make the best-seller lists, and advertisements for simple solutions for weight control abound. In this chapter, an overview of energy balance is presented, and treatment approaches for obesity, anorexia nervosa, and bulimia are discussed to enable you to help patients separate fact from fiction in the field of eating disorders.

ENERGY BALANCE

Kilocalorie Intake

Kilocalorie intake is determined by the food we eat. More specifically, it is determined by the protein, fat, carbohydrate, and alcohol content of the food. Fat is the most dense source of kilocalories, followed closely by alcohol (Table 15-1). Contrary to popular belief, vitamins and minerals do not contribute to caloric intake.

Food intake is regulated by complex and incompletely understood physiological and psychological factors. The master control of appetite is the hypothalamus, which responds to various body stimuli, including chemical and hormonal signals (1). The role of the hypothalamus in intake regulation was delineated by classic studies of feeding behavior in rats. Destruction of the ventromedial hypothalamus (VMH) resulted in hyperphagia and an increase in fat stores. The VMH has, therefore, been called the satiety center. Destruction of the lateral hypothalamus (LH) resulted in a cessation of eating behavior to the point of starvation and a decrease in fat stores. As a result, the LH is referred to as the feeding center, although this is a misnomer because it has been learned that the LH is involved in all motivated behavior, including the maternal instinct, muscular activity, and thirst. It appears that the centers are never inactive but respond more or less vigorously depending on the body state.

Theories have evolved regarding the action of body chemicals and hormones on the hypothalamus. One theory emphasizes the presence of a glucose receptor, possibly the VMH, in the brain. The VMH is insulin-sensitive and appears to monitor the availability of and the body's ability to use glucose. An increase in blood glucose (which occurs after eating) stimulates the VMH and inhibits the nerve fibers in the LH (the feeding center) from firing. Low glucose levels are suspected to inhibit the VMH signals and stimulate the LH to initiate feeding behavior. Neurotransmitters may also be involved in regulating food intake. Hypothalamic infusions of norepinephrine have been found to increase food intake and fat stores, and drugs that block serotonin increase food intake and body weight (2).

Psychological and social factors also play a role in food intake. Some individuals turn to food to deal with loneliness, anger, guilt, and happiness. Also, many of our social customs revolve around eating. (See Chapter 1 for a discussion of the impact of various factors on food intake.)

Kilocalorie Expenditure

Kilocalorie expenditure includes basal metabolism, physical activity, and diet-induced thermogenesis. Basal metabolism energy needs are influenced by body size and composition, which are determined by gender and age. The greater the body size, the greater the energy needed for basal metabolism because there is a greater amount of body tissue to maintain. Muscle requires greater energy for tissue integrity than does fat, so that individuals with a higher proportion of muscle

Table 15-1. KILOCALORIES IN MACRONUTRIENTS

MACRONUTRIENT	KILOCALORIES/GRAM
Protein	4
Carbohydrate	4
Fat	9
Alcohol	7

have an increased basal metabolism. Females usually have a smaller body size than males and a higher proportion of body fat. Their basal-metabolic needs are, therefore, less than those for males. As we age, the ratio of lean tissue to fat tissue declines, resulting in a lower basal-metabolic rate (BMR). After 20 years of age, the approximate rate of decline in BMR is 2% per decade.

Basal needs are also influenced by the environment and physiological state. Environmental extremes influence the amount of kilocalories expended to keep the body at a constant temperature. In the United States, the environment does not play a significant role in basal-metabolic needs for the majority of individuals because we compensate for lower or higher temperatures by heating or air-conditioning our homes, cars, and working environments. The physiological state of the individual can alter metabolic needs considerably. The energy needs of burn victims are extremely high as a result of the energy cost of tissue repair. The greater body surface area affected, the greater the kilocalorie needs. Fever also increases basal metabolism because much energy is expended as heat. For each single degree rise in temperature above 98.6°F, the body's metabolic rate increases 7%. (Refer to Chapter 6 for a discussion of physiological stress.) Cancer patients can have higher or lower metabolic rates and, therefore, require continuous assessment (see Chapter 12).

Physical activity is variable from individual to individual, and is under our direct control. (See Table 15-2.) As with BMR, body size contributes to the kilocalories expended during exercise. Individuals of greater body weight expend more energy doing weight-bearing exercises than individuals of

Table 15-2. CALORIC COST OF PHYSICAL ACTIVITY

ACTIVITY	MALE (155 lbs.)	FEMALE (115 lbs.)
	kilocalories/minute	
Sleeping, reading	1.0–1.2	0.9–1.1
Very light Seated and standing activities, auto and truck driving, lab work, typing, sewing, ironing, playing musical instruments	up to 2.5	up to 2.0
Light Walking on level, 2.5–3 mph, tailoring, pressing, garage work, electrical trades, carpentry, restaurant trades, cannery workers, washing clothes, shopping with light load, golf, sailing, table tennis, volleyball	2.5–4.9	2.0–3.9
Moderate Walking 3.5–4 mph, plastering, weeding and hoeing, loading and stacking bales, scrubbing floors, shopping with heavy load, cycling, skiing, tennis, dancing	5.0–7.4	4.0–5.9
Heavy Walking with load uphill, tree felling, work with pick and shovel, basketball, swimming, climbing, football	7.5–12.0	6.0–10.0

Source: FDA Consumer, June 1984.

normal weight because it takes more energy to move a greater mass. Some research findings support a positive effect of physical activity on BMR that extends beyond the exercising period itself.

Diet-induced thermogenesis is the third factor that determines energy expenditure. It includes the energy expended in the digestion and absorption of food and amounts to approximately 10% of the total energy needs for basal metabolism and physical activity: Diet-induced thermogenesis = (BMR + physical activity) times 10%.

Kilocalorie intake does not always balance kilocalorie expenditure, and obesity results when the imbalance exists for long periods of time. In our society today, the problem of energy imbalance in the form of obesity is a major public health problem.

OBESITY

Obesity is an excess of body fat. Classification of obesity is based on measurements of body fat or comparisons with measurements in standard height-weight tables. Females are considered to be obese when their fat content exceeds 30% of body weight. The percentage is lower for males: 20%–25%. Using height-weight tables as a guide, an individual is considered obese if body weight exceeds by 20% or more the standard weight for sex, height, and frame size (3). It is estimated that more than one-fourth of the U.S. adult population is 20% above desirable weight (4). More disturbing are statistics that support the growing problem of childhood obesity (5). Why and how do individuals become overfat and obese?

The Metabolic Picture in Obesity

It is accepted that obesity results from a complex interaction between genetics and the environment. The precise role that each plays is far from settled, however. Considerable evidence supports that the fatness level in children reflects the fatness level of their parents (6). The risk of the child becoming obese is approximately 7% if both parents are lean. This figure rises to 40% with one obese parent and to 80% when both parents are obese. Still, it is difficult to implicate only genetics, since environ-

mental factors, such as overfeeding, inactivity, and socioeconomic status, certainly contribute to the problem. Two major physiological theories have been advanced to explain the metabolic picture of obesity: the fat-cell theory and the set-point theory.
Fat Cell Theory. Originally, it was thought that there were certain critical periods during which fat cell numbers could increase: for the fetus, during the last trimester of pregnancy; at one to two years of age; and during early adolescence. It was believed that overfeeding during these critical periods would result in an excessive number of fat cells (hyperplastic obesity). Outside of the critical periods, it was believed that the fat cells could only increase in size (hypertrophic obesity). According to this theory, then, children and adolescents would be prone to developing a combination of hyperplastic and hypertrophic obesity. Individuals that increased weight only during adulthood would develop hypertrophic obesity. The former type of obesity was deemed more difficult to treat because weight loss results in a decrease in fat cell size only, and not a decrease in fat cell number. Thus, the potential for regaining weight is ever present, even after considerable weight loss.

Today, the theory has been modified somewhat. It is currently believed that when fat cells reach a peak size, a stimulus occurs that results in the production of even more fat cells. In response to highly palatable diets, therefore, adults may develop new fat cells producing the long-term possibility of weight gain through fat-cell addition (3). Because the body can add but never decrease fat-cell number, the ability always exists to increase weight but to decrease weight only to a certain level (6).
Set-Point Theory. The set-point theory advocates the existence of an ideal biological weight for individuals from which change in either direction (loss or gain) is resisted. While animal data supports the set-point theory, human data is less supportive. A modification of the set-point theory that is more flexible is the buffer-control system (7). According to this view, the body opposes and minimizes any imposed weight changes. Overfeeding is a stimulus initiating changes in the body that resist or limit

weight gain, such as an increase in the thermic effect of food and endocrine changes.

Another physiological mechanism suggested to play a role in the development of obesity is brown-fat thermogenesis. According to this theory, individuals with obesity are believed to have a defect in brown-adipose-tissue metabolism. Brown adipose tissue, or "brown fat," provides heat to the body via nonshivering (maintaining body temperature when exposed to cold) and diet-induced thermogenesis (8). The daily contribution of brown-fat metabolism to overall energy balance is questionable, and the theory continues to be debated.

Assessment of Obesity

Numerous methods exist for determining the existence of obesity, the percentage of body fat, and percentage of excess weight. Some methods are used more often in the clinical setting, while others, due to lack of equipment and personnel needs, are restricted to the laboratory. Visual assessment, simple rules of thumb, height-weight measurements, the body-mass index, skinfold measurements, girth measurements, ultrasonic assessment, and bioelectrical impedance are examples of assessments completed often in the clinical setting. Underwater weighing, total-body-potassium measurement and total-body-electrical conductivity are methods often restricted to specialized laboratories.

Visual Assessment. Obesity can be categorized based on anatomical distribution of adipose tissue. Excess body fat located in the abdominal area is classified as android obesity. Gynoid obesity refers to excess fat in the gluteal-femoral area. Individuals with android obesity are more likely to exhibit insulin resistance, hyperinsulinemia, Type II diabetes mellitus (NIDDM), hyperlipidemia, hypertension, cancer, gout, and possibly some joint diseases (9). It also appears that android obesity is influenced more by environmental factors than genetic factors.

Simple Rules of Thumb. Height and weight measurements are often done at or soon after hospital admission. The recorded height and weight can be compared with the results from a quick and easy method that requires no charts. In this method, women are assigned 100 lb for their first 60 in of height, and 5 lb are added for each inch over 60. Thus, for a woman who is 5'3" the ideal weight estimate is 115 lb. Male standards differ. For males, 106 lb are assigned for the first 60 in, and then 6 lb are added for each inch over 60. For example, the ideal weight estimate for a male who is 6'2" is 190 lb. It is obvious from the calculations that the results obtained through the use of this method are estimates that do not take into account individual variations in frame size. Although the figures obtained may be "in the ball park," more exact measures are preferable if possible.

Height-Weight Tables. Comparison of measured height and weight can also be made using height-weight tables. The major assumption of the desirable weight tables is that once growth in height has ceased, there is no biological need to gain weight. The best health, therefore, would be found in individuals of average or less than average weight in their early twenties (10). The most commonly used tables are from the Metropolitan Life Insurance Company. The first table was based on data in the Build and Blood-Pressure Study of 1959 (see Table 15-3). In 1983, new tables were issued (see Table 15-4). In the latest version, an attempt to approximate frame size was made. As the data in tables clearly shows, the 1983 tables list weights that are higher than those for 1959 for the same heights. Authorities in the health profession are not convinced that higher weights should be advocated and continue to rely on the 1959 tables. The National Institutes of Health recommends that weight loss be considered in patients who are 120% or more of their desirable weight using the 1959 insurance tables and the midpoint of the medium frame (4). While the tables are slightly more individualized than the rules of thumb, they have definite limitations. The subjects on whom the information for the tables is based were self-selected and weighed in clothes and shoes and the frame size is not accurate (11). While a comparison with these standards gives an estimate of degree of overweight, it is impossible to use the standards to

Table 15-3. HEIGHT AND WEIGHT TABLES FOR ADULTS (1959)

Desirable Weights for Persons Aged 25 and Over Weight in pounds according to frame (in indoor clothing)								
MEN				WOMEN*				
Height (with shoes on) 1-inch heels		Small Frame	Medium Frame	Large Frame	Height (with shoes on) 2-inch heels		Small Frame	Medium Frame	Large Frame
Feet	Inches	(lb)	(lb)	(lb)	Feet	Inches	(lb)	(lb)	(lb)
5	2	112–120	118–129	126–141	4	10	92–98	96–107	104–119
5	3	115–123	121–133	129–144	4	11	94–101	98–110	106–122
5	4	118–126	124–136	132–148	5	0	96–104	101–113	109–125
5	5	121–129	127–139	135–152	5	1	99–107	104–116	112–128
5	6	124–133	130–143	138–156	5	2	102–110	107–119	115–131
5	7	128–137	134–147	142–161	5	3	105–113	110–122	118–134
5	8	132–141	138–152	147–166	5	4	108–116	113–126	121–138
5	9	136–145	142–156	151–170	5	5	111–119	116–130	125–142
5	10	140–150	146–160	155–174	5	6	114–123	120–135	129–146
5	11	144–154	150–165	159–179	5	7	118–127	124–139	133–150
6	0	148–158	154–170	164–184	5	8	122–131	128–143	137–154
6	1	152–162	158–175	168–189	5	9	126–135	132–147	141–158
6	2	156–167	162–180	173–194	5	10	130–140	136–151	145–163
6	3	160–171	167–185	178–199	5	11	134–144	140–155	149–168
6	4	164–175	172–190	182–204	6	0	138–148	144–159	153–173

Courtesy Metropolitan Life Insurance Company.

*For girls between 18 and 25, subtract 1 lb for each year under 25.

compute an index of body fatness. As a result, individuals may be overweight according to the standard because of large musculature and yet not be obese. Conversely, individuals may be of the correct weight yet excessively fat if they have small musculature (10).

Body-Mass Index. A final measurement that requires the measurement of height and weight for its calculation is the body-mass index (BMI). BMI is the ratio of weight in kilograms to height in meters squared: weight (kilograms)/height^2 (meters). BMI minimizes the effect of height and has a good correlation with total body fat. A BMI greater than 35 indicates that an individual is significantly obese (12). Still other measurements can determine the risk of disease or body fatness.

Skinfold Measurements. Skinfold measurements reflect the amount of subcutaneous fat present at various body sites. Approximately one-half of the body fat is subcutaneous; therefore, these measurements have merit in the estimation of fatness. The procedure for measuring fatfold thickness is to grasp firmly between the thumb and forefinger a fold of skin and subcutaneous fat. The fatfold should be pulled away from the muscle to avoid including it in the measurement. The width of the fatfold is then measured with a caliper. Three readings are usually taken at the same site, and the

Table 15-4. HEIGHT AND WEIGHT TABLES FOR ADULTS (1983)

MEN					WOMEN				
Height		Small Frame	Medium Frame	Large Frame	Height		Small Frame	Medium Frame	Large Frame
Feet	Inches				Feet	Inches			
5	2	128–134	131–141	138–150	4	10	102–111	109–121	118–131
5	3	130–136	133–143	140–153	4	11	103–113	111–123	120–134
5	4	132–138	135–145	142–156	5	0	104–115	113–126	122–137
5	5	134–140	137–148	144–160	5	1	106–118	115–129	125–140
5	6	136–142	139–151	146–164	5	2	108–121	118–132	128–143
5	7	138–145	142–154	149–168	5	3	111–124	121–135	131–147
5	8	140–148	145–157	152–172	5	4	114–127	124–138	134–151
5	9	142–151	148–160	155–176	5	5	117–130	127–141	137–155
5	10	144–154	151–163	158–180	5	6	120–133	130–144	140–159
5	11	146–157	154–166	161–184	5	7	123–136	133–147	143–163
6	0	149–160	157–170	164–188	5	8	126–139	136–150	146–167
6	1	152–164	160–174	168–192	5	9	129–142	139–153	149–170
6	2	155–168	164–178	172–197	5	10	132–145	142–156	152–173
6	3	158–172	167–182	176–202	5	11	135–148	145–159	155–176
6	4	162–176	171–187	181–207	6	0	138–151	148–162	158–179

Weights at ages 25–59 based on lowest mortality. Weight in pounds according to frame (in indoor clothing weight 5 lbs for men and 3 lbs for women; shoes with 1" heels).

TO MAKE AN APPROXIMATION OF FRAME SIZE . . .

Extend arm and bend the forearm upward at a 90 degree angle. Keep fingers straight and turn the inside of wrist toward your body. If a caliper is available, use it to measure the space between the two prominent bones on *either side* of elbow. Without a caliper, place thumb and index finger of other hand on these two bones. Measure the space between fingers against a ruler or tape measure. Compare it with these tables that list elbow measurements for *medium-framed* men and women. Measurements lower than those listed indicate a small frame. Higher measurements indicate a large frame.

Height in 1" heels Men	Elbow Breadth
5'2"–5'3"	2½"–2⅞"
5'4"–5'7"	2⅝"–2⅞"
5'8"–5'11"	2¾"–3"
6'0"–6'3"	2¾"–3⅛"
6'4"	2⅞"–3¼"
Women	
4'10"–4'11"	2¼"–2½"
5'0"–5'3"	2¼"–2½"
5'4"–5'7"	2⅜"–2⅝"
5'8"–5'11"	2⅜"–2⅝"
6'0"	2½"–2¾"

Courtesy Metropolitan Life Insurance Company.

average reading for the particular site is reported. Various sites in the body have been identified for measuring skinfolds, the most common being the triceps (back of the upper arm) (Figure 15-1), the supra-iliac (the vertical fold above the hip bone), the subscapula (just below the tip of the right scapula), and the abdominal skinfold (one inch to the right of the umbilicus (13). The skinfold measurements can be compared with reference tables to assess the degree of obesity or can be used to compute percentage of body fat based on a series of equations.

The skinfold procedure has the following limitations (14): The amount of tissue picked up to form

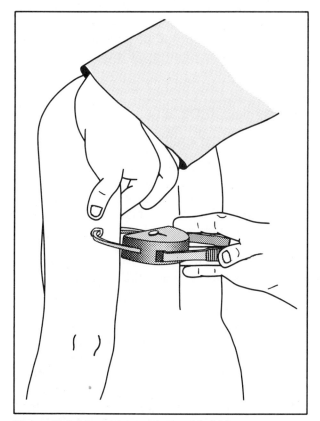

Figure 15-1. Measuring a triceps skinfold.
Source: S.J. Fomon, *Nutritional Disorders of Children. Prevention, Screening, and Followup.* U.S. Department of Health, Education and Welfare, Public Health Service, DHEW Publication No. (HSA) 76-5612, 1976.

the skinfold can vary; the skinfold thickness is sometimes impossible to measure at some sites on the obese individual because the skinfold can be greater than the caliper opening; compression of the body tissue can occur that would give an inaccurate reading; the presence of ascites or edema gives inaccurate results; and differences occur depending on the person doing the measurement.

Girth Measurements. The only equipment required to take girth measurements is a flexible measuring tape. Tables converting specific girth measurements (e.g., for the neck, waist, hip) to body fat have been published. Although rather easy to do, girth measurements may be invalid for very thin, very fat, or athletic individuals. Additionally, as with most standards, the reference tables are based on girth measurements of healthy individuals, invalidating results from patients with ascites or edema (15). If repeated girth measurements are required, mark the skin where the tape should be placed so that all persons measure the same area.

Ultrasonic Assessment. This rather new method, which operates on similar principles as skinfold measurements, involves the use of a portable ultrasound meter. The meter is used to measure the distance between skin to fat tissue, fat to muscle tissue, and muscle to bone. A panel on the meter automatically displays the measured distances that are used to compute total body fat.

Bioelectrical Impedance. The bioelectrical impedance method for measuring body fat is based on the fact that nonfat tissue has greater conductivity than fat tissue. A small, harmless amount of electrical current (via electrodes placed on various body sites) is uniformly applied to the body. Lean body mass, with its high water and electrolyte content, is very conductive. Fat tissue, on the other hand, contains little water and electrolytes and is less conductive. The benefits of bioelectrical impedance are that it is rapid, safe, noninvasive, moderate in cost, convenient, and painless. It remains controversial because it is based on the assumption that the body has a uniform distribution of body fluids (16); gender, age, height, activity, and frame size are not taken into account (15); and most validation studies were completed on healthy subjects (17). Disease states in which fluid and/or electrolytes are not normal invalidate the bioelectrical impedance method.

Laboratory Procedures. Laboratory methods are more precise than the clinical procedures just described; however, they usually involve costly, specialized, and, sometimes, cumbersome equipment (18, 19). Measurements of body potassium, total body water, and body density from which total body fat can be determined are included in this category. The theoretical bases for the measurements are based on assumptions of body composition that may not be true. Most body-fat assessment methods are based on the assumption that two distinct body compartments with constant compositions exist: the lean-body or fat-free mass and the fat mass. We know that age and disease states alter the composition of water and potassium in the fat-free mass, thus making the computations less accurate. Additionally, gender, race, and diet can affect the composition of the fat-free mass (18).

As you can see, all methods of body-fat measurements or percentage of overweight computations have limitations. The choice of the method in a particular institution is a result of careful consideration of the costs versus the benefits.

Complications of Obesity

Most physiological complications of obesity appear at weights greater than 110% of desirable body weight. As previously discussed, individuals with the android type of obesity are especially at risk for complications. Blood-pressure readings above 160/95 are nearly three times more prevalent in obese individuals than in persons of normal weight (4). Type II diabetes prevalence is also greatly increased; in fact, the chance of developing the disease more than doubles for each 20% increase of excess body weight (20). Until age 45, the risk of hypercholesterolemia (cholesterol greater than 250 gm/dl) is twice as likely to be found in the obese individual. Hypertriglyceridemia, osteoarthritis, high uric-acid levels (gout), and higher mortality rates also plague individuals carrying excess body fat.

Surgical procedures carry an extra risk for obese patients. Five major problems are faced by the nurse when surgery is performed on these patients (20): technical problems related to airway management and vascular access; increased risk of aspiration pneumonitis due to a lower than normal pH of gastric fluid; increased volume of gastric fluid, higher intra-abdominal pressure, and greater incidence of hiatal hernia with reflux of gastric contents; alterations in drug metabolism; and oxygenation.

Psychological complications in obese individuals are more likely to be a consequence rather than a cause of obesity. The emphasis on thinness in the American society has resulted in subtle and overt social prejudice against overfat individuals, even among young children. Self-esteem is often poor, and the prevalence of suicide is reportedly higher in obese persons than in individuals of normal weight (21).

Management of Obesity

There are actually two components to consider in the management of obesity: weight loss and weight maintenance. It is actually easier to lose weight than to maintain the loss over time. Permanent maintenance of a decreased weight requires lifetime changes in food intake and activity patterns. Individuals must, therefore, have a high level of commitment to any program.

Commitment is higher when individuals want to lose weight; that is, when the motivation comes from within, rather than when they feel they should lose weight. Frequently, pressure to lose weight is applied by the physician, nurse, or dietitian. One way to encourage patient commitment and responsibility in the process of weight loss and maintenance is to involve the patient in setting treatment goals. Answers to the following questions often aid in guiding the type of treatment plan developed: What does the individual want to achieve? What is it about his/her medical condition that makes it important to lose weight? What past attempts have been made at weight loss, and how successful were they?

It is important to note that physiological improvements can occur well before achievement of ideal body weight. A 10%–15% weight loss in an individual with a BMI greater than 30 results in an improvement of heart function, blood pressure, respiratory function, glucose tolerance, and sleep disorders (12). Concentrating on ideal body weight is therefore not appropriate and can be discouraging. Current treatments for obesity are outlined in Table 15-5.

Diets

The rationale for the dieting approach is that obesity is caused by taking in an excessive amount of kilocalories relative to expenditure; therefore, intake is restricted. Diets can be classified into three categories: the self-treatment fad diets, very-low-kilocalorie diets, and low-kilocalorie diets.

Self-Treatment Fad Diets. The continued popularity of fad diets can be ascribed to the eternal hope that a magic formula exists that will result in weight loss without extensive effort. It is very difficult for people to accept that weight gain occurred over a number of years through small imbalances between intake and expenditure. Just 50-100 kcal per day beyond bodily needs can result in an increase in weight of several pounds over the course of a year. When people want to lose weight, however, immediate results are desired.

Fad diets are not based on sound nutritional principles. Often, one or more food groups is entirely deleted, and kilocalorie intake is terribly unbalanced. Some weight loss can occur when these diets are followed, because daily kilocalorie intake is usually 1200 or less. Also, the diets force drastic changes in eating habits (which usually cannot be maintained). For example, the diet may require eating certain combinations of foods or drastically reducing carbohydrate intake. Usually the loss is not permanent because as soon as the old eating habits are resumed, the weight is regained. The initial weight loss is often a result of water rather than fat loss. Some of the fad diets have resulted in illness and death, and most have the potential for inducing serious nutritional deficiencies if followed for an extensive period (22, 23). The reason that more negative consequences are not seen is most likely due to lack of adherence. Most people go off the diet for one reason or another (usually, to try a new one).

Very-Low-Kilocalorie Diets. When obesity is life-threatening, or if an individual has failed repeatedly on a low-kilocalorie diet (described below) and must lose weight prior to surgery, drastic measures are used for limited periods and always under medical supervision. Total fasts are extremely dangerous, and deaths can be attributed to protein undernutrition affecting vital organs. In order to spare body protein, fasts are supplemented with high-quality protein. This approach provides for a very-low-kilocalorie diet. The amount of high-quality protein needed in the diet to maintain nitrogen balance is still controversial. The following points are considered to ensure the safety of patients who are placed on a very-low-kilocalorie diet (23):

- Medical supervision is required on a weekly basis. This includes regular monitoring of blood pressure, electrolytes, uric acid, and heart functions.
- The very low kilocalorie diet is prescribed only for those persons who are moderately or massively obese. The plan is not appropriate for pregnant women, adolescents, or the elderly. It is also contraindicated in patients

Table 15-5. CURRENT TREATMENTS FOR OBESITY

Diets	Drug Therapy	Surgery	Exercise	Behavioral approaches
Self-treatment Fad Very low kilocalorie Low kilocalorie	Prescription Nonprescription	Malabsorptive Gastric restrictive		

who have an abnormal ECG, hepatic or renal disease, severe cerebrovascular disease, or IDDM.

- Only protein of good to excellent biological value, such as eggs or meats, should be used. The diet normally contains at least 1.5 g of high-biological-value protein per kilogram ideal body weight and 400-800 kcal; 1500 ml or more of water is required daily. Vitamin, mineral, and trace-element supplementation is a must.
- This type of diet is only a temporary measure. Prolonging the very-low-kilocalorie diet is a lethal risk. The rate of weight loss slows considerably if a very low kilocalorie diet is prolonged. Very-low kilocalorie diets (depending on the type) are prescribed for 4 weeks, 12 weeks, or 16 weeks (22–24). At the completion of the very-low-kilocalorie phase, a refeeding phase begins, during which the patients are taught how to change their eating behaviors.
- In addition to behavioral guidance, moderate exercise (walking) is incorporated.

The short-term results of very-low-kilocalorie diets are excellent and reproducible. Individuals can lose about 16 lb in 3–4 weeks (22, 23). Temporary possible side effects reported include amenorrhea, hair loss, constipation, dizziness, mild cold intolerance, skin dryness, and mild fatigue (22). The major drawback to the very-low-kilocalorie diet is lack of weight loss maintenance. It has been reported that more than half the patients who follow a very-low-kilocalorie diet gain back 50% or more of the weight lost (23).

Low Kilocalorie Diets. Nutritionally balanced low-kilocalorie diets must be adequate in all nutrients with the exception of energy (kilocalories). Therefore, foods from all of the basic food groups are included, protein content ranges from 0.8-1.2 g per kilogram ideal body weight, and carbohydrate is not less than 100 g (3). Fat is restricted because of its caloric density, but it is not deleted entirely because it adds satiety value to the diet. Kilocalorie levels are normally no less than 1200 kcal for women and 1500–1800 for men. Medical supervision and vitamin and mineral supplementation is necessary for diets that contain less than 1200 kcal, because it is virtually impossible to satisfy nutritional needs below that level.

Anyone who has followed a low-kilocalorie diet can identify with the inevitable "plateau stage," when weight loss slows or ceases despite rigid adherence to the diet. This is thought to be due to the lower energy cost of normal physical activity and a lower BMR. Recall that kilocalorie expenditure in any physical activity is greater at high weights because a larger mass must be moved. As weight decreases, less energy is needed to perform the same tasks. Also, weight gain or loss never involves just adipose tissue. Lean body mass increases along with fat when weight is gained and decreases along with fat when weight is lost. Balanced diets are designed to minimize lean body mass loss, but some loss is unavoidable. The lower physical-activity expenditures and lower BMR result in fewer kilocalories expended. Fewer kilocalories are therefore needed to maintain weight. In order to continue losing weight, activity must be increased in the form of regular exercise to increase kilocalorie expenditure, or kilocalorie intake must be further reduced.

Following low-kilocalorie diets does result in weight loss. As with very-low-kilocalorie diets, the major problem is weight maintenance after the initial loss. People often do not make the permanent life-style changes; instead, they go on and off diets.

Drug Therapy

Prescription anorectic agents act on the hypothalamus to diminish hunger. *Amphetamines* are an example of anorectic agents. Their use is not advocated due to the dependance that occurs and the devastating weight gain resulting once the drugs are discontinued. Possible side effects include nervousness, irritability, insomnia, blurred vision, dizziness, palpitations, hypertension, sweating, nausea, vomiting, diarrhea, and constipation. These drugs are contraindicated for persons with existing hypertension or glaucoma.

Related to amphetamines but with a lesser effect on the appetite is *phenylpropanolamine* (PPA), the active ingredient in most nonprescription weight control products. Side effects include nervousness, insomnia, headache, nausea, tinnitus, and hypertension. FDA has declared PPA safe and effective for short-term weight control at specified doses. *Starch blockers* are supposed to work by blocking the action of amylase, the carbohydrate-splitting enzyme. They also supposedly prevent carbohydrate absorption. No clinical studies have shown starch blockers to be useful in the treatment of obesity. The FDA has received complaints from users, and these include nausea, vomiting, diarrhea, and stomach pains. The drugs were ordered off the market (25).

Promoters for *arginine and ornithine* capsules claim that these substances stimulate human growth hormone and burn fat. No data exists to support this claim (26). *Spirulina* is promoted as containing an agent (the amino acid phenylalanine) that supposedly switches off hunger pains. The FDA found no evidence of its safety or effectiveness (1).

While the amphetamine and amphetaminelike drugs can result in short-term weight loss, weight rebounds sharply after discontinuing use. Worse than the lack of success in maintaining weight loss is the message that drugs convey. Taking drugs to combat obesity encourages the idea that the person who is obese has a disease over which he or she has no control. Drugs mystify the process of weight loss, and probably do more harm than good in this respect.

Surgery

The only class of obesity for which surgical treatment should even be considered is morbid obesity; that is, when weight is 100 lb in excess of ideal body weight or the individual is at least 200% of ideal body weight. Surgery is very hazardous and guidelines have been published that outline patient eligibility and the role of the hospital in the procedure (27). Only patients who have a history of repeated failures to lose weight, have been mor-

bidly obese for three to five years, and can tolerate operative trauma and anesthesia are even considered. The hospital must have standards for treatment, the surgeons must be knowledgeable and have experience in the field of obesity surgery, and nutritional support must be available.

Surgical treatment for obesity falls into two major categories: malabsorptive and gastric restrictive procedures. The malabsorptive procedures (jejunocolic, jejunoileal bypass, biliopancreatic bypass, duodenoileal bypass) have essentially been abandoned due to serious complications. Renal problems, diarrhea, severe malabsorption, malnutrition, and liver disease are common problems associated with these procedures (28). After a time, the remaining portion of the intestine seems to adapt and weight loss slows by the second or third year postoperatively.

The gastric restrictive procedures (gastric stapling or partitioning, insertion of an intragastric balloon) work by forcing a limitation of food consumed. The procedures involve the construction of a small gastric pouch with only a 10-15 cc capacity that empties slowly, thus resulting in satiety. Patients are thoroughly instructed about the size of the pouch and encouraged to strictly adhere to the prescribed diet. The post-op diet has four stages, gradually progressing from pure liquids to solid foods. The type of food, even in the final stage, is extremely limited, and portion sizes are very small. If patients eat foods that are not permitted (such as high fat or concentrated sweets), or eat too much food, vomiting results. Initially a loss of 1% of body weight is expected on a weekly basis with this type of surgery (29). Weight loss slows as the body adapts. Patient complaints include dizziness, nausea, vomiting, stomach pains, headache, and orthostatic hypotension.

The deflated intragastric balloon is inserted into the stomach through an endoscope. When inflated, the balloon is about the size of a six ounce fruit juice can. The mechanism of action may be stimulation of the gastric nerves to produce satiety. The balloon is an adjunct to diet and behavioral therapy. It must be removed every three months to prevent complications such as pyloric obstruction.

The balloon may be reinserted as often as necessary.

Exercise

Exercise focuses on output. The rationale is that weight loss will occur when more kilocalories are expended than ingested. It has been found that exercise does not usually result in significant weight loss unless coupled with a reduction in caloric intake. Exercise is therefore considered to be an essential adjunct to weight-loss methods rather than a primary intervention method. Research indicates that weight loss is more likely to be maintained over the long term when an exercise program is incorporated as a permanent part of the life-style.

Behavioral Methods

The assumption of traditional behavioral-therapy approaches is that obesity is due to disordered eating behaviors (30). Eating behaviors are classified as acts that can then be observed, counted, evaluated, and changed. Self-monitoring of eating behaviors, controlling the environment for eating, restructuring counterproductive thoughts related to food intake, using techniques to control eating, such as slowing the speed of eating by chewing food more thoroughly, and reinforcing oneself for achieving goals are some of the elements of the behavioral approach. The advantage of the behavioral approach is that it is a learning model. Eating behaviors are viewed as learned responses rather than as character flaws of the individual (31). Only modest weight loss has been achieved with behavioral programs, but maintenance of loss is superior compared with other methods (30).

Today, the behavioral approach is somewhat modified. Programs that began as strictly behavioral have incorporated components of other approaches, and the reverse has occurred as well (30). It appears that treatment success is enhanced when a combination of approaches is used. The most promising combination is a behavioral program that incorporates physical activity and nutrition education. The first step in this approach is identifying the problems and then changing them into positive, behavioral goals. This approach is detailed by Danish and D'Augelli and is called "Goal Assessment" (32). Patients assess the importance of achieving the goals, and the health professional and patient work together to determine the obstacles hindering goal achievement. Only four obstacles exist that inhibit goal achievement when the goal is important: lack of knowledge, lack of skills, inability to take risks, and lack of support. Once the obstacle(s) is (are) identified, steps can be taken towards goal achievement.

As an example, although a person's problem may be obesity, there are many facets to the problem that need to be explored. After a discussion with the patient, you may discover that the person has problems with eating a large portion of high-kilocalorie (high-fat) foods, too many kilocalories at lunch and dinner, snacking excessively at night, eating in the afternoons, and not exercising on a regular basis. The patient then turns each of the problems into a positive, behavioral goal. For example, the problem, "eating too many kilocalories at lunch and dinner" can be changed to the positive, behavioral goal: "I would like to eat just one portion of what is served at lunch and dinner rather than two or three." Notice that a specific diet is not the approach taken.

Once all of the problems are changed into goals, it is important to prioritize the goals. The patient begins with the goal of highest priority. The health professional helps the patient determine what obstacles (if any) stand in the way of goal achievement. In the previous example, the person may lack knowledge about what an appropriate portion size is or may lack the skill of self-control. The person may also be afraid to risk hurting the cook's feelings if only one portion is eaten or may live in a nonsupportive environment. A combination of these obstacles may also exist.

Once the obstacles have been identified, the health professional can work with patients to develop steps for goal achievement. (See Figure 15-2.) It is important to help individuals acquire the necessary nutrition knowledge or teach the skills that are lacking. If the person is afraid to take a risk, it is possible to help the individual weigh the costs and the benefits of the action. A lack of support at home may require researching the community to identify support groups or resources. Once the first goal is reached, steps can be taken to reach the other goals, following the same procedures. The achievement of each goal brings the patient closer to the ultimate goal of weight loss and weight maintenance.

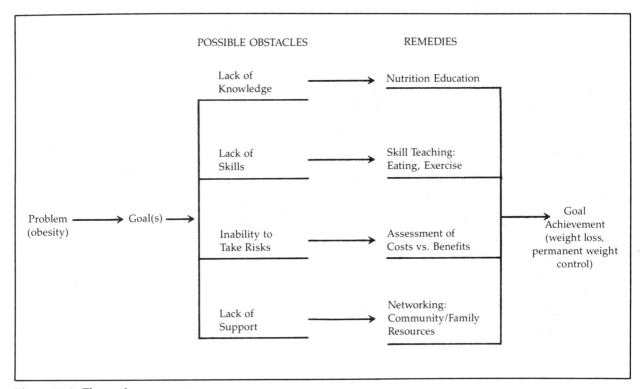

Figure 15-2. The goal assessment process.

POSSIBLE NURSING DIAGNOSES

Alteration in nutrition; more than body requirements related to
- food intake greater than metabolic needs.
- possible decrease in physical activity.

Ineffective individual coping related to use of food intake to mediate stress response(s).

Knowledge deficit related to
- dietary needs.
- hazards of obesity.

NURSING INTERVENTIONS
FOR NUTRITIONAL DISORDERS

Work closely with the patient, physician, and dietitian to develop a dietary plan that will enable the patient to lose weight and maintain the weight loss.

Alteration in nutrition; more than body requirements related to food intake greater than metabolic needs and possible decrease in physical activity.

- Recommend that food intake include choices from each of the four food groups. Remind the individual that fewer than 1200 kcal will not provide the body with essential nutrients.
- Discuss low-kilocalorie (low-fat) cooking ideas. Patients can broil, bake, or steam rather than fry foods.
- Explain how to cut extra kilocalories by choosing leaner cuts of meat (see Chapter 9), and removing the skin from chicken prior to cooking and eating, and trimming all visible fats prior to cooking or eating.

Ineffective individual coping related to use of food intake to mediate stress response(s).

- Suggest that the individual keep a record of what is eaten for a period of one week. The food record should include what was eaten, the amount eaten, when it was eaten, and what feelings were being experienced.

- Review the record with the person to target problem areas, set goals for each problem, and help the individual write out exactly how each goal will be achieved.

Knowledge deficit related to
- **dietary needs.**
- **hazards of obesity.**

- Instruct the patient in the importance of medical supervision during periods of dieting.
- Help the person plan ahead for social occasions and set goals prior to the event.
- Help the person explore ways to incorporate exercise into everyday life. It can begin with simple increases, such as using the stairs instead of the elevator or parking a little further from the store entrance to encourage walking.
- Encourage the use of "nonfood" items as rewards for successful behavior.

ANOREXIA NERVOSA

Anorexia nervosa is characterized by relentless food restriction that results in life-threatening emaciation (6). No specific cause of anorexia has been identified; however, it appears to be the result of individual and family variables. Anorexia usually begins during puberty or later in adolescence. Females seem to be more prone to developing the disorder than males, and the typical anorectic patient had been described as a white adolescent female from a middle- to upper-middle-class family with parental pressures to achieve. She can be described as a "perfect" child who tends to be obedient, a perfectionist, overly compliant, highly motivated, very successful academically, well liked by her peers, and athletic (33).

Assessment of the Patient with Anorexia Nervosa

Anorexia nervosa is defined in the revised Diagnostic and Statistical Manual of Medical Disorders by four criteria (34): (a.) an intense fear of becoming obese, which does not diminish as weight loss progresses; (b.) disturbance in the way in which one's body weight, size, or shape is experienced; (c.) refusal to maintain body weight appropriate for age and height; and (d.) in females, amenorrhea. Anorexia nervosa patients can be subdivided into those who binge and purge (bulimia symptoms), and those who only restrict food intake to lose weight (35). It has been estimated that 30%–50% of anorectic patients also develop bulimia symptoms. When anorectic patients are emaciated, they are often depressed and irritable. They show an inability to concentrate and often have sleep disturbances.

Amenorrhea is a common problem in anorexia nervosa. Surprisingly, 30% of anorectic patients develop amenorrhea prior to significant weight loss, which has led some researchers to consider the role of stress in the development of the disorder (33). Lanugo, or the growth of soft, fine hair covering the skin, may be apparent. Body stature may be decreased due to loss of bone mass as a result of osteoporosis and/or delayed skeletal maturation. Anorectic patients often exhibit cold intolerance due to loss of body fat, and cardiac abnormalities such as bradycardia or tachycardia, hypotension, and electrocardiographic changes. Constipation is common, and dehydration may be apparent due to the impairment of the renal-concentrating mechanism (35).

Many anorectic patients demonstrate an elevated serum cholesterol and hypercarotinemia. Abnormalities in nutrient metabolism (such as iron, copper, and zinc) have also been reported (35). Basal metabolism is slow because of a loss of total body mass, including lean body mass. Hematological changes, such as severe leukopenia, relative lymphocytosis, and hypocellularity of the bone marrow are also common (35).

Management of the Patient with Anorexia Nervosa

A combined approach including nutritional rehabilitation, psychotherapy, behavioral therapy, and medication (if needed) is optimal. The very nature of the approach requires a multidisciplinary health-care team. Treatment is usually on an outpatient basis and can last for three to four years. Psychologically, the goals include the resolution of psychological misperceptions and improvement in family relations. Individual- and family-counseling sessions are the approach used to achieve the goals. Antidepressants are sometimes used if warranted. Physiologically, the goal is to return the body to a normal homeostatic state. Because the clinical and biochemical abnormalities are a result of malnutrition, their resolution occurs when nutritional status improves. Return of the menses requires regaining of 90% of the initial weight; however, menstrual irregularities are common problems even after weight gain.

The goals of nutritional treatment are to encourage the cessation of weight loss, improve nutritional status, and gradually increase weight through regular self-feeding (36). If the nutritional treatment is to be successful, the health professional must recognize that patients are extremely fearful of gaining weight rapidly and becoming fat. Therefore, certain physiological phenomena that occur with refeeding should be described so that patients know what to expect. Patients may feel some discomfort after eating even small amounts because their stomachs are not used to having food. They may experience rapid weight gain initially due to water retention; therefore, patients need to be reassured that weight gain will slow as they become rehydrated. A slow increase in kilocalories on a weekly basis will result in better acceptance of food. Weight gain expectations need to be clearly stated and understood.

Hospitalization occurs when weight loss is severe, outpatient treatment fails after a reasonable period (6–12 months), metabolic abnormalities occur, the patient is suicidal, or the family is in crisis (33). Using parenteral or enteral feeding in the hospital until the patient is out of acute danger is controversial. Some researchers feel these drastic measures are unnecessary due to increased morbidity and failure of long-term benefit. Often weight gain that occurs during hospitalization is lost quickly once the patient is released, unless outpatient counseling is part of the treatment.

Of all anorectic patients treated, 18% remain chronically anorectic and 7% die of anorexia and suicide (6). At this time, recovery rates are worse for males than females. Better outcomes are associated with shorter duration of illness, early initiation of treatment, lack of bulimia symptoms, and a supportive family environment.

POSSIBLE NURSING DIAGNOSES

Disturbance in self-concept related to distorted view of thinness.

Alteration in nutrition; less than body requirements related to
- anorexia.
- vomiting, self-induced.
- laxative abuse.

Potential fluid-volume deficit related to
- self-induced vomiting.
- inadequate intake.
- laxative abuse.

Activity intolerance; fatigue related to inadequate nutrition.

Alteration in bowel elimination; constipation related to insufficient food and fluid intake.

Ineffective individual coping related to
- self-induced vomiting.
- denial of hunger.
- inadequate nutritional intake.

NURSING INTERVENTIONS
FOR NUTRITIONAL DISORDERS

Work closely with the patient and the patient's family and the physician, dietitian, and other members of the health team to develop a realistic approach to this complex problem.

Disturbance in self-concept related to distorted view of thinness.

- Record weight daily. Be nonjudgmental and straightforward.

Alteration in nutrition; less than body requirements related to
- **anorexia.**
- **vomiting, self-induced.**
- **laxative abuse.**

- Reinforce the nutrition plan prescribed by the physician and set up by the dietitian.
- Offer small quantities of food at more frequent intervals to prevent the feeling of bloating and fullness.
- Supervise and record the quantities of food and fluids that are ingested.
- Explain the rationale for use of nasogastric tube feeding, if appropriate. Tube feedings may be used to promote weight gain and correct electrolyte imbalances.

Potential fluid-volume deficit related to
- **self-induced vomiting.**
- **inadequate intake.**
- **laxative abuse.**

- Monitor fluid intake and output.
- Monitor vital signs.
- Monitor laboratory reports and administer electrolyte replacements as prescribed.

Activity intolerance; fatigue related to inadequate nutrition.

- Limit exercise, initially to conserve strength; encourage the patient to gradually increase exercise tolerance as prescribed.

Alteration in bowel elimination; constipation related to insufficient food and fluid intake.

- Provide high-fiber foods (as prescribed) if the patient has had a history of laxative abuse (see Chapter 7).

Ineffective individual coping related to
- **self-induced vomiting.**
- **denial of hunger.**
- **inadequate nutritional intake.**

- Correct inadequate knowledge regarding binge/purge behaviors. The use of laxatives will not prevent the absorption of kilocalories.
- Reinforce healthful behaviors that may be a substitute for the binge eating and purging.

BULIMIA

Bulimia is characterized by recurrent episodes of binge eating often followed by self-induced vomiting or laxative abuse. It is most often seen in young women of normal weight or who have a history of being slightly overweight. The age range is from the late teenage years to the midthirties. The onset commonly begins in late adolescence and often follows a period of dieting to lose weight. Feelings of self-deprivation result in a binge, a rapid consumption of large quantities of high-kilocalorie, easily-eaten foods. Binges can last from 15 minutes to several hours, occur with varying frequencies (from daily to twice weekly), and are done in private. Binges are then followed by intense guilt resulting in fasting or severe dieting and may include self-induced vomiting and/or abuse of laxatives or diuretics. Regurgitation is the most common evacuation technique (37). The gag reflex is stimulated by sticking fingers, toothbrushes, or silverware down the throat, or using external pressure to the neck. Over time, patients with this disorder develop the ability to vomit simply by contracting the abdominal muscles. The entire process of binge eating and purging becomes a vicious cycle that is difficult for the patient to interrupt or control.

The exact incidence of bulimia is unknown due to the elusive nature and lack of obvious clinical signs. Estimates of prevalence range from a low of 1% to a high of 20% in college-aged females (37, 38). The cause of bulimia is unknown, but several models have been advanced (37). The psychosocial models implicate the pressure in today's society to be thin. This often results in excessive dieting that eventually backfires and drives the patient to binge on "forbidden" foods, feeling completely out of control. Binge severity is significantly and positively correlated with dietary restraint, compulsive dieting, and weight preoccupation. Consistently, the onset of evacuation techniques occurs about one year after initiation of binge behavior (33). No distinct personality variables or family patterns have emerged; however, clinical reports suggest greater risk among individuals who are not assertive, have a poor self-image, are depen-

dent, have a high need for approval, and are unable to deal with negative emotions.

Biological models link bulimia with a form of depression, neurological disturbance, or metabolic disturbance involving neurotransmitter defects. The biopsychosocial model is a blending of the two models and is deemed most appropriate. According to this model, bulimia is a result of a biological predisposition to overweight or metabolic disturbance, psychological risk factors, and the social pressure for thinness.

Assessment of the Patient with Bulimia

There are four criteria for the diagnosis of bulimia (34): (1) recurrent episodes of binge eating; (2) fear of an inability to stop eating during the binges; (3) regularly engaging in self-induced vomiting, use of laxative, or rigorous dieting or fasting to counteract the effects of binge eating; and (4) a minimum average of two binge-eating episodes per week for at least three months.

Common complaints of individuals with bulimia include chronic indigestion, facial puffiness, menstrual disturbances, sore throats, constipation, and weakness. The parotid gland becomes enlarged due to chronic vomiting. Vomiting or diuretic abuse can cause dehydration. Abuse of laxatives can cause colon damage. Dental caries and enamel erosion can result from the effects of vomiting.

Self-induced vomiting and abusive use of purgatives and diuretics can cause electrolyte disturbances, particularly hypokalemic alkalosis, as a result of excessive potassium loss. The electrolyte disturbance results in weakness, lethargy, and cardiac arrhythmias (35). Metabolic acidosis can be present if laxatives are abused.

Complications

Acute gastric dilation, pancreatitis, renal failure, and esophageal strictures are some of the possible complications of this disorder. If severe, the electrolyte disturbance can result in seizures.

Management of the Patient with Bulimia

As with anorexia nervosa, there is no single-treatment approach for bulimia. The complex nature of the disorder requires a multidisciplinary approach involving psychotherapy, behavioral therapy, and medication (antidepressants). The goals are to normalize the eating pattern and work for changes in attitudes towards food, eating, and body size. Most treatment is through outpatient services and must be continued on a long-term basis. Suicide is the most common cause of death in individuals with bulimia. Prognosis is better for normal weight bulimia patients than for bulimia individuals who are also anorectic, abuse alcohol, abuse drugs, or have severe disorders.

POSSIBLE NURSING DIAGNOSES

Disturbance in self-concept related to distorted view of thinness.

Alteration in nutrition; less than body requirements related to
- anorexia.
- self-induced vomiting.
- laxative abuse.

Potential fluid-volume deficit related to
- self-induced vomiting.
- inadequate intake.
- laxative abuse.

Activity intolerance; fatigue related to inadequate nutrition.

Alteration in bowel elimination; constipation related to insufficient food and fluid intake.

Ineffective individual coping related to
- self-induced vomiting.
- denial of hunger.
- inadequate nutritional intake.

NURSING INTERVENTIONS
FOR NUTRITIONAL DISORDERS

Work closely with the patient and the patient's family, the physician, dietitian, and other members of the health team to develop a realistic approach to this complex problem.

(Refer to the section on anorexia nervosa in this chapter for suggested "Nursing Interventions".)

TOPIC OF INTEREST

Most people are very familiar with nutritive (aspartame) and nonnutritive (saccharin) sweeteners, and the impact they have had on product development. Now, fat substitutes are fast becoming a reality. Fat substitutes replace some of the fat in food and have either fewer kilocalories or no kilocalories, resulting in a net reduction of the caloric value of food. Two fat substitutes include Simplesse and Olestra.

Simplesse, from the NutraSweet Company, is made with protein from whey or egg whites. The protein is blended and heated to form tiny particles which feel like fat in the mouth. One gram of Simplesse contains only 1.33 kcal compared with 9 kcal from fat (39). Some or all of the fat in ice cream, yogurt, butter, margarine, cheese foods, cream cheese, and sour cream could be replaced with Simplesse, resulting in a substantial kilocalorie reduction. Simplesse can only be used in products that are not heated.

Olestra, from the Proctor and Gamble Company, is another fat substitute that looks like fat and has the same texture as fat. Olestra is sucrose polyester, a modified triglyceride (40). It is a carbohydrate backbone (sucrose) to which fatty acids are added. Unlike Simplesse, Olestra is not absorbed; therefore, it contributes zero kilocalories to food. In addition, it can be used in cooking and frying, and Proctor and Gamble is proposing that it partially replace the fat in shortening and oils used in fried and baked foods. Because Olestra is not absorbed, scientists have questioned its impact on the fat-soluble vitamins, A, D, E, and K.

SPOTLIGHT ON LEARNING

A patient picked up a copy of the latest fad diet book and asks your opinion about it. She seems convinced that this diet will work, and you sense she will not be swayed if you simply preach about good nutritional principles. You agree to review the diet and get back to her with your assessment. On review, you note that the diet is extremely unbalanced. In good conscience, you cannot recommend that she follow it. How can you prepare yourself to approach the patient?

1. Search for the facts on which the dietary recommendations are based. Sometimes, fad diets base claims on actual studies, but draw inappropriate conclusions or overgeneralize the results. In other instances, the recommendations are misinterpretations of physiology.
2. Check to see how many of the reported results are based on testimonials or anecdotal evidence rather than solid clinical studies.
3. Realize that many individuals who write diet books do not have appropriate credentials. If possible, try to find out where the author received his or her degree. It may be from a nonaccredited institution.

4. See if you can find any reviews of the book. The American Dietetic Association and The Society for Nutrition Education may be of help.
5. Analyze the nutritional adequacy of the diet by writing out the suggested meal plan. Note any food groups that are deleted. Do a nutrient analysis, using food composition tables, and compare the results with the RDA (see Appendix B). Ascertain where possible problems lie.
6. Take the time to outline specific rather than vague criticisms of the plan for the patient.

REVIEW QUESTIONS

1. Which of the following is not a component of energy expenditure?
   a. kilocalorie intake
   b. physical activity
   c. diet-induced thermogenesis
   d. basal metabolic rate

2. Which of the following factors results in a decrease in basal metabolic rate?
   a. age
   b. fever
   c. high ratio of muscle to fat
   d. large body size

3. Which of the following is not a complication of obesity, or excess body fat?
   a. Type II diabetes mellitus
   b. hypertension
   c. hypercholesterolemia
   d. hyperthyroidism

4. Which of the following is positive goal?
   a. I would like to design and follow an exercise program
   b. My husband doesn't support my weight-loss efforts
   c. I eat a large number of snacks throughout the day
   d. I will offend my friends if I take just one portion

5. Anorexia nervosa is characterized by which of the following?
   a. an intense fear of obesity, even after weight loss
   b. a loss of appetite
   c. nausea as a result of eating
   d. an increase in basal metabolic rate

6. Which of the following is the goal of nutritional treatment of anorexia nervosa?
   a. to resolve misperceptions of body size
   b. to encourage the cessation of weight loss
   c. to gradually increase metabolic rate
   d. to improve family relations

7. What is the most common evacuation technique in bulimia?
   a. laxative abuse
   b. regurgitation
   c. diuretic abuse
   d. enema abuse

8. What does a binge mean with respect to bulimia?
   a. eating a large meal with family and friends
   b. rapid consumption of large quantities of high-kilocalorie foods
   c. snacking throughout the day
   d. self-induced vomiting

9. What is the exact cause of eating disorders?
   a. an unhappy family environment
   b. a metabolic abnormality
   c. depression, guilt, and anxiety
   d. unknown

10. Which of the following characterize safe nutritional plans for permanent weight control?
   a. require minimal effort
   b. promise quick results
   c. are adequate in all nutrients but energy
   d. restrict complex carbohydrates

ACTIVITIES

1. Keep a food record for three days using the following setup:

Day	Time	Food Eaten	Amount	Feelings

   a. How much of the food was eaten for comfort, out of anger, out of boredom?
   b. Using a food composition table, calculate the total kilocalories eaten.
   c. How does your kilocalorie intake compare with the RDA for energy? (See Appendix A for the RDA for energy.)
   d. If you had to reduce your kilocalorie intake, what areas would you target?
   e. Write three goals based on the problem areas identified.

2. Invite a member of a health-care team responsible for working with individuals with anorexia nevosa or bulimia. Have the person explain his or her responsibilities.

3. Review popular magazines for weight-loss advertisements and critique the advertisements.

4. Go to a neighborhood bookstore and count the books on weight loss. Choose one book and review it for accuracy. Assess the chances for permanent weight loss if the recommendations in the book are followed.

5. Compare your height and weight with the ideal body weights listed in the 1959 and 1983 Metropolitan Life Insurance Height and Weight Tables and with the ideal body weight calculated using the simple rules of thumb.

REFERENCES

1. Ballentine, C.L. Hunger is more than an empty stomach. HHS Pub. No. (FDA) 84-2182. Dept. HHS, PHS, February 1984. Reprinted in 1986.
2. Bray, G.A. Obesity—A disease of nutrient or energy balance? *Nutrition Reviews* 45(1987):33–43.
3. Council for Agricultural Science and Technology. *Diet and health.* Report No. 111. Ames: CAST, 1987.
4. NIH Consensus Development Conference Statement. *Health implications of obesity.* Volume 5, Number 9. Bethesda: U.S. Dept. HHS, PHS, NIH Office of Medical Applications of Research, 1985.
5. Community Nutrition Institute. Childhood obesity increasing in U.S.; Many factors cited. *Nutrition Week* 27, no. 28 (1987).
6. Peck, E.B., and H.D. Ulrich. *Children and weight: A changing perspective. As identified by ad hoc interdisciplinary committee on children and weight.* Berkeley: Nutrition Communications Associates, 1985. Update, 1988.
7. Garrow, J.S. Energy balance in man—An overview. *American Journal of Clinical Nutrition Supplement* 45(1987):1114–19.
8. Shulz, L.O. Brown adipose tissue: Regulation of thermogenesis and implications for obesity. *Journal of the American Dietetic Association* 87(1987):761–64.
9. Bjorntorp, P. Classification of obese patients and complications related to the distribution of surplus fat. *American Journal of Clinical Nutrition Supplement* 45(1987):1120–25.
10. U.S. Department of Health, Education, and Welfare, Public Health Service. Definitions and methods: Definitions of obesity and methods of assessment. In *Behavioral treatments of obesity,* edited by J.P. Foreyt, New York: Pergamon Press, 1977.

11. Sims, E.A.H. Definitions, criteria, and prevalence of obesity. In *Obesity in America,* edited by G.A. Bray. U.S. Department of Health, Education, and Welfare, NIH Publication No. 79-359, November 1979.
12. Blackburn, G.L. Guest editorial. *Topics in Clinical Nutrition* 2(1987):viii-ix.
13. Katch, F.I., and W.D. McArdle. Nutrition, weight control, and exercise. Philadelphia: Lea and Febiger, 1983.
14. Kuczmarski, R.J., M.T. Fanelli, and G.G. Koch. Ultrasonic assessment of body composition in obese adults: Overcoming the limitations of the skinfold caliper. *American Journal of Clinical Nutrition* 45(1987):717–24.
15. Fox, E.A., L.M. Boylan, and L. Johnson. Clinically applicable methods for body fat determination. *Topics in Clinical Nutrition* 2(1987):1–9.
16. ———. Bioelectric impedance to measure body fat. *Nutrition and the MD* 13, no. 3 (March 1987):4–5.
17. Cohn, S.H. How valid are bioelectric impedance measurements in body composition studies? *American Journal of Clinical Nutrition* 42(1985):889–90.
18. Bandini, L.G., and W.H. Dietz. Assessment of body fatness in childhood obesity: Evaluation of laboratory and anthropometric techniques. *Journal of the American Dietetic Association* 87(1987):1344–48.
19. Salans, L.B. Natural history of obesity. *Obesity in America*, edited by G.A. Bray. U.S. Department of Health, Education, and Welfare, NIH Publication No. 79-359, 1979.
20. McDonough, A.B. Health implications of obesity. *Topics in Clinical Nutrition* 2(1987):5–13.
21. Pasulka, P.S. Is there a risk in recurrent dieting? *Topics in Clinical Nutrition* 2(1987):1–4.
22. Haggerty, P.A., and G.L. Blackburn. A critical evaluation of popular low-calorie diets in America: Part 2. *Topics in Clinical Nutrition* 2(1987):37–46.
23. Apfelbaum, M., J. Fricker, and L. Igoin-Apfelbaum. Low- and very-low-calorie diets. *American Journal of Clinical Nutrition Supplement* 45(1987):1126–34.
24. Fenhouse, D. The OPTIFAST program: A viable treatment for obesity. *Topics in Clinical Nutrition* 2(1987):69–73.
25. Hirsch, J. New treatments for obesity. *Current Concepts and Perspectives in Nutrition* 1, no. 4. New York: The Nutrition Information Center, 1982.
26. Willis, J. How to take weight off (and keep it off) without getting ripped off. Dept. HHS, PHS. HHS Pub. No. (FDA) 85–1116, 1987.
27. Task Force of the American Society for Clinical Nutrition: Van Itallie, T.B., et al. Guidelines for surgery for morbid obesity. *American Journal of Clinical Nutrition* 42(1985):904–5.
28. Randall, S., and W.W. Zeffiro. Surgical management of the morbidly obese. *Topics in Clinical Nutrition* 2(1987):55–58.
29. Cronin, B.S., and A.B. McDonough. Nutritional management of morbid obesity in conjunction with surgical intervention. *Topics in Clinical Nutrition* 2(1987):59–68.
30. Stunkard, A.J. Conservative treatments for obesity. *American Journal of Clinical Nutrition Supplement* 45(1987):1142–54.

31. Stuart, R.B. A three-dimensional program for the treatment of obesity. In *Behavioral treatments of obesity,* edited by J.P. Foreyt. New York: Pergamon Press, 1977.
32. Danish, S.J., and A.R. D'Augelli. *Helping skills II: Life development intervention.* New York: Human Sciences Press, Inc., 1983.
33. Eating disorders. *Dairy Council Digest* 56, no. 1 (January-February 1985).
34. American Psychiatric Association. *Diagnostic and statistical manual of medical disorders.* Washington, D.C.: ASA, 1980.
35. Halmi, K.A. Nutritional state and behavior of anorexia nervosa and bulimia nervosa patients. *Current Concepts and Perspectives in Nutrition* 4, no. 2. New York: Nutrition Information Center, 1985.
36. Huse, D.M., and A.R. Lucas. Dietary treatment of anorexia nervosa. *Journal of the American Dietetic Association* 83(1983):687–90.
37. Kirkley, B.G. Bulimia: Clinical characteristics, development and etiology. *Journal of the American Dietetic Association* 86(1986):468–72.
38. ———. Bulimia cases overstated new research indicates. *Nutrition Week* 18, no. 34 (1988):6.
39. ———. A better "fat" than butterfat? *Dairy Foods* 89(1988):35–36.
40. LaBarge, R.G. The search for a low-calorie oil. *Food Technology* 42(1988):84, 86–88, and 90.

CHAPTER
16

NUTRITION AND THE PATIENT WITH AN ALTERATION IN THE IMMUNE RESPONSE

Objectives

After studying this chapter, you will be able to

- differentiate between food allergy and food sensitivity or intolerance.
- identify the role of the immune response in the development of a food allergy.
- identify the clinical manifestations that may be associated with a food allergy.
- discuss the importance of dietary management in the control of food allergy.
- identify nursing interventions that may help alleviate nutritional problems associated with food allergy.
- list the nutritional problems that develop in a patient with acquired immunodeficiency syndrome (AIDS).
- identify the nursing interventions for nutritional disorders associated with an altered immune response.

Overview

The immune system is composed of specialized cells and tissues that respond to protect the body from invasion by foreign substances. The immune response is a complex mechanism in which the body reacts to the introduction of specific antigens or allergens (usually proteins) by producing antibodies to protect the body against that foreign substance. Allergies (hypersensitive reactions) are exaggerated responses of the immune system to an antigen or allergen (a substance that does not normally cause a reaction). Manifestations of the allergic response are frequently noted in those organs that are readily exposed to the antigens. The skin, the respiratory tract, and the gastrointestinal system are particularly affected (1).

When there is a malfunction of the immune system, the person may become susceptible to a number of life-threatening diseases, including infections and malignant disease. Acquired immunodeficiency syndrome is included in this category.

The focus of this chapter pertains to food allergy, in contrast to other forms of allergic response. The nutritional implications of AIDS are also discussed.

FOOD ALLERGY

Food allergy refers to a reaction caused as a result of an immunological mechanism; that is, one that can be reproduced with a blind food challenge (the offending substance is offered without the knowledge of the individual), and one that precipitates physiological changes in the target organ(s), the skin, respiratory tract, or the gastrointestinal tract (2). It is important that the true meaning of food allergy be understood and used appropriately (3).

The true food allergy response must be differentiated from food sensitivity or intolerance. Many times, the terms are used interchangeably with allergy to describe the adverse reaction to food but are used incorrectly by the patient or health professional. Adverse reactions to food may occur as the result of bacterial contamination (see Chapter 1) or chemical irritants and do not involve the immune response (4).

When the body manifests a hypersensitive response to an antigenic substance (protein) in food, both the T-cells and B-cells (lymphocytes present in the bone marrow) may become involved in the reaction (2). The T-lymphocytes, which are formed in the thymus gland, produce more T-cells (cell-mediated immunity) to help fight the offending substance. These cells may play a role in the intestinal involvement (diarrhea) in persons who are sensitive to gluten (protein in wheat, rye, oats, and barley).

In addition, antibodies or immunoglobulins, such as IgE, are formed by the B-lymphocytes and circulate in the plasma and lymph and may be attached to the surface of the mast cells. Antibody formation is referred to as humoral response. Once the cells have been sensitized to a substance, antibodies are formed that bind to the specific antigen on the surface of the mast cells and lead to the destruction of the offending substance.

The mast cells are specialized cells found in the skin, the mucous membranes of the respiratory and gastrointestinal tracts, and in connective tissue. When the mast cells are sensitized, histamine, heparin, and other chemical substances that are involved in the hypersensitive response are released. The histamine release precipitates a number of symptoms. Dilation and congestion of the peripheral blood vessels may lead to edema of the tissues and mucous membranes. A patient may manifest a number of systemic symptoms, such as rhinitis (runny nose), itching, skin rashes, eczema, gastrointestinal upset, wheezing, and anaphylactic reaction (an extreme hypersensitive response leading to shock and death, if not reversed).

Sources of Allergens

The most common allergenic foods are among those that are high in protein content and are more commonly consumed, including those of plant, animal, or marine origin (5). Environmental factors will usually influence the likelihood of allergic sensitization to certain food proteins. Milk is frequently an allergen for infants because it is almost exclusively consumed, especially during the early months of life (6). People who live near the seacoast and eat larger quantities of fish and shellfish are more likely to develop allergic reactions to those substances.

In most persons, the food allergens are destroyed in the gastrointestinal tract. However, in those persons who are predisposed to allergies, after repeated exposure, the allergens enter the circulation after being absorbed from the gastrointestinal tract (7).

The offending allergens for adult and pediatric populations may differ. Research has shown that infants and children are more likely to develop allergic reactions to cow's milk, chicken eggs, legumes (peanuts and soybeans), wheat, tree nuts (cashews, filberts, pecans, and or walnuts), and fish. However, children are also more likely to "outgrow" the allergies as they get older. Studies involving adult populations are more limited in scope but indicate that shellfish, peanuts, tree nuts, and grains frequently cause problems (2, 6). Chocolate, fruits such as apples, peaches and strawberries, celery, tomatoes, potatoes, and spices have been found to precipitate an allergic response in a sensitive person (6, 8, 9). Fruit and vegetable allergies may be caused by a cross-reaction with the antigens of pollens from the plant. For example, persons with an allergy to apples or hazelnuts may develop allergic symptoms when the pollen of apple or hazelnut flowers are present in the air while the plant is in bloom.

Other substances in food have been found to create problems for some persons. Individuals who are allergic to aspirin (salicylates) often have a reaction to the food additive FD&C Yellow Number 5 (tartrazine). Preservatives such as sulfites can also cause an allergic response in sensitive individuals. Particularly susceptible to life-threatening reactions are asthmatic individuals who are sulfite-sensitive. As a result of sulfite sensitivity, the FDA has prohibited its use on raw fruits and vegetables. Further, the FDA requires that manufacturers declare sulfites on the label when the sulfite is used as an antioxidant, regardless of the amount present in the finished product, and when the level of sulfite is 10 ppm or more regardless of its function.

One flavor enhancer that has been extensively researched is monosodium glutamate (MSG). MSG is a safe additive for the vast majority of the population; however, some individuals react negatively to it. The unpleasant transient reactions are often referred to as "Chinese restaurant syndrome" due to the widespread use of MSG in Chinese food preparation. The current research has been summarized as follows (10):

- Symptoms characteristic of Chinese restaurant syndrome can be provoked in a limited number of individuals about one-third of the time;
- Symptom experience varies from day to day and is not related to plasma glutamate levels; and
- Subjective symptoms of warmth, tingling, and tightness or pressure in skin and muscles are not reflected in altered skin temperature or muscle tone.

Sensitivity to MSG may be related to vitamin-B_6 deficiency, excess sodium (MSG is 12.3% sodium), and stimulation of the esophageal receptors (10).

Other food additives to which individuals may be sensitive include texturizing agents, flavorings, and some synthetic sweeteners (2, 6, 11, 12).

Symptoms or clinical manifestations of food allergy are varied and may occur within a few seconds to several hours after food ingestion (Table 16-1). In some instances, delayed reactions may occur several days later. A study of 68 children by

Table 16-1. CLINICAL MANIFESTATIONS THAT MAY BE ASSOCIATED WITH FOOD ALLERGY

Skin and Connective Tissue
itching
rash
eczema
angioedema (edema around lips, nose, eyes)
arthritis

Respiratory Tract
rhinitis
cough
asthma
bronchitis
otitis media (middle-ear infection)

Gastrointestinal Tract
nausea
vomiting
diarrhea
pain (cramps or colic)
distention
malabsorption

Nervous System
fatigue
behavior disorders: anxiety, irritability, sleep disturbances, depression, psychotic manifestations
headaches, including migraine
anaphylaxis: tachycardia, hypotension, respiratory distress, shock

Minford and associates found that 70% of the patients developed gastrointestinal symptoms, 24% developed skin reactions, and 4% reported respiratory problems (2).

Central-nervous-system involvement is also possible and may be manifested by innocuous symptoms, such as fatigue, to behavior problems, migraine headaches, and severe manifestations including anaphylactic reactions (13, 14). Some individuals manifest symptoms only during the "allergy seasons," spring and fall, when there are a greater number of pollens and molds present in the environment (6, 15).

Diagnosis of food allergy is difficult and is highly controversial. A variety of tests are used to determine the presence of an allergy. The history and physical exam are components of all diagnostic workups. In addition, a patient who may be suspected of having a food allergy is frequently asked to keep a two-week diary to record all foods eaten, the time and amount; the time symptoms, if any, appeared; and the type of medication used to control the symptoms. Skin tests (prick or scratch) may also be used to detect the offending foods.

When a list of foods that may precipitate allergic manifestations is compiled, an elimination diet may be prescribed. The patient again keeps a record of any offending foods and subsequent symptoms that develop during the time that the foods that are known to be provocative are avoided.

Some physicians may use a food-challenge test, during which foods that are known to provoke a response are added to the diet one at a time, in very small quantities (one-half to one teaspoon) and increased gradually until the patient can tolerate the food (2). Blind food challenges are used for some patients, but this is a controversial diagnostic procedure because it is possible to precipitate an anaphylactic reaction.

Usually, no single test provides conclusive evidence. The history, however, is an important factor in determining the cause of the allergic reaction (16).

Treatment of food allergy is difficult. Prevention of the allergic manifestations is of extreme importance. Avoidance of the offending substance is the only way to prevent the recurrence of symptoms.

For some patients, this is very difficult. If multiple foods are implicated, the diet must be analyzed to determine whether it is nutritionally adequate. Patients must be cautioned to read all labels on foods to determine the presence of possible allergens. Depending on the severity of the allergy, it may be necessary for the person to write to the manufacturing company to obtain more detailed information on the ingredients contained in the product.

Breast feeding of infants and delaying the introduction of solid foods in infants with a familial predisposition to allergy may be of benefit. In addition, the infant is supplied with the protective immunity through the mother's milk (17). Treatment modalities may change in the future as continuing research into this complex phenomenon provides additional information as to cause and control of food allergies.

POSSIBLE NURSING DIAGNOSES

Potential for injury related to the possible damage to the cells of the skin, respiratory tract, and gastrointestinal system.

Potential alteration in nutrition; less than body requirements related to dietary restriction.

Potential alteration in bowel elimination; diarrhea related to gastrointestinal irritation.

Potential alteration in comfort; pain related to abdominal bloating or headache.

NURSING INTERVENTIONS FOR NUTRITIONAL DISORDERS

Work closely with the patient, dietitian, and physician to help plan a diet that will prevent the allergic response.

Potential for injury related to the possible damage to the cells of the skin, respiratory tract, and gastrointestinal system.

- Instruct the patient to:
  avoid foods that precipitate an allergic response;

  read all labels carefully to determine the presence of food allergens;

  write to the manufacturer, if necessary, to secure more detailed information on the ingredients used in the product.

- Stress that different terms may be used to refer to a substance. For example, a person with a milk allergy would not only avoid products containing milk but also products containing compounds derived from milk, such as whey, casein, or sodium caseinate.
- Encourage mothers to breast feed infants to prevent the introduction of allergens and provide protective immunity.
- Advise patients who have controlled the allergic manifestations to abstain from the provocative foods during allergy seasons (spring and fall) when additional environmental allergens (pollens and molds) may be present in the air.
- Encourage the patient to adhere to the prescribed diet and avoid the offending foods.

Potential alteration in nutrition: less than body requirements related to dietary restriction.

- Arrange for a nutritional consultation with the dietitian to:
  determine the nutritional adequacy of the diet;

  obtain suggestions for alternate food sources that will not act as allergens;

  obtain recipes and suggestions for preparing foods at home.

Potential alteration in bowel elimination; diarrhea related to gastrointestinal irritation.

- Instruct the patient to seek medical advice to determine the possibility of food allergy as the precipitating factor for severe diarrhea.
- Encourage the patient to consume adequate fluid during periods of diarrhea to prevent fluid imbalance, especially with infants and young children.

Potential alteration in comfort; pain related to abdominal bloating or headache.

- Encourage the patient to avoid those food allergens that tend to cause the unpleasant symptoms.

ACQUIRED IMMUNODEFICIENCY SYNDROME

Acquired immunodeficiency syndrome is characterized by a loss of T-cell function (cell mediated immunity), which leaves the person susceptible to developing life-threatening, opportunistic infections such as pneumonia and certain malignancies such as Kaposi's sarcoma. AIDS is characterized by weakness, anorexia, weight loss, fever, and leukopenia (decreased white blood cell count).

Populations susceptible to the development of AIDS include homosexuals and bisexuals, IV drug users, hemophiliacs, and recipients of blood transfusions prior to screening for the human immunodeficiency virus (HIV).

This discussion focuses on the nutritional needs of the AIDS patient. Malnutrition is a major factor in the mortality of the patient because malabsorption syndromes develop and cause an inability to utilize nutrients (18). The role of good nutrition in maintaining the function of the immune system is well established in preventing infection in patients who are manifesting physiological stress (refer to the preceding section of this chapter and also to Chapter 6). Specific nursing interventions that may be helpful in working with the AIDS patient in the hospital and in the home are listed under the appropriate nursing diagnoses in the following section.

POSSIBLE NURSING DIAGNOSES

Potential alteration in nutrition; less than body requirements related to
- anorexia, nausea, vomiting, diarrhea, and malnutrition secondary to gastrointestinal complications.
- inability to swallow or impaired motor ability secondary to central nervous system involvement.

Potential alteration in comfort; pain related to oral or esophageal irritation.

Knowledge deficit related to the importance of adequate nutrition.

Social isolation related to the fear of disease transmission.

NURSING INTERVENTIONS FOR NUTRITIONAL DISORDERS

Work closely with the patient, dietitian, and physician to develop a diet that will meet the metabolic needs of the patient and prevent malnutrition.

Potential alteration in nutrition; less than body requirements related to

- **anorexia, nausea, vomiting, diarrhea, and malnutrition secondary to gastrointestinal complications.**
- **inability to swallow or impaired motor ability secondary to central nervous system involvement.**

Continued

NURSING INTERVENTIONS (continued)

- Offer small meals at more frequent intervals (five to six meals per day).
- Use conventional dishes rather than disposable dishes. If tray and eating utensils should become contaminated with blood, vomitus, urine, or feces, follow the infectious disease protocols of the institution for handling soiled objects.
- Offer nutritious snacks in between meals, milk-based drinks, instant breakfast drinks, lactose-free canned supplements, or protein-fortified fruit juices (19).
- Give medications at least 30 minutes to one hour prior to meals to prevent nausea (20).
- Arrange for a consultation with the physical or occupational therapist, if specialized feeding utensils are required due to neurological involvement.
- Feed the patient if necessary.
- Assess the patient's swallowing reflex; request that a nasogastric tube be inserted if necessary.

Potential alteration in comfort; pain related to oral or esophageal irritation.

- Offer foods that are bland and nonirritating, and avoid highly acidic or highly seasoned foods.
- Avoid temperature extremes in foods and beverages.
- Modify the texture of the food by blending or pureeing to reduce the amount of chewing required.

- Offer nutrient-dense liquid supplements, such as instant breakfast or lactose-free canned supplements (19).
- Assess the patient for difficulty in swallowing, and request an order for a nasogastric tube if necessary.

(Additional suggestions may be found in Chapter 12.)

Knowledge deficit related to the importance of adequate nutrition.

- Instruct the patient in the importance of consuming nutritious foods and beverages in order to prevent malnutrition.
- Arrange for the patient to meet regularly with the dietitian so that dietary modifications can be made as soon as necessary.
- Suggest that the patient discuss unproven food therapies, such as macrobiotic diet practices, and the use of such therapies as lecithin, orange juice and butter mixtures with the dietitian to ensure adequate nutritional intake (19).

Social isolation related to the fear of disease transmission.

- Use conventional dishes rather than disposable dishes. If tray and eating utensils should become contaminated with blood, vomitus, urine, or feces, follow the infectious disease protocols of the institution for handling soiled objects.

TOPIC OF INTEREST

Numerous theories on hyperactivity exist. One in particular is the Feingold hypothesis, which attributes hyperactivity to the presence of artificial colors and flavors, as well as salicylates in foods. In 1980, the Nutrition Foundation published a critical review of Dr. Feingold's claims. The conclusion of the review was that controlled studies provide sufficient evidence to refute the claim that artificial colorings, flavorings, and salicylates produce hyperactivity or learning disabilities (21).

A National Institutes of Health panel also reviewed the relationship between food additives and hyperactivity. The panel felt that studies indicated a limited positive association between the Feingold diet and a decrease in hyperactivity in a small proportion of patients; however, the decreases in hyperactivity were not consistently observed. The panel concluded that the diet should not be universally applied in all cases of hyperactivity; however, an initial trial of the diet after a thorough evaluation of the child, family, and therapeutic options may be warranted (22).

In summary then, it appears that much more needs to be learned about hyperactivity. Although the relationship between food additives and behavior is not completely clear, it appears that diet plays a minor role (23).

SPOTLIGHT ON LEARNING

Trent Haley, age three, has had repeated episodes of otitis media (middle-ear infections). The pediatrician referred the family to a pediatric allergist for consultation.

After the initial visit to the allergist, the child was diagnosed as having multiple allergies. Skin testing indicated allergic responses to a number of inhalants, such as molds, pollens, and dust. In addition, a variety of foods were found to be allergens: milk, egg white, tuna fish, peanuts, string beans, tomatoes, apples, grapes, pecans, and chocolate.

The parents were instructed to create an environment that would be as dust free as possible and to avoid the offending foods in the diet.

You are the Haley's next door neighbor. Trent's mother calls you on the phone with numerous questions about the dietary restrictions. How would you respond to these?

1. "I don't want Trent to think that he is different from the other children. How can I avoid all these foods in his diet? These are all his favorite foods!"
2. "What should I tell the teachers at the preschool? Should I send the morning snack with him everyday?"
3. "If Trent is invited to a birthday party, should I let him go? Should I tell him he can eat anything at the party?"

REVIEW QUESTIONS

1. What is the treatment of choice for food allergy?
   a. desensitizing injections
   b. hypoallergenic diet
   c. elimination of offending food
   d. antihistamine drugs prior to eating

2. Which of the following is not likely to cause an allergic reaction?
   a. chicken eggs
   b. milk
   c. tree nuts and peanuts
   d. rice

3. Severe reactions to sulfites most frequently occur in which group?
   a. AIDS patients
   b. asthmatics
   c. children under age three
   d. the elderly

4. Which of the following factors may not be involved in developing a sensitivity to a food?
   a. heredity
   b. prior exposure
   c. cooking procedures
   d. immune responsiveness

5. Which is the most common symptom associated with food allergy?
   a. dermatitis
   b. nausea and vomiting
   c. wheezing
   d. bizarre behavior

6. Food allergy in children is usually associated with which of the following?
   a. prolonged breast feeding
   b. a better prognosis if the food allergy develops after age six
   c. improper food processing
   d. a greater prevalence if there is a family history of food allergy

7. "Chinese restaurant syndrome" has been frequently associated with which of the following?
   a. rice
   b. soy sauce
   c. monosodium glutamate
   d. tea

8. Which of the following is not appropriate in instructing the patient to prevent an allergic response?
   a. avoid known food allergens
   b. discourage breast feeding of infants
   c. carefully read the label
   d. write to the manufacturer for a list of ingredients

9. With respect to food allergies, which of the following is outside of a dietitian's expertise?
   a. determine the nutritional adequacy of the diet
   b. provide suggestions for alternate food sources of nutrients
   c. provide recipes and suggestions for preparing foods at home that omit offending ingredients
   d. test for food sensitivity

10. Which of the following is not included in the nutritional aspects of care for a patient with AIDS?
   a. using isolation precautions for the food tray (e.g., disposable dishes)
   b. providing snacks between meals
   c. giving antiemetic drugs 30 minutes before meals if required
   d. arranging for regular consultation visits with the dietitian

ACTIVITIES

1. Make a list of all the possible ways milk or milk constituents may be identified in the list of ingredients on a food package.

2. Look through the selection of cookies at the supermarket. Read the ingredients to find a cookie that does not contain chocolate, nuts, coconut, apples, or raisins. How many brands were you able to find? What suggestions could you give to a mother who is looking for cookies to include in a school lunch for a child with multiple allergies?

3. Visit the drug store or supermarket. What brands of infant formula are available for the infant who may be allergic to cow's milk? How does the cost compare with standard formula preparations?

4. Eliminate one item such as wheat or milk from your diet for one day. What foods did you substitute? Did your diet contain adequate nutrients? What foods would need to be substituted if you eliminated that foodstuff for a long period of time?

5. Some food additives are likely to cause serious problems for sensitive persons. Read the labels on packages of cake mix. What food additives (colorings, preservatives) are listed on the package? What can you do if you need more information than that which is provided on the package?

REFERENCES

1. Bullock, B.L., and P.P. Rosendahl. *Pathophysiology: Adaptations and alterations in function*, 2d ed. Glenview: Scott, Foresman and Company, 1988.
2. Butkus, S.N., and L.K. Mahan. Food allergies: Immunological reactions to food. *Journal of the American Dietetic Association* 86 (1986):601–8.
3. Taylor, S.L. Food allergies and sensitivities. *Journal of the American Dietetic Association* 86 (1986):599–600.
4. Lessof, M.H., and M.H. Brueton. Gastrointestinal reactions and food intolerance. In *Allergy: Immunological and clinical aspects*, edited by M.H. Lessof. New York: John Wiley and Sons, 1984.
5. Taylor, S.L., et al. Chemistry of food allergens. In *Food allergy*, edited by R.K. Chandra. St. John's, Newfoundland, Canada: Nutrition Research Education Foundation, 1987.
6. Moneret-Vautrin, D.A. Food antigens and additives. *Journal of Clinical Immunology* 78 (1986):1039–46.
7. Robinson, C.H., et al. *Normal and therapeutic nutrition.* New York: Macmillan Publishing Company, 1986.
8. von Toorenenbergen, A.W., and P.H. Dieges. Demonstration of spice-specific IgE in patient with suspected food allergies. *Journal of Allergy and Clinical Immunology* 79 (1987):108–13.
9. Check, W. Eat, drink, and be merry—or argue about food allergy. *Journal of the American Medical Association* 250 (1983):701–11.
10. Institute of Food Technologists' Expert Panel on Food Safety and Nutrition. Monosodium glutamate (MSG). A scientific status summary. *Food Technology* 41 (1987):143–54.
11. Kniker, W.T., and L.M. Rodriguez. Non-IgE-mediated and delayed adverse reactions to food or additives. In *Handbook of food allergies*, edited by J.C. Breneman. New York: Marcel Dekker, Inc., 1987.
12. Schultz, C.M. Sulfite sensitivity. *American Journal of Nursing* 86 (1986):914.
13. Perkins, J.E., and J. Hartje. Diet and migraine: A review of the literature. *Journal of the American Dietetic Association* 83 (1983):459–63.
14. Steinberg, M., et al. Food induced migraine with increased cerebral blood flow. *Annual Meeting Abstracts, The Journal of Allergy and Clinical Immunology* 81 (1988):167–89.
15. Krause, M.V., and L.K. Mahan. *Food, nutrition and diet therapy: A textbook of nutritional care.* Philadelphia: W.B. Saunders Company, 1984.
16. Halpern, G.M., and J.R. Scott. Non-IgE antibody mediated mechanisms in food allergy. *Annals of Allergy* 58 (1987):14–27.
17. Hamburger, R.N., and G.A. Cohen. New and promising treatments. In *Handbook of food allergies*, edited by J.C. Breneman. New York: Marcel Dekker, Inc., 1987.
18. ———. Clinical nutrition cases: Severe malnutrition in a young man with AIDS. *Nutrition Reviews* 46 (1988):126–32.

19. Resler, S.S. Nutrition care of AIDS patients. *Journal of the American Dietetic Association* 88 (1988):828–32.
20. Baer, C.L., and B.R. Williams. *Clinical pharmacology and nursing.* Springhouse: Springhouse Publishing Company, 1988.
21. National Advisory Committee on Hyperkinesis and Food Additives. *Final report to the nutrition foundation* (October 1980).
22. ———. NIH Panel sees limited positive association for Feingold diet, hyperactivity. *Food Chemical News* (January 18, 1982):54–56.
23. Stare, F.J., E.M. Whelan, and M. Sheridan. Diet and hyperactivity: Is there a relationship? *Pediatrics* 66 (1980):521–25.

CHAPTER
17
SELECTED NURSING-CARE PLANS

The nursing-care plans in this chapter have been adapted from plans developed by nursing students and faculty in baccalaureate- and associate-degree nursing programs. In addition, a standardized plan used by a hospital nursing-service depart- ment is included. In the original care plans, the nursing diagnoses were identified and prioritized. Those nursing diagnoses that pertained to the nutritional priorities were selected for inclusion in this chapter for illustrative purposes.

THE PATIENT WITH
CIRRHOSIS OF THE LIVER

Mr. John F. is a 74-year-old male who was admitted with massive ascites, secondary to cirrhosis of the liver as revealed by CT scan. His chief complaint was abdominal fullness and sudden weight gain. A paracentesis was performed, and the results indicated no evidence of malignancy.

Mr. F.'s past history indicates that he suffers from right-sided congestive heart failure and has experienced episodes of upper gastrointestinal bleeding. He does not drink alcohol or smoke cigarettes.

Mr. F. has abdominal ascites and edema of the lower extremities and complains of "unbearably cold feet at night." His physician's orders include fluid restriction (800 ml/24 hours), sodium restriction, and 2500 kcal per day.

The focus of this portion of the nursing plan deals with fluid alteration, nutritional alteration, and knowledge deficit.

(Adapted from a Nursing Management Plan developed by Stephanie Moser as a senior nursing student at Medical College of Georgia School of Nursing, Athens, GA.)

NURSING CARE PLAN

NURSING DIAGNOSIS

Alteration in fluid volume; excess related to ascites secondary to increased intraabdominal pressure.

DESIRED OUTCOMES/EVALUATION	INTERVENTIONS
The patient will have no increase in fluid volume as evidenced by: No weight gain	Weigh daily and compare with previous determinations; report weight gain or loss of more than one pound per day. Compare weight with intake and output.
No increase in abdominal girth	Measure abdominal girth. Elevate head of bed as tolerated to minimize dyspnea.
Output greater than intake	Measure intake and output. Monitor laboratory reports, especially electrolytes. Encourage sodium and fluid restriction (800 ml/24 hours).

Continued

NURSING DIAGNOSIS *(continued)*

DESIRED OUTCOMES/EVALUATION	INTERVENTIONS
No increase in peripheral edema	Elevate edematous extremities (if possible).
Vital signs (blood pressure and pulse) within normal limits	Monitor vital signs.

NURSING DIAGNOSIS

Alteration in nutrition; less than body requirements related to anorexia and epigastric pressure.

DESIRED OUTCOMES/EVALUATION	INTERVENTIONS
The patient will have adequate nutritional intake and positive nitrogen balance to support metabolic needs as evidenced by: Weight within normal range after fluid volume excess is resolved	Assess for signs of malnutrition. Arrange for a dietary consultation. Offer frequent small meals (six to eight per day). Explain rationale for 2500 kcal intake, allow patient to select foods. Encourage sodium restriction. Weigh daily and compare with intake and output to note possible fluid loss. Encourage intake of food high in vitamin and mineral content. Encourage the use of herbs, spices, and salt substitutes (if prescribed) to increase palatability of food.
Improved activity tolerance	Encourage rest periods before meals. Encourage maximum kilocalorie intake early in day.
Improved serum albumin and protein as well as HCT, Hbg, vitamin-B_{12}, folic-acid, and cholesterol levels	Monitor laboratory reports; note levels of serum albumin, protein, HCT, Hbg, vitamin B_{12}, folic acid, and cholesterol. Provide vitamin and mineral supplementation (as prescribed).
No evidence of stomatitis	Assess for signs of stomatitis. Provide mouth care prior to meals.

NURSING DIAGNOSIS

Knowledge deficit related to nutritional needs; fluid and sodium retention.

DESIRED OUTCOMES/EVALUATION	INTERVENTIONS
The patient will consume the required nutrients and observe fluid and sodium restrictions as evidenced by: Consuming prescribed kilocalories (2500 kcals) but avoiding sodium	Assess patient's ability and willingness to learn. Encourage eating six to eight smaller meals per day. Encourage rest periods, especially before meals. Teach patient about foods high in sodium and those with "hidden" sodium (e.g., soups, canned vegetables, processed meats, and condiments). Teach patient to use spices, herbs, and salt substitutes (if prescribed) to increase palatability of foods. Instruct patient to take multivitamin and mineral supplements as prescribed.
Drinking no more than 800 ml/24 hours	Record daily weight and intake and output; report weight gain or loss of more than one pound per day. Teach patient to convert ounces to milliliters. Pour 800 ml in a container to illustrate quantity.

THE PATIENT WITH
SICKLE-CELL DISEASE

Cissy T. is an 11-year-old girl who is in the fifth grade. She is small for her age; her height and weight are in the 10th–25th percentile (height = 4'6"; weight = 70 lb). She is currently hospitalized with a diagnosis of sickle-cell disease with "numerous pain crises." Her past hospitalizations include a cholecystectomy in 1984 and left lower lobe pneumonia in 1987.

At home, Cissy eats a regular diet (three meals per day with three snacks). Her parents reported that in the past, Cissy has also been on Ensure (enteral supplement) because of "poor growth." The initial assessment revealed that although Cissy and her parents were well informed about sickle-cell disease in general, they lacked knowledge of the importance of adequate hydration and its role in sickle-cell crisis. The dietary assessment indicated that Cissy lacks sufficient calcium in her diet. She dislikes milk and prefers to drink colas. She also tends to refuse green vegetables, and she dislikes liver.

Admission orders included regular diet, minimum intake of approximately 4000 ml, activity as tolerated, and codeine for pain crises.

(*Note.* In addition to the nutritional priorities, Cissy was monitored for signs and symptoms of sickle-cell crisis.)

(Adapted from a Nursing-Care Plan developed by Anne B. Karch as a junior nursing student at Kennesaw State College, GA.)

NURSING CARE PLAN

NURSING DIAGNOSIS

Potential fluid-volume deficit related to decreased oral intake.

DESIRED OUTCOMES/EVALUATION	INTERVENTIONS
The patient will restore, maintain, and promote hydration (fluid balance) as evidenced by: Exhibiting no signs of dehydration	Assess for signs of dehydration every four hours (skin turgor, mucous membranes, temperature, level of consciousness).
Consuming at least 100 ml/kg every 24 hours of hospitalization	Monitor intake, output and daily weight. Determine minimum fluid intake (body weight 70 lb). Encourage oral fluids (minimum 3200 ml/24 hours).

Continued

NURSING DIAGNOSIS (continued)

DESIRED OUTCOMES/EVALUATION	INTERVENTIONS
	Offer oral fluids or fluid substitutes (e.g., jello, popsicles, ice slush, every one to two hours). Assess for knowledge deficit related to importance of adequate fluid intake, especially during periods of crisis. Teach Cissy to record fluid intake. Encourage parents to discuss increased fluid needs with teachers so that liberal fluid intake may be achieved while at school.
Electrolyte levels remaining within normal limits	Monitor laboratory results for signs of electrolyte imbalance and hemoglobin and hematocrit.

NURSING DIAGNOSIS

Alteration in nutrition; less than body requirements related to inadequate nutrient intake.

DESIRED OUTCOMES/EVALUATION	INTERVENTIONS
The patient will maintain an optimum oral intake as evidenced by: Understanding basic nutritional concepts (patient and family)	Encourage frequent intake of high-kilocalorie, high-protein foods and fluids. Arrange for nutrition consultation.
Demonstrating an understanding of correct food choices (patient and family)	Allow Cissy to record food and fluid intake as appropriate.
No weight loss	Weigh weekly; daily during sickle-cell crises.

NURSING DIAGNOSIS

Knowledge deficit related to nutritional requirements and food choices.

DESIRED OUTCOMES/EVALUATION	INTERVENTIONS
The patient will maintain optimum weight and height for age by eating foods that will promote adequate nutrition as evidenced by: Understanding basic nutritional concepts (patient and family)	Arrange for dietary consultation to instruct Cissy and her parents about the components of an adequate diet. Instruct Cissy to follow diet prescription to gain necessary weight. Instruct Cissy to avoid foods high in iron because of the increased supply and store resulting from red-blood-cell destruction. Advise Cissy of the importance of consuming vitamin-C-containing foods but ingesting these foods and fluids between meals to prevent additional uptake of iron. Encourage frequent intake of high-kilocalorie high-protein foods and fluids. Talk with parents about encouraging teachers to allow for additional nutritious snack intake throughout the school day.
Demonstrating an understanding of correct food choices (patient and family)	Plan a two-day balanced menu using food models, incorporating the basic food groups and optimum hydration.

THE PATIENT WITH
METASTATIC CANCER

At age 57, Bertha M. was diagnosed as having uterine cancer. She underwent a cesium implant, total abdominal hysterectomy, radiation, and chemotherapy. After a period of years, Bertha was considered "cured." At age 67, Bertha developed an intestinal obstruction that necessitated a colostomy. She adjusted well to the procedure and cares for the colostomy with skill.

Currently, Bertha is 72 years old and is complaining of continuous, intense back pain, fatigue, nausea, vomiting, and weight loss. She was admitted to the hospital for a bone scan and needle biopsy, which confirmed metastatic carcinoma (paraspinal mass involving the first lumbar vertebra). She was given 10 radiation treatments to reduce the growth of the mass, but she refuses all other treatments. Bertha continues to smoke two packages of cigarettes per day.

The nursing priority for Bertha at this time is relief of pain. The following segment of the care plan focuses on the nutritional alterations.

(Adapted from a Nursing-Care Plan developed by Denise B. Larsen as a sophomore nursing student at University of South Carolina, Aiken, SC.)

NURSING CARE PLAN

NURSING DIAGNOSIS

Alteration in nutrition; less than body requirements related to nausea, vomiting, and anorexia secondary to chronic pain.

DESIRED OUTCOMES/EVALUATION	INTERVENTIONS
The patient will: 　Maintain present weight	Encourage six smaller meals at evenly spaced intervals throughout the day. Obtain a dietary consultation. Encourage intake of eight ounces of Ensure, four times a day (as prescribed), if unable to consume adequate kilocalories through usual food intake.
Experience relief from nausea (frequency and duration)	Administer antiemetic drugs as prescribed, after breakfast and evening meal. Maintain an odor-free environment.

Continued

NURSING DIAGNOSIS (continued)

DESIRED OUTCOMES/EVALUATION	INTERVENTIONS
	Encourage rest periods before meals. Maintain semi-Fowler's position for at least two hours after meals to prevent pressure on the distended stomach.
Be able to consume oral foods and fluids	Offer fluids between meals to reduce gastric distention and allow for more concentrated intake of kilocalories at mealtime. Offer fluids in the form of clear liquids (cool tea, apple juice, jello, popsicles). Encourage family members to bring "favorite" foods to serve at mealtime. Serve food at a cool or cold temperature to reduce odor. Encourage intake of protein and carbohydrates; avoid fatty foods.

THE PATIENT WITH
DEPRESSION AND OBESITY

Ronald W. is a 25-year-old male who was admitted to the psychiatric unit of a local hospital following ingestion of butabarbital sodium (11 capsules). He has been hospitalized on three previous occasions for depression and attempted suicide.

Ronald is obese; he is 6'2" tall and weighs 270 lb. He has a low self-esteem and states, "I feel self-conscious about my weight. I eat when I'm anxious."

In addition to his psychiatric problems, Ronald fell at work and suffers from chronic pain resulting from a herniated disk. He also has a history of migraine headaches, kidney stones, and intermittent elevated blood pressure.

Nursing priorities focus on his potential for self-harm, disturbance in self-concept, comfort alteration, and ineffective coping techniques. This portion of the plan highlights the nutritional alteration related to increased food intake.

(Adapted from a Nursing-Management Plan developed by Monica Mathis as a junior nursing student at Medical College of Georgia School of Nursing, Athens, GA.)

NURSING CARE PLAN

NURSING DIAGNOSIS

Alteration in nutrition; more than body requirements related to increased food intake secondary to relief of anxiety.

DESIRED OUTCOMES/EVALUATION	INTERVENTIONS
The patient will: Attain a desirable body weight within four to six months as evidenced by loss of two pounds per week	Obtain a dietary consultation; collaborate with the patient and the dietitian in developing a dietary plan. Help the patient set realistic goals for weight loss. Instruct the patient to keep a weekly weight record. Instruct the patient in the importance of medical supervision while dieting.
Identify behaviors that precipitate increased food intake and modify behavior when recognized	Discuss perception of food and the act of eating. Encourage the use of a food record; record the foods eaten (time and amount) and activities and feelings that preceded food intake.
Demonstrate a change in eating patterns and food choices and quantity after instruction	Help calculate caloric intake. Encourage the use of "non-food" items as rewards for successful behavior. Note whether food choices include foods from the basic food groups. Assess understanding of calculating kilocalories from food intake. Provide positive reinforcement and encouragement for weight loss.

NURSING DIAGNOSIS

Knowledge deficit related to dietary needs and hazards of obesity.

DESIRED OUTCOMES/EVALUATION	INTERVENTIONS
The patient will maintain optimal individual diet and exercise plan following hospitalization	Work closely with the patient (and family), dietitian, and physician in implementing a weight-loss plan. Explore ways to increase exercise in daily activities. Involve wife in planning for ways to cut calories in food selection and preparation: choose lean cuts of meat; remove skin from chicken before cooking and eating; trim all visible fats from meats prior to cooking; broil, bake or steam foods.

THE PATIENT WITH
SURGICAL INTERVENTION FOR MORBID OBESITY

Harry B. is a 43-year-old male who was admitted for surgical repair of fistula that developed at the superior portion of a vertical-banded gastroplasty (performed five months ago). His diagnosis is acute morbid obesity.

Harry has a lifelong history of being overweight. His maximum weight was 460 lb in 1981. He has undergone two previous gastric bypass procedures because diet and weight reduction strategies had been unsuccessful. At no time following the surgical procedures did Harry modify the type, amount, or frequency of his intake. Complications including formation of chronic cal-culi throughout the lower urinary tract and the current fistula necessitated a Roux-en-Y procedure.

At this time, the fistula was repaired, the stomach totally resected, and the esophagus anastomosed to the jejunum. The recovery period was uneventful. Harry is now being prepared for discharge from the hospital.

The focus of this portion of the nursing-care plan deals with the nutritional aspects of preparation for discharge.

(Adapted from a Nursing-Care Plan developed by Robert Cone as a sophomore nursing student at University of South Carolina, Aiken, SC.)

NURSING CARE PLAN

NURSING DIAGNOSIS

Potential fluid-volume deficit related to inability to consume large quantities of fluid secondary to absence of gastric reservoir.

DESIRED OUTCOMES/EVALUATION	INTERVENTIONS
The patient will: Be alert for signs of dehydration and electrolyte imbalance	Instruct the patient to monitor fluid intake and output (including diarrhea). Instruct the patient to drink small quantities of low-caloric fluids at frequent intervals (broth; unsweetened tea with artificial sweetener, if necessary; noncaloric drink mixes; water). Instruct the patient to detect signs of dehydration (poor skin turgor, dry mouth, elevated body temperature). Instruct the patient to take electrolyte replacements as prescribed; potassium loss is associated with diarrhea.
Avoid consuming high-carbohydrate, high-kilocalorie fluids in excess of body needs.	Instruct the patient about the hazards of weight gain.

NURSING DIAGNOSIS

Alteration in nutrition; more than body requirements related to dysfunctional eating habits.

DESIRED OUTCOMES/EVALUATION	INTERVENTIONS
The patient will: Attain a desirable body weight as evidenced by a weight loss of two pounds per week	Obtain a dietary consultation. Collaborate with the patient and dietitian to develop a dietary plan not to exceed 1300 kcal as prescribed.

Continued

NURSING DIAGNOSIS (continued)

DESIRED OUTCOMES/EVALUATION	INTERVENTIONS
Demonstrate a change in eating patterns and food choices and quantity following dietary instruction	Instruct Harry and his wife on how to translate caloric intake from solid foods to semisolid or liquid forms. Reinforce diet teaching to include food choices from the basic food groups. Assess knowledge of calculating kilocalories. Suggest joining a support group such as Overeaters Anonymous.
Experience minimal discomfort associated with gastric bypass procedure	Discuss the importance of continued medical supervision. Instruct Harry to report persistent vomiting, bloating, esophagitis, excessive or persistent diarrhea, and dehydration. Instruct Harry to consume small amounts of fluid or semi-solid food at frequent intervals, but not to exceed 1300 kcal per day. Instruct Harry to take multivitamin supplements, as prescribed, since intestinal absorption from food sources may not be sufficient to meet the RDAs.

NURSING DIAGNOSIS

Knowledge deficit related to dietary needs; alterations required because of surgery and hazards of obesity.

DESIRED OUTCOMES/EVALUATION	INTERVENTIONS
The patient will: Maintain optimal, individualized diet and exercise plan following hospitalization	Collaborate with patient, dietitian, and physician to implement weight-loss plan. Help explore ways to increase exercise in daily activities. Involve wife in helping to plan meals requiring alteration in consistency and adhering to prescribed kilocalorie count.

THE PATIENT WITH
CYSTIC FIBROSIS

Eric is a four-year-old who was diagnosed with cystic fibrosis at 18 months of age. He has been hospitalized several times for respiratory infections. He is pale, with slight cyanosis of the nailbeds and slight clubbing of the fingers. His mother is a 28-year-old, obese, single parent. She gave the following 24-hour dietary recall for Eric:

Breakfast
Grilled cheese sandwich (1 slice American cheese, 2 slices bread, 1 tbs mayonnaise, 4 slices bacon); 4 oz soda

Snack
3 Vienna sausages

Lunch
1 hot dog on bun; 1 oz potato chips; 8 oz cola.

Dinner
2 fried chicken legs; ½ cup fried potatoes; 8 oz sweetened icea tea

The mother reports, "Eric is hungry all the time. Nobody has ever said anything about what Eric needs to eat. He takes pancrease pills in the mornings but not with other meals or snacks." She reports that Eric has 3–4 foul smelling stools per day. Eric's weight is approximately 28 lb (13 kg); height is 38 in (95 cm). His percentile weight for height is below the fifth percentile. His hemoglobin is 11 g; his hematocrit is 33%; all other values are within normal limits.

This section of the care plan focuses on the lack of parental knowledge about optimum nutrition.

(Adapted from a Nursing-Care Plan developed by Susan S. Kronberg, M.S., R.N., Assistant Professor, Maternal Child Nursing, University of South Carolina, Aiken, SC.)

NURSING CARE PLAN

NURSING DIAGNOSIS

Alteration in nutrition; less than body requirements related to lack of knowledge (parental).

DESIRED OUTCOMES/EVALUATION	INTERVENTIONS
Within three months: Eric's weight will be at the 10th percentile weight for height; hemoglobin will measure 12g	Obtain a dietary consultation and collaborate with the dietitian and Eric's mother in planning an optimum diet for Eric: 2600 kcal (80 g protein, 80 fat, 390 g carbohydrate, 500 IU vitamin A, 45 mg vitamin C, 18 mg iron)

Continued

NURSING DIAGNOSIS *(continued)*

DESIRED OUTCOMES/EVALUATION	INTERVENTIONS
Eric's mother will: State the relationship of pancreatic enzymes and utilization of food intake	Stress the importance of administering pancrease at least 30 minutes prior to meals and snacks to improve the absorption of fat and fat-soluble vitamins.
Plan a two-day balanced menu using food models and incorporating the basic food groups	Stress the importance of offering meals at frequent intervals (at least four) plus several snacks. Reinforce the importance of dietary balance, incorporating the basic food groups. Instruct Eric's mother to offer new food gradually to determine tolerance; avoid foods that cause diarrhea (response is individual); administer vitamin and mineral supplements as prescribed.
Identify specific foods that are high in protein, iron, vitamins A and C	Reinforce the knowledge of foods that are sources of protein, iron, vitamins A and C.
Understand the importance of maintaining optimum nutrition, especially during periods of stress	Encourage Eric to consume the prescribed kilocalories, especially during times of illness (fever or infection).

THE PATIENT WITH
AIDS

(Adapted from a standardized Nursing-Care Plan, St. Mary's Hospital, Athens, GA.)

NURSING CARE PLAN

NURSING DIAGNOSIS

Alteration in nutrition; less than body requirements related to
- **anorexia, nausea, vomiting and malnutrition secondary to gastrointestinal complications.**
- **inability to swallow or impaired motor ability secondary to central-nervous-system involvement.**

DESIRED OUTCOMES/EVALUATION	INTERVENTIONS
Achieve adequate nutrition as evidenced by: Weight maintenance or stabilization, increased activity tolerance, and absence of nausea and vomiting	Assess for difficulty in swallowing. Document dietary intake. Arrange for a dietary consultation. Offer small meals at frequent intervals (five to six meals per day). Offer nutritious between-meal snacks. Administer antiemetic drugs 30 minutes prior to meals, if prescribed. Offer foods that are bland and nonirritating.

NURSING DIAGNOSIS

Potential alteration in comfort; pain related to oral or esophageal irritation.

DESIRED OUTCOMES/EVALUATION	INTERVENTIONS
Oral and/or esophageal mucous membranes are intact (restored or maintained in optimum condition).	Assess the patient for difficulty in swallowing. Offer mouth care prior to and after meals, use non-irritating solution such as saline. (Note: always wear gloves when handling body fluids or excrement.) Request a dietary consultation. Offer foods that are bland and nonirritating. Avoid temperature extremes in foods and fluids. Request food texture be modified if chewing is difficult. Avoid use of acidic or carbonated beverages.

NURSING DIAGNOSIS

Potential fluid-volume deficit related to nausea, vomiting, diarrhea.

DESIRED OUTCOMES/EVALUATION	INTERVENTIONS
Hydration will be restored, maintained and promoted.	Monitor fluid intake and output. (Note: Always wear gloves when handling body fluids or excrement.) Weigh and record daily. Monitor number and consistency of stools. (Note: Always wear gloves when handling body fluids or excrement.) Assess for signs of dehydration (skin turgor, mucous membranes, vital signs, level of consciousness). Monitor laboratory results for electrolytes; assess for changes noting imbalance. Offer fluids at frequent intervals; every time someone enters the room. Provide bulk-forming foods. Administer antiemetic and/or antidiarrheal drugs as prescribed.

APPENDICES

APPENDICES

APPENDIX A
Median Heights and Weights and Recommended Energy Intake[a]

Category	Age (years) or Condition	Weight (kg)	Weight (lb)	Height (cm)	Height (in)	REF[b] (kcal/day)	Multiples of REE	Average Energy Allowance (kcal)[c] Per kg	Per day[d]
Infants	0.0–0.5	6	13	60	24	320		108	650
	0.5–1.0	9	20	71	28	500		98	850
Children	1–3	13	29	90	35	740		102	1,300
	4–6	20	44	112	44	950		90	1,800
	7–10	28	62	132	52	1,130		70	2,000
Males	11–14	45	99	157	62	1,440	1.70	55	2,500
	15–18	66	145	176	69	1,760	1.67	45	3,000
	19–24	72	160	177	70	1,780	1.67	40	2,900
	25–50	79	174	176	70	1,800	1.60	37	2,900
	51 +	77	170	173	68	1,530	1.50	30	2,300
Females	11–14	46	101	157	62	1,310	1.67	47	2,200
	15–18	55	120	163	64	1,370	1.60	40	2,200
	19–24	58	128	164	65	1,350	1.60	38	2,200
	25–50	63	138	163	64	1,380	1.55	36	2,200
	51 +	65	143	160	63	1,280	1.50	30	1,900
Pregnant	1st trimester								+0
	2nd trimester								+300
	3rd trimester								+300
Lactating	1st 6 months								+500
	2nd 6 months								+500

[a]The data in this table has been assembled from the observed median heights and weights of children, together with desirable weights for adults for the mean heights of men (70 in) and women (64 in) between the ages of 18 and 34 years as surveyed in the U.S. population.

The energy allowances for the young adults are for men and women doing light work. The allowances for the two older age groups represent mean energy needs over these age spans, allowing for a 2% decrease in basal (resting) metabolic rate per decade and a reduction in activity of 200 kcal/day for men and women between 51 and 75 years, 500 kcal for men over 75 years, and 400 kcal for women over 75 years. The customary range of daily energy output is shown in parentheses for adults and is based on a variation in energy needs of ± 400 kcal at any one age, emphasizing the wide range of energy intakes appropriate for any group of people.

Energy allowances for children through age 18 are based on median energy intakes of children of these ages followed in longitudinal growth studies. The values in parentheses are 10th and 90th percentiles of energy intake, to indicate the range of energy consumption among children of these ages.

[b]Calculation based on FAO equations, then rounded.

[c]In the range of light to moderate activity, the coefficient of variation is ±20%.

[d]Figure is rounded.

Reproduced from the Recommended Dietary Allowances, 10th Edition, © 1989 by the National Academy of Sciences, National Academy Press, Washington, D.C.

APPENDIX B
Food and Nutrition Board, National Academy of Sciences–National Research Council
Recommended Dietary Allowances,[a] Revised 1989
Designed for the maintenance of good nutrition of practically all healthy people in the U.S.A.

Category	Age (years) or Condition	Weight[b] (kg)	(lb)	Height[b] (cm)	(in)	Protein (g)	Vitamin A (μg RE)[c]	Vitamin D (μg)[d]	Vitamin E (mg α-TE)[e]	Vitamin K (μg)
Infants	0.0–0.5	6	13	60	24	13	375	7.5	3	5
	0.5–1.0	9	20	71	28	14	375	10	4	10
Children	1–3	13	29	90	35	16	400	10	6	15
	4–6	20	44	112	44	24	500	10	7	20
	7–10	28	62	132	52	28	700	10	7	30
Males	11–14	45	99	157	62	45	1,000	10	10	45
	15–18	66	145	176	69	59	1,000	10	10	65
	19–24	72	160	177	70	58	1,000	10	10	70
	25–50	79	174	176	70	63	1,000	5	10	80
	51 +	77	170	173	68	63	1,000	5	10	80
Females	11–14	46	101	157	62	46	800	10	8	45
	15–18	55	120	163	64	44	800	10	8	55
	19–24	58	128	164	65	46	800	10	8	60
	25–50	63	138	163	64	50	800	5	8	65
	51 +	65	143	160	63	50	800	5	8	65
Pregnant						60	800	10	10	65
Lactating	1st 6 months					65	1,300	10	12	65
	2nd 6 months					62	1,200	10	11	65

[a] The allowances, expressed as average daily intakes over time, are intended to provide for individual variations among most normal persons as they live in the United States under usual environmental stresses. Diets should be based on a variety of common foods in order to provide other nutrients for which human requirements have been less well defined.

[b] Weights and heights of Reference Adults are actual medians for the U.S. population of the designated age, as reported by NHANES II. The median weights and heights of those under 19 years of age were taken from Hamill et al. (1979). The use of these figures does not imply that the height-to-weight ratios are ideal.

[c] Retinol equivalents. 1 retinol equivalent = 1 μg retinol or 6 μg β-carotene.

[d] As cholecalciferol. 10 μg cholecalciferol = 400 IU of vitamin D.

[e] α-Tocopherol equivalents. 1 mg d-α tocopherol = 1 α-TE.

APPENDIX B *(continued)*

	Water-Soluble Vitamins							Minerals						
	Vita-min C (mg)	Thia-min (mg)	Ribo-flavin (mg)	Niacin (mg NE)[f]	Vita-min B$_6$ (mg)	Fo-late (μg)	Vitamin B$_{12}$ (μg)	Cal-cium (mg)	Phos-phorus (mg)	Mag-nesium (mg)	Iron (mg)	Zinc (mg)	Iodine (μg)	Sele-nium (μg)
Infants	30	0.3	0.4	5	0.3	25	0.3	400	300	40	6	5	40	10
	35	0.4	0.5	6	0.6	35	0.5	600	500	60	10	5	50	15
Children	40	0.7	0.8	9	1.0	50	0.7	800	800	80	10	10	70	20
	45	0.9	1.1	12	1.1	75	1.0	800	800	120	10	10	90	20
	45	1.0	1.2	13	1.4	100	1.4	800	800	170	10	10	120	30
Males	50	1.3	1.5	17	1.7	150	2.0	1,200	1,200	270	12	15	150	40
	60	1.5	1.8	20	2.0	200	2.0	1,200	1,200	400	12	15	150	50
	60	1.5	1.7	19	2.0	200	2.0	1,200	1,200	350	10	15	150	70
	60	1.5	1.7	19	2.0	200	2.0	800	800	350	10	15	150	70
	60	1.2	1.4	15	2.0	200	2.0	800	800	350	10	15	150	70
Females	50	1.1	1.3	15	1.4	150	2.0	1,200	1,200	280	15	12	150	45
	60	1.1	1.3	15	1.5	180	2.0	1,200	1,200	300	15	12	150	50
	60	1.1	1.3	15	1.6	180	2.0	1,200	1,200	280	15	12	150	55
	60	1.1	1.3	15	1.6	180	2.0	800	800	280	15	12	150	55
	60	1.0	1.2	13	1.6	180	2.0	800	800	280	10	12	150	55
Pregnant	70	1.5	1.6	17	2.2	400	2.2	1,200	1,200	320	30	15	175	65
Lactating	95	1.6	1.8	20	2.1	280	2.6	1,200	1,200	355	15	19	200	75
	90	1.6	1.7	20	2.1	260	2.6	1,200	1,200	340	15	16	200	75

[f] 1 NE (niacin equivalent) is equal to 1 mg of niacin or 60 mg of dietary tryptophan.

APPENDIX C
Estimated Safe and Adequate Daily Dietary Intakes of Selected Vitamins and Minerals[a]

		Vitamins	
Category	Age (years)	Biotin (μg)	Pantothenic Acid (mg)
Infants	0–0.5	10	2
	0.5–1	15	3
Children and Adolescents	1–3	20	3
	4–6	25	3–4
	7–10	30	4–5
	11+	30–100	4–7
Adults		30–100	4–7

		Trace Elements[b]				
Category	Age (years)	Copper (mg)	Manganese (mg)	Fluoride (mg)	Chromium (μg)	Molybdenum (μg)
Infants	0–0.5	0.4–0.6	0.3–0.6	0.1–0.5	10–40	15–30
	0.5–1	0.6–0.7	0.6–1.0	0.2–1.0	20–60	20–40
Children and Adolescents	1–3	0.7–1.0	1.0–1.5	0.5–1.5	20–80	25–50
	4–6	1.0–1.5	1.5–2.0	1.0–2.5	30–120	30–75
	7–10	1.0–2.0	2.0–3.0	1.5–2.5	50–200	50–150
	11+	1.5–2.5	2.0–5.0	1.5–2.5	50–200	75–250
Adults		1.5–3.0	2.0–5.0	1.5–4.0	50–200	75–250

[a] Because there is less information on which to base allowances, these figures are not given in the main table of RDA and are provided here in the form of ranges of recommended intakes.

[b] Since the toxic levels for many trace elements may be only several times usual intakes, the upper levels for the trace elements given in this table should not be habitually exceeded.

Estimated Sodium, Chloride, and Potassium Minimum Requirements of Healthy Persons[a]

Age	Weight (kg)[a]	Sodium (mg)[a,b]	Chloride (mg)[a,b]	Potassium (mg)[c]
Months				
0–5	4.5	120	180	500
6–11	8.9	200	300	700
Years				
1	11.0	225	350	1,000
2–5	16.0	300	500	1,400
6–9	25.0	400	600	1,600
10–18	50.0	500	750	2,000
>18[d]	70.0	500	750	2,000

[a] No allowance has been included for large, prolonged losses from the skin through sweat.

[b] There is no evidence that higher intakes confer any health benefit.

[c] Desirable intakes of potassium may considerably exceed these values (~3,500 mg for adults).

[d] No allowance included for growth. Values for those below 18 years assume a growth rate at the 50th percentile reported by the National Center for Health Statistics (Hamill et al., 1979) and averaged for males and females.

Reproduced from the Recommended Dietary Allowances, 10th Edition, © 1989 by the National Academy of Sciences, National Academy Press, Washington, D.C.

APPENDIX D
Growth Charts: Length and Weight Percentiles for Girls and Boys, Birth to 36 Months

APPENDIX D-1
Girls length by age percentiles: ages birth–36 months

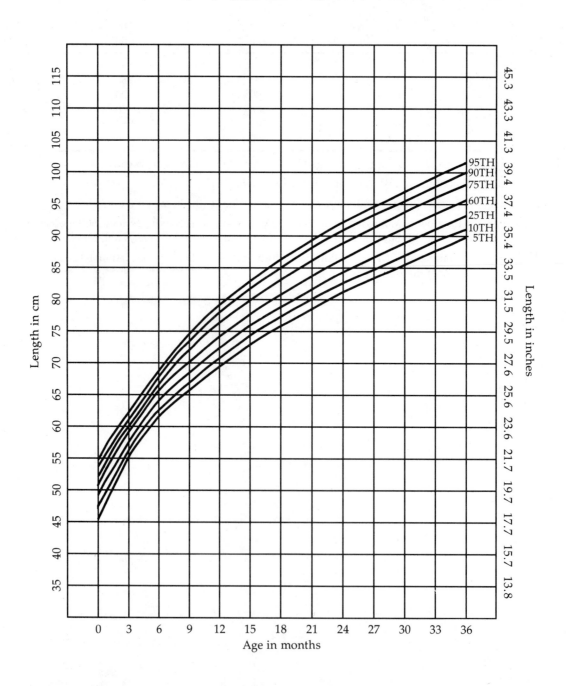

APPENDIX D-2
Boys length by age percentiles: ages birth–36 months

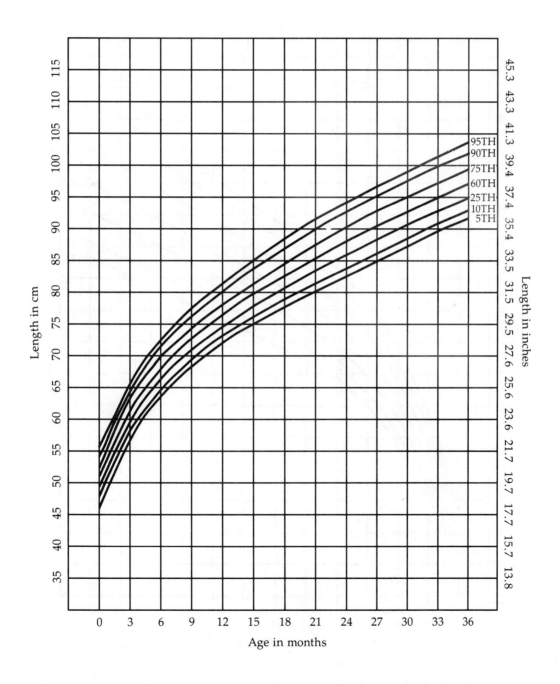

APPENDIX D-3
Girls weight by age percentiles: ages birth–36 months

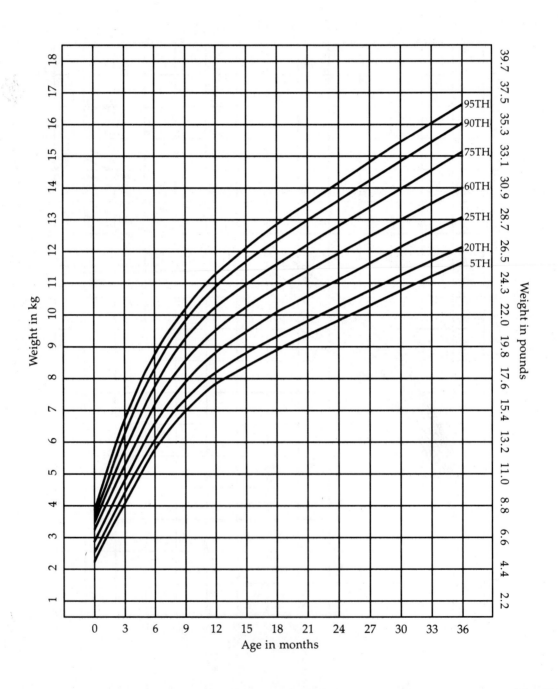

APPENDIX D-4
Boys weight by age percentiles: ages birth–36 months

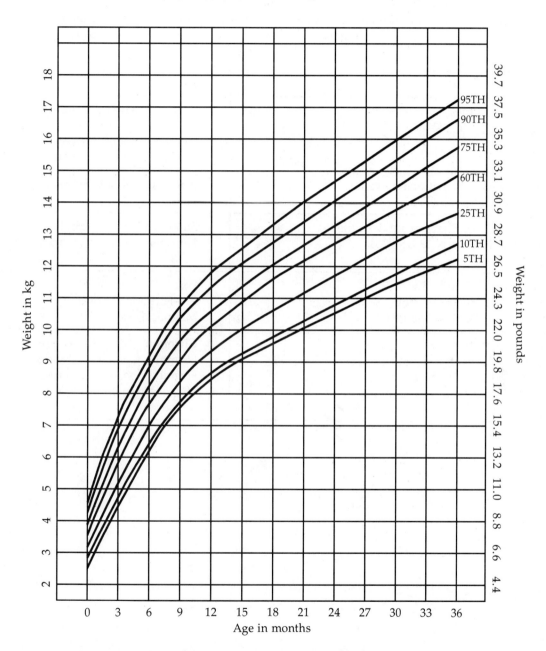

Source: National Center for Health Statistics: NCHS Growth Charts. 1976. Monthly Vital Statistics Report, Volume 25, No. 3. Supplement (HRA) 76-1120. Health Resources Administration. Rockville, MD, June 22, 1976.

APPENDIX E
Examples of Enteral Formulas for Tube or Oral Feeding

The following products are available for tube or oral feeding and can be used as a total source of kilocalories and nutrients or as a supplement. The listing is not intended to be complete.

MANUFACTURER	PRODUCT
Ross Laboratories Columbus, Ohio 43216	Enrich, Ensure, Ensure HN, Ensure Plus, Ensure Plus HN, Jevity, Osmolite, Osmolite HN, Pulmocare Vital High Nitrogen
Mead Johnson Nutritional Division Evansville, Indiana 47721	Isocal, Isocal HN, Sustacal, Traumacal
Norwich-Eaton Pharmaceuticals, Inc. Norwich, New York 13815-0231	Standard Vivonex, High Nitrogen Vivonex, Vivonex T.E.N.
Chesebrough-Ponds, Inc. Hospital Products Division Greenwich, Connecticut 06830	Fortison, Fortison L.S., Pre-Fortison Fortical, Magnacal, Pepti 2000
Sandoz Nutrition Clinical Products Division Minneapolis, MN 55416	Citrotein, Compleat—Regular Formula, Compleat—Modified Formula, Isosource, Isosource HN, Meritene, Resource, Resource Plus

INDEX

Note that italic page numbers indicate that an entry comes from a table or figure.

A

Achalasia, 153–54
  nursing interventions, 154
  possible nursing diagnoses, 153
Acquired immunodeficiency syndrome
    (AIDS), 378
  nursing care plan for patients with,
    400–401
  nursing interventions for nutritional
    disorders, 378–79
  possible nursing diagnoses, 378
Addison's disease, 330
  nursing interventions for nutritional
    disorders, 331
  possible nursing diagnoses,
    330
Adolescent nutrition, 92–93
  daily dietary intakes of vitamins
    and minerals, 408
  daily food guide, 92
  during pregnancy, 66, 69
Adrenal disorders, 328–31
  Addison's disease, 330–31
  Cushing's syndrome, 328–29
Adult nutrition, 101–14. See also Older
    adults
  aging, myths of, 102–3
  daily dietary intakes of vitamins
    and minerals, 408
  early years, 102
  older adults, 102, 103–4,
    107–9
Aging. See Older adults
AIDS. See Acquired
    immunodeficiency syndrome
Alcohol consumption, 33
  and blood pressure, 231
  and diabetes mellitus, 308
  during pregnancy, 61–62
  and thiamin, 40
Alcoholic beverages, 6

kilocalories and alcohol content of
    beverages, 232
Allergies. See Food allergies
American Academy of Pediatrics'
    infant nutrition guidelines,
    82–83
Amphetamines, 356, 357
Anemia, 250–61
  blood-loss, 260–61
    nursing interventions for
      nutritional disorders,
      261
  folic-acid deficiency, 257–58
  hemolytic, 258–60
  iron deficiency, 46, 252–55
    nursing interventions for
      nutritional disorders,
      254–55
  nutritional, 252–58
  pernicious, 255–57
  possible nursing diagnoses, 252
  sickle-cell, 258–60
  stages of, 47
  types and causes of, 251
  vitamin B_{12} deficiency, 255–57
    nursing interventions for
      nutritional disorders, 256
Anorexia nervosa, 361–63
  nursing interventions for nutritional
    disorders, 363
  possible nursing diagnoses, 362
Anthropometry, 111
Arthritis, 334–37
  nursing interventions for nutritional
    disorders, 336–37
  possible nursing diagnoses, 336
Asian cultural influences on dietary
    intake, 13
Aspartame, 308
Atherosclerosis, 218–29
  drug therapy, 227

lipoproteins, 219–23
  nursing interventions for nutritional
    disorders, 228–29
  nutritional therapy, 223–27
  possible nursing diagnoses, 227
  risk factors, 219–23

B

Baby boomer generation, aging of,
    114
Baby food, commercial, 86
  analysis of label, 85
Behavioral methods of treating
    obesity, 358–59
Beriberi, 40
Biochemical indices of nutrition in
    older adults, 111
Bioelectrical impedance to determine
    obesity, 353–54
Biotin, 41
Black American cultural influences on
    dietary intake, 12
Blood disorders and nutrition,
    250–61. See also Anemia
Blood pressure
  and alcohol consumption, 231
  and calcium, 231
  classification of, 230
  and diet, 230
  and fat, 231
  and fiber, 230–31
  hypertension. See Hypertension
  and obesity, 231
  potassium and, 232
  sodium and, 232, 234–36
Body-mass index, 351
Bone disorders. See Joint and bone
    disorders
Botulism, 18
  infant botulism, 84

Breast-feeding. *See* Lactation
Bronchitis, chronic, 267
Bulimia, 364–65
   assessment of patient, 364
   complications, 364
   management of patient, 365
   nursing interventions for nutritional
      disorders, 365
   possible nursing diagnoses, 365
Burns
   nursing interventions for nutritional
      disorders, 134
   nutritional implications related to,
      132–34
   possible nursing diagnoses, 133

C

Caffeine
   amount in common items, *62–63*
   during pregnancy, 62
Calcium, 42–43
   and blood pressure, 231
   dietary sources, 42
   foods high in, *195*
   and magnesium, 44
   and phosphorus, 42
   supplements, 341
   and vitamin D, 34
Caloric cost of physical activity, *348*
Campylobacterosis, 16
Cancer, metastatic; nursing care plan,
      392–93
Cancer and nutrition, 279–93
   clinical assessment of patient, 283
   dietary guidelines to prevent
      cancer, 291–92
   drug therapy, 283
   enteral nutrition, 285–86, *287*
   home parenteral nutrition, 286–87
   management of the patient, 283–90
   metabolism, effect of cancer on,
      280, 283
   nursing interventions, 289–90
   nutrition therapy, 284
   possible nursing diagnoses, 288
   radiation therapy, 284
   side effects and their management,
      284–85
   surgery and, 285
   terminally ill patients, 288
   total parenteral nutrition, 286
CAPD, 203
Carbohydrates, 30, 306
   complex, *225,* 227

diabetics' guidelines for supplemen-
      tation during exercise, *309*
Cardiovascular disease and nutrition,
      217–45
   atherosclerosis, 218–29
   congestive heart failure, 242–43
   hypertension, 229–40
   ischemic heart disease, 240–42
Care, nurses' approach to, 20–21
Carotene, 34
Catabolism, *122*
Celiac sprue, 170
   nursing interventions for nutritional
      disorders, 171
   possible nursing diagnoses, 171
Childhood nutrition, 76. *See also*
      Preschool nutrition
   of cystic fibrosis patients, 271–72
   government feeding programs, 93
   nursing interventions, 95
   possible nursing diagnoses, 76
   preschool years, 89–91
   school-age years, 91–92
   school lunch patterns, *93–94*
Children
   chronic renal failure, 210
   daily dietary intakes of vitamins
      and minerals, *408*
   growth charts (0–36 months),
      410–13
   median height-weight tables, *405*
   normal growth and development in
      relation to nutrition, 76
   recommended dietary allowances,
      406–7
Chinese restaurant syndrome, 374
Chloride, estimated minimum
      requirements, *409*
Cholecystitis, 178–80
   nursing interventions for nutritional
      disorders, 180
   possible nursing diagnoses, 180
Cholelithiasis, 178–80
   nursing interventions for nutritional
      disorders, 180
   possible nursing diagnoses, 180
Cholera, 17
Cholesterol, 219–23, 226, 307
   food labeling proposal, 243
   food sources of, *225*
   National Cholesterol Education
      Program, 244
Chromium, 46
Chronic obstructive lung disease
      (COLD), 267–70

nursing interventions, 269–70
   possible nursing diagnoses, 269
Chronic obstructive pulmonary
      disease (COPD), 267–70
   nursing interventions, 269–70
   possible nursing diagnoses, 269
Cirrhosis, 175–76
   nursing care plan, 386–88
   nursing interventions for nutritional
      disorders, 176
   possible nursing diagnoses, 176
COLD. *See* Chronic obstructive lung
      disease
Colic, 81, 88
Complex carbohydrates, 227
   food sources of, *225*
Congestive heart failure, 242–43
   nursing interventions for nutritional
      disorders, 243
   possible nursing diagnoses, 242
Constipation, 145–46, 284
   during pregnancy, 64
   nursing interventions for nutritional
      disorders, 146
   possible nursing diagnoses, 146
   recommended dietary fiber,
      sources of, *146–51*
COPD. *See* Chronic obstructive
      pulmonary disease
Copper, 47–48
   deficiency, 47–48
   dietary sources, 47
Cultural awareness in nursing, 13
Cultural factors influencing dietary
      intake, 11–13
Cushing's syndrome, 328
   nursing interventions for nutritional
      disorders, 329
   possible nursing diagnoses, 328
Cystic fibrosis, 271–74
   nursing care plan, 398–99
   nursing interventions related to
      nutritional disorders, 273–74
   possible nursing diagnoses, 272
   study involving nutrition
      counseling of patients, 275

D

Dairy products. *See* Milk products
Diabetes, gestational, 65
Diabetes mellitus and nutrition,
      297–315
   alcohol, 308
   alternate sweeteners, 308

blood glucose values (normal and diabetic), *303*
carbohydrate, 306
cholesterol, 307
classification of diabetes mellitus, 298
complications of diabetes, 302–4
dietary fiber and, 306
dietary recommendations, *307*
dietetic foods, 308
education of patients, 310
exercise and, 309
fat, 307
glycemic index, 313
hypoglycemia, 302–3
illness and, 310
insulin, 304–5
kilocalories, 306
laboratory assessment, 302
meal plan, 310–11
medication, 304–5
minerals, 307–8
nursing interventions, 312–13
nutrition therapy, 305–8
oral agents, 305
possible nursing diagnoses, 311
protein, 307
sodium, 307
sucrose, 306–7
surgery and, 310
untreated diabetes; clinical picture, *301*
vitamins, 307–8
Dialysis, 202
  chronic ambulatory peritoneal dialysis (CAPD), 203
  chronic intermittent peritoneal, 203
  nutritional therapy prior to, 204–8
Dialysis Unit for Pennsylvania State University Students (DUPSUS), 211
Diarrhea, 17, 19, 144–45, 285
  in infancy, 87
  nursing interventions for nutritional disorders, 145
  possible nursing diagnoses, 145
Dietary guidelines, 6–7
  adolescent years, *92*
  for cancer prevention, 291–92
  for daily intake, *60*
  for diabetes mellitus patients, *307*
  National Academy of Sciences' Committee on Diet and Health, 9

for pregnant adolescents, *66*
preschool years, *89*
recommended allowances, *406–7*
  for women, *57*
in renal failure, *205*
selected liver diseases, *173*
Surgeon General's, *8*
Dietary intake
  cultural factors, 11–13
  economic factors, 8–10
  factors influencing, 7–13
  psychosocial factors, 7–8
  religious factors, 10–11
Dietary management, nursing interventions, 68–69, 95
Dietetic foods and diabetes mellitus, 308
Dietitian (registered), role of, 19–20
Digestive tract, age-related changes, *106*
Disease
  chronic, in older adults, 109
  prevention through diet, 7
Diverticular disease, 167–68
  nursing interventions for nutritional disorders, 168
  possible nursing diagnoses, 168
Drug-nutrient interactions, 109–11
Drugs during pregnancy, 62
Drug therapy
  of cancer patients, 283, 284–85
  for obesity, 356–57
Dumping syndrome, 164
DUPSUS, 211

E
Eating disorders and nutrition, 346–66
  anorexia nervosa, 361–63
  bulimia, 364–65
  energy balance, 347–49
  obesity, 349–60
Economic factors influencing dietary intake, 8–10
Electrolytes, 48
Emphysema, pulmonary, 267
Enteral therapy
  of cancer patients, 285–86
  examples of formulas, *414*
  indications for use and possible complications, *287*
Exercise
  caloric cost of, *348*

during pregnancy, 61
obesity and, 358

F
Fad diets (self-treatment), 355
Fat, *6*, 31–32, 307
  and blood pressure, 231
  digestion of, 32
  food sources of, *225*
  metabolism of, 32
  monounsaturated, *225*, 226
  polyunsaturated, *225*, 226
  saturated, 223, *225*, 226
  substitutes for, 366
Fat cell theory of obesity, 349
Feingold hypothesis on hyperactivity, 380
Fetal development, 56. *See also* Pregnancy
Fever
  catabolic response to, *129*
  nursing interventions for nutritional disorders, 131–32
  nutritional implications related to, 128–30
  possible nursing diagnoses, 131
Fiber, dietary, 183, 306
  and blood pressure, 230–31
  plant fiber, classification of, *147*
  sources of, *147–51*
Fish, *5*
Flatus, 152–53
  nursing interventions, 153
  possible nursing diagnoses, 152
Fluoride, 45
Folate
  anemia caused by deficiency of, 257–58
    nursing interventions, 258
  deficiency, 37
  dietary sources, *37*
  and vitamin B_{12}, 38, *39*
Folic acid. *See* Folate
Food allergies, 373–77
  altered immune response, 373–77
  clinical manifestations, *375*
  Feingold hypothesis, 380
  food sensitivities in infants, 87
  introduction of solid foods to infants, 83
  nursing interventions for nutritional disorders, 377
  possible nursing diagnoses, 376

sources of allergens, 374–77
to infant formula, 81
Food aversions, 284
during pregnancy, 64
Food cravings and aversions during
pregnancy, 64
Food and Drug Administration (FDA),
food labeling program, 21–22
Food, fortified, 49
Food groups, 4–6
fats, sweets, alcoholic beverages, 6
fruits, 5
grain products, 4
meat, poultry, fish, 5
milk products, 6
protein values, 206
vegetables, 5
Food guides. See Dietary guidelines
Food labeling program, 21–22
cholesterol content, 243
Food safety, 14–19
food-borne illnesses, 16–19
Food sensitivities. See Food allergies
Food stamps, 112
Fortified foods, 49
Fractures
nursing interventions for nutritional
disorders, 136
nutritional implications related to,
135–36
possible nursing diagnoses, 136
Fructose, 308
Fruits, 5
Full liquid diets, 143

G
Gallbladder, 29–30
dysfunctions of, 178–80
Gastritis, 156–57
nursing interventions for nutritional
disorders, 156–57
possible nursing diagnoses, 156
Gastroenteritis, 17
Gastrointestinal disorders and
nutrition, 141–87
achalasia, 153
constipation, 145–46
diarrhea, 144–45
flatus, 152–53
heartburn, 151–52
inflammation, 156–61
intestinal obstruction, 154–56
malabsorption, 170–72
muscle weakness, 165–68

nausea and vomiting, 142–44
nursing interventions, 144
obstruction of the GI tract, 153–54
possible nursing diagnoses, 143
ulceration, 161–65
weakness in blood vessels, 169
Gastrointestinal tract, 28–30
accessory organs, relationship of,
179
exocrine pancreas, 29
gallbladder, 29–30
large intestine, 30
liver, 29–30
mouth, 28
obstruction of, 153–54
small intestine, 29
stomach, 28–29
Girth measurements to determine
obesity, 353
Glomerulonephritis, 188, 192–93
nursing interventions for nutritional
disorders, 192
possible nursing diagnoses, 192
Glucose
blood glucose values (normal and
diabetic), 303
laboratory assessment, 302
measurement of blood glucose
control, 310
metabolism, disturbances in,
300–304
Glycemic index, 313
Gout, 337–39
nursing interventions for nutritional
disorders, 339
possible nursing diagnoses, 338
Grain products, 4
Growth charts (0–36 months),
410–13
Gums, bleeding, 284

H
HDL. See Lipoproteins
Health-care team
dietitian, 19–20
nurse's role in, 19–20
pharmacist, 20
physician, 19
social worker, 20
therapists, 20
Health and nutrition, 3–22. See also
specific subjects, i.e.,
Malnutrition
evolution of nutrition's role, 4, 6–7

overview, 3
Heartburn, 151–52
during pregnancy, 64
nursing interventions, 152
possible nursing diagnoses, 151
Heart failure, congestive, 242–43
Height-weight tables
median, 405
used to measure obesity, 350–60,
352
Hemodialysis, 202–3
nutritional therapy, 208–9
Hemorrhoids, 169
nursing interventions for nutritional
disorders, 169
possible nursing diagnoses, 169
Hepatic encephalopathy, 177–78
nursing interventions for nutritional
disorders, 177–78
possible nursing diagnoses, 177
Hepatitis, 172–75
nursing interventions for nutritional
disorders, 174–75
possible nursing diagnoses, 174
Hiatal hernia, 165–66
nursing interventions for nutritional
disorders, 166–67
possible nursing diagnoses, 166
Hispanic cultural influences on dietary
intake, 12–13
Home health care, 112
Home parenteral nutrition (HPN),
286–87
Housing options for older adults,
112–13
HPN, 286–87
Hyperactivity, 380
Hypercalcemia, 332
nursing interventions for nutritional
disorders, 332–33
possible nursing diagnoses, 332
Hyperglycemia, 300–304
Hyperinsulinism. See Hypoglycemia
Hyperlipoproteinemia, dietary
modifications for, 224
Hypertension, 229–40. See also Blood
pressure
drug therapy, 236
nursing interventions for nutritional
disorders, 239–40
possible nursing diagnoses, 239
Hyperthyroidism, 323–24
nursing interventions for nutritional
disorders, 324–25
possible nursing diagnoses, 324

Hypocalcemia, 333
  nursing interventions for nutritional
    disorders, 334
  possible nursing diagnoses, 333
Hypoglycemia, 302–3, 321–23
  nursing interventions for nutritional
    disorders, 322–23
  possible nursing diagnoses, 322
Hypothyroidism, 326
  nursing interventions for nutritional
    disorders, 327
  possible nursing diagnoses, 326

I
Ileostomies, potential problem foods
    for persons with, 160
Illness
  and diabetics, 310
  food-borne, 16–19
  role of nutrition in, 13–14
Immune response, altered, 372–80
  AIDS, 378
  food allergies, 373–77
Indians, American. See Native
    Americans
Infancy
  colic, 88
  growth charts (0–36 months),
    410–13
  median height-weight tables, 405
Infant nutrition, 76–88, 376. See also
    Lactation
  amount of formula recommended,
    81–82
  commercial baby food, 86
    label analysis, 85
  commercial infant formulas, 78–82
  cow's milk, 82–83
  daily dietary intakes of vitamins
    and minerals, 408
  diarrhea, 87
  food sensitivities, 87
  human milk, 77–78
  iron supplementation, 82
  low-birth-weight infants, 88
  modified adult period, 86
  nursing-bottle syndrome, 87–88
  nursing interventions, 95
  nursing period, 77–83
  nutrient content of human milk,
    formula, and cow's milk,
    79–80
  nutrient supplementation, 78
  obesity, 87
  recent dietary modifications, 88

recommended dietary allowances,
    406–7
solid foods, 83–84, 86
soy-protein formulas, 80–81
transitional period, 83–84, 86
Infection, 125–28
  nursing interventions for nutritional
    disorders, 127–28
  possible nursing diagnoses, 127
Inflammatory bowel disease, 157–59
  nursing interventions for nutritional
    disorders, 158–59
  possible nursing diagnoses, 158
Insulin
  action in normal metabolism,
    299–300
  effect of lack of, 300
  formulations, 305
  as medication, 304–5
  reaction (hypoglycemia), 302–3
Interactions
  among nutrients, 49–50
  drug-nutrient, 109–11
Intestinal obstruction, 154–56
Intestines, 29–30
  obstruction of, 154–56
    nursing interventions for
      nutritional disorders, 155–56
    possible nursing diagnoses, 155
Iodine, 45
Iron, 44–46
  anemia caused by deficiency of,
    252–55
  deficiency, 46
  dietary sources, 44–45
  pregnancy and, 59, 61
  supplements in infant nutrition, 82
  toxicity, 46
Ischemic heart disease, 240–42
  nursing interventions for nutritional
    disorders, 241–42
  possible nursing diagnoses, 241

J
Jewish dietary rules, 10
Joint and bone disorders, 334–41
  arthritis, 334–37
  gout, 337–39
  osteoporosis, 339–41

K
Kidney. See also Renal disease and
    nutrition; Renal failure
  nephron, 190
  normal function, 188

protein intakes at various levels,
    206
renin-angiotensin system, 189
role in vitamin D metabolism, 190
Kidney stones. See Renal calculi
Kilocalories, 306
  expenditure, 347–49
  intake, 347
  low kilocalorie diets, 355–56
  very-low-kilocalorie diets, 355–56

L
Lactation, 67–68. See also Infant
    nutrition
  colostrum, 77
  food guide for daily intake, 60
  government programs, 68
  human milk, 77, 79–80
    nutrient content of, 79–80
  median height-weight tables, 405
  recommended dietary allowances,
    406–7
Lactose intolerance, 170
  nursing interventions for nutritional
    disorders, 171
  possible nursing diagnoses, 171
Large intestine, 30
LDL. See Lipoproteins
Lipoproteins, 219–23
Listeriosis, 16
Liver, 29–30
  dietary guidelines for selected
    diseases of, 173
  dysfunctions of, 172–78

M
Magnesium, 43–44
  and calcium, 44
  deficiency, 44
  dietary sources, 44
Malnutrition, 14
  among COPD patients, 268
  of cystic fibrosis patients, 272
  and infection, 126
  physical signs of, 15
Manganese, 45
Mannitol, 308
Maple-syrup urine disease, 95, 96
Meat, 5
Media's role in dissemination of
    information, 7
Medications
  for diabetes mellitus, 304–5
  during pregnancy, 62
  for hypertension, 236

Men
  median height-weight tables, *405*
  recommended dietary allowances,
    406–7
Metabolic disorders and nutrition,
    320–41
  adrenal disorders, 328–31
  hyperthyroidism, 323–24
  hypoglycemia, 321–23
  hypothyroidism, 326
  joint and bone disorders, 334–41
  parathyroid disorders, 332–33
Metabolic response to physiological
    stress, 122–24, *126*
  catabolism, *122*
  nutritional implications related to
    surgery, 123–24
  supplements used for patients, *137*
Metabolism, 95–96
  in cancer, 280, 283
  glucose, 300–304
  insulin action in normal
    metabolism, 299–300
  in obesity, 349–50
  in starvation, 280
Milk products, *6*
  commercial infant formulas, 78–82
  cow's milk for infants, 82–83
  nutrient content of human milk,
    formula, and cow's milk,
    79–80
Minerals, 42–44. *See also names of
    specific minerals, i.e.,*
    Calcium
  daily dietary intakes, *408*
  and diabetes mellitus, 307–8
  needs of older adults, 109
Molybdenum, 46
Morning sickness during pregnancy,
    64
Moslem dietary rules, 10–11
Mouth, 28
MSG, 374
Myocardial infarction. *See* Ischemic
    heart disease

N
National Academy of Sciences,
    Committee on Diet and
    Health, dietary
    recommendations, *9*
National Cholesterol Education
    Program (NCEP), 244
Native American cultural influences on
    dietary intake, 13

Nausea and vomiting, 142–44, 284
NCEP, 244
Nephrosis, 193–94
  nursing interventions for nutritional
    disorders, 194
  possible nursing diagnoses, 194
Niacin, 40–41
  deficiency, 40
  dietary sources, 40
  toxicity, 41
Nursing-bottle syndrome, 87–88
Nursing care plans, 385–401
  AIDS, 400–401
  cirrhosis of the liver, 386–88
  cystic fibrosis, 398–99
  depression and obesity, 393–95
  metastatic cancer, 392–93
  sickle-cell disease, 389–91
Nursing process, 20–21
Nutrients, interactions among, 49–50
Nutritional therapy, special considera-
    tions for cancer patients,
    285–86
Nutrition principles, 27–50
  overview, 27–28
Nutrition. *See specific types, i.e.,*
    Childhood nutrition; Infant
    nutrition

O
Obesity, 349–60
  assessment of, 350–54
  behavioral methods of treatment,
    358–59
  and blood pressure, 231
  complications of, 354
  depression and; nursing care plan,
    393–95
  dieting approach, 355–56
  drug therapy, 356–57
  exercise and, 358
  fat cell theory, 349
  in infancy, 87
  management of, 354–55
  metabolic picture, 349–50
  morbid; nursing care plan for
    patient with surgical
    intervention, 395–97
  nursing interventions for nutritional
    disorders, 360
  possible nursing diagnoses, 359
  of school-aged children, 91
  set-point theory, 349–50
  surgical treatment for, 357–58
Occupational therapist, role of, 20

Older adults
  biological changes, *105*
  chronic disease, 109
  drug-nutrient interactions, 109–11
  economic changes, 107
  housing options, 112–13
  nursing interventions related to
    dietary management, 113
  nutritional needs, 107–9
  nutrition assessment, 111–12
  nutrition and health concerns,
    103–4
  physiological changes, 105–7
  possible nursing diagnoses, 104
  psychosocial changes, 107
  support services, 112
Older Americans Act, Title, III-C, 112
Olestra, 366
Osteomalacia, 35
Osteoporosis, 43, 339–41
  nursing interventions for nutritional
    disorders, 340–41
  possible nursing diagnoses, 340
Ostomies, 159–60
  nursing interventions for nutritional
    disorders, 161
  possible nursing diagnoses, 160
  potential problem foods for
    persons with ileostomies,
    160
Oxalates, foods high in, *195*

P
Pancreas
  dysfunctions of, 181–82
  exocrine, 29
Pancreatitis, 181–82
  nursing interventions for nutritional
    disorders, 182
  possible nursing diagnoses, 181
Pantothenic acid, 41–42
  deficiency, 41–42
  dietary sources, 41
Parathyroid disorders, 332–33
Pellagra, 40
Peptic-ulcer disease, 161–65
  nursing interventions for nutritional
    disorders, 163
  possible nursing diagnoses, 163
  surgical treatment, 164
    nursing interventions for
      nutritional disorders, 165
    possible nursing diagnoses, 165
Perfringens food poisoning, 17
Pernicious anemia, 255–56

Pharmacist, role of, 20
Phenylketonuria (PKU), 95
Phenylpropanolamine (PPA), 357
Phosphorus, 43
  and calcium, 42
  dietary sources, 43
Physical activity, caloric cost of, *348*
Physical therapist, role of, 20
Physician, role of, 19
Physiological stress, 121–38
  metabolic response, 122–24
  nursing interventions for nutritional
      disorders, 124–25
  nutritional implications related to
      surgery, 123–24
  overview, 121
  possible nursing diagnoses, 124
PKU, 95
Potassium, 48
  blood pressure and, 232
  deficiency, 48
  estimated minimum requirements,
      409
  in foods, *233–34*
Poultry, *5*
PPA, 357
Pregnancy, 55–69
  adolescent, 65–66, 69
  alcohol and, 61–62
  caffeine and, 62
  common discomforts, 64
  complications, 65
  energy needs, 57–58
  exercise and, 61
  food guide for daily intake, *60*
  government programs, 68
  labor, nutrition implications during,
      67
  life-style factors, 61–62
  median height-weight tables, *405*
  medications and drugs during, 62
  multipara, 67
  nursing interventions, 68–69
  nutrient needs during, 57–61
  overview, 56
  possible nursing diagnoses, 56
  primigravida (older), 67
  recommended dietary allowances,
      406–7
  smoking and, 62
  weight gain, 58, *59*
Preschool nutrition
  characteristics of food commonly
      accepted, *90*
  common feeding problems, 90–91

substitutions for disliked foods, *91*
Principles of nutrition, 27–50
Protein, 30–31, 307
  digestion, 31
  metabolism, 31
  sources, strengths and weaknesses
      of, *12*
Psychosocial factors influencing
      dietary intake, 7–8
Purines, foods high in, *195*

R

Radiation therapy of cancer patients,
      284
  side effects and their management,
      284–85
Religious factors influencing dietary
      intake, 10–11
Renal calculi, 195–97
  nursing interventions for nutritional
      disorders, 196–97
  possible nursing diagnoses, 196
Renal disease and nutrition, 187–211
      See also Renal failure
  of children, 210
  dietary adherence, 210
  dietary recommendations, *205*
  glomerulonephritis, 188, 192–93
  hemodialysis, 202–3
  keto analogues of essential amino
      acids, 211
  nephrosis, 193–94
  nutritional therapy, 203–10
  renal calculi, 195–97
  renal failure, 197–210
  transplantation as treatment, 203
Renal failure, 197–210. *See also* Renal
      disease and nutrition
  acute, 197–98
    nursing interventions for
        nutritional disorders, 198
    possible nursing diagnoses, 198
  chronic, 199–210, 211
    nursing interventions for
        nutritional disorders, 209–10
    possible nursing diagnoses, 199
    treatment of, 201–10
  dialysis, 202, 203
  medication to treat, 201–2
  treatment of, 201–10
Respiratory disorders and nutrition,
      266–75
  COPD patients, dietary manage-
      ment of, 268
  cystic fibrosis, 271–74

obstructive pulmonary diseases,
      267–74
Riboflavin, 40
Rickets, 35
Roman Catholic dietary rules, 10

S

Saccharin, 308
Saliva, decreased production of, 284
Salmonellosis, 16
Salt substitutes
  flavor enhancers, 244–45
  herb blends, recipes for, 245
School lunch patterns, *93–94*
Scurvy, 36
Selenium, 45
Septicemia, 17
Set-point theory in obesity, 349–50
Seventh-Day Adventist dietary rules,
      11
Shigellosis, 16
Sickle-cell anemia, 258–60
  nursing care plan, 389–91
  nursing interventions for nutritional
      disorders, 259
Simplesse, 366
Skinfold measurements to determine
      obesity, 351–52
Small intestine, 29
Smoking during pregnancy, 62
Social worker, role of, 20
Sodium, 48, 307
  in baby food, 84
  blood pressure and, 232, 234–36
  estimated minimum requirements,
      409
  in foods, *237–38*
  natural (in foods), *235*
Soft diets, *143*
Sorbitol, 308
Speech therapist, role of, 20
Staphylococcal food poisoning, 18
Starch blockers, 357
Starvation
  adaptation to, *282*
  initial stage, *281*
  metabolism in, 280
Stomach, 28–29
Stomatitis, 284
Stress
  and calcium, 43
  physiological. *See* Physiological
      stress
Sucrose, 306–7
Supplements, 48–49

Surgeon General, dietary
   recommendations from, *8*
Surgery
   cancer patients, special considera-
      tions for, 285
   on diabetics, 310
   nutritional implications related to,
      123–24
   as treatment for obesity, 357–58,
      395–97
Sweeteners, alternate, 308
Sweets, *6*

T
Taste, alterations in, 284
Thiamin, 39–40
   deficiency, 40
Thyroid disorders, 323–27
Toddler nutrition, 86
Tooth formation and calcium, 43
Total parenteral nutrition (TPN), 286
Toxemia during pregnancy, 65
TPN, 286
Trace elements, 44–48, *45–46*. *See
   also names of specific
   elements, i.e.,* Iron
Transplant, nutritional therapy
   following, 209

U
Ulcerations. *See* Peptic-ulcer disease

V
Vegetables, *5*
Vegetarians, and vitamin B$_{12}$, 38
Very-low-kilocalorie diets, 355–56
Vitamin A, 33–34
   toxicity, 34
Vitamin B$_{12}$, 37–39, *38*
   anemia caused by deficiency of,
      255–57
      nursing interventions, 256
   deficiency, 38
   dietary sources, 37
   and vitamin C, 261
Vitamin B$_1$. *See* Thiamin
Vitamin B$_2$. *See* Riboflavin
Vitamin B$_6$, 41
Vitamin C
   deficiency, 36
   dietary sources, *36*
   and vitamin B$_{12}$, 261
Vitamin D
   and calcium, 34
   deficiency, 35
   dietary sources, 34
   metabolism of, *190*

toxicity, 35
Vitamin E, 35
Vitamin K, 35–36
Vitamins, 33–42. *See also names of
   specific vitamins, i.e.,*
   Vitamin A
   daily dietary intakes, *408*
   and diabetes mellitus, 307–8
   fat-soluble, 33–36
   older adults, needs of, 108–9
   water-soluble, 36–42
VLDL. *See* Lipoproteins
Vomiting, 142–44, 284

W
Water, 48
   baseline fluid requirements in
      temperate climate, *130*
Weight gain during pregnancy, 58, *59*
Weight loss, 285
Women
   median height-weight tables, *405*
   postmenopausal, 341
   recommended dietary allowances
      for, *57, 406–7*

Z
Zinc, 46–47